When the Dream is Shattered

When the Dream is Shattered

Judith and Michael Murray

Coping with child-bearing difficulties:
- infertility • miscarriage • premature birth
- loss of a newborn • abnormality

Lutheran Publishing House

Cover design by Wolfgang Rogge.

National Library of Australia
Cataloguing-in-publication entry

Murray, Judith, 1958 —
    When the dream is shattered.

    Bibliography.
    Includes index.
    ISBN 0 85910 448 6.

    1. Pregnancy, Complications of. 2. Pregnancy,
    Complications of — Religious aspects — Christianity.
    3. Infertility. 4. Infertility — Religious
    aspects — Christianity. 5. Abnormalities, Human.
    6. Abnormalities, Human — Religious aspects —
    Christianity. I. Murray, Michael, 1955 —
    II. Title.

306.8'8

First printing March 1988.
Second printing October 1988.

Printed and published by
Lutheran Publishing House,
205 Halifax Street, Adelaide, South Australia   87-1642

For our daughter Kate whose
short life provided the
inspiration and meaning for
this book.

Contents

Acknowledgments

The writing of this book is credited to Judith and Michael Murray, but in actuality we simply wrote the words. Many others have provided the information, the experience, and the practical hard work that brought about its creation. Here we salute their efforts. The order in which such persons are mentioned here is not necessarily indicative of the value we have placed upon their contribution.

Dr Margaret Franklin not only provided her support from the inception of this project, but she also gave willingly of her medical experience and knowledge to ensure that the information presented here is accurate and current at the time of publication. Her own first-hand knowledge of child-bearing difficulties has given her valuable unique insights from which this book has benefited.

Our sister, Dr Suzanne Miller, who herself experienced the fears accompanying the delivery of our niece Lauren at 28 weeks' gestation, further added her medical and emotional support and knowledge.

It would be impossible to mention by name all the individuals and couples who willingly shared with us their experiences of such difficulties. For many, painful memories were rekindled. They are the vital binding of this book, and their assistance and honesty are sincerely appreciated.

In a similar manner, we acknowledge the valuable information and moral support offered by the many support groups mentioned in the final section of this book.

Pastor Paul Renner was instrumental in ensuring that this whole project began and was eventually completed. Neither he nor we realized that a discussion held in pain in a labour room would lead to such a mammoth task.

The staff of the Mater Misericordiae Hospital Brisbane, and in particular the former chaplain of that hospital, Father John Chalmers, provided invaluable assistance. Their sharing of knowledge and experiences during discussion helped to highlight issues and attitudes. The pain they shared with us at Kate's death, and their joy when *their* baby Peter was born, went well beyond professional bounds.

Mrs Pamela Bruun took on the most demanding task of typing this manuscript. Her efforts are most sincerely appreciated.

Our families and friends must also be thanked publicly for their support in this venture. Particular mention must be made of Mrs Eunice Bruun, without whose practical support this whole project would have stagnated.

The other professionals — including doctors, nurses, social workers, psychologists, chaplains, and University of Queensland staff, who also provided valuable input and are too numerous to mention individually — are remembered here.

We acknowledge the authors and researchers in this area of child-bearing difficulties who have gone before us and provided us and others with food for thought.

A final special thought is given to our children: two we never held, our Kate whom we loved in life and love in death, and our precious Peter and Benjamin. Without them this book would never have been.

Foreword

My meeting with Judith some four years ago was precipitated by the very premature labour of my friend and Judith's sister. Happily, in the fullness of time and after an uncertain outcome, a healthy baby (and her parents!) survived. During this stressful time, I was impressed by Judith's compassion and common sense. Little did I know, at that stage, of Michael and Judith's own grief and frustration, nor that they were to suffer another ill-fated pregnancy before Peter Robert was born.

Most of this book was written during those long six months of the pregnancy spent in hospital. Despite the great care and expertise given by their specialist, no guarantee could be given to Judith and Michael that this baby would survive. In many ways, I look on the gestation of Peter Robert as a twin pregnancy, and it is heartening to look back on that time and know that Judith and Michael have achieved their dual goals of a much-wanted baby and a worthwhile book.

However, many readers will know, sadly, that long periods of time and effort are not necessarily rewarded as they should be. It is mainly for you that this book is written. Also, as one of the 'helping professionals', I found these pages valuable reading, and recommend them to anyone who would wish to comfort those suffering from the protracted and less tangible forms of grief associated with childbearing difficulties or survival of a healthy infant.

What a beautiful gift for Kate and the other non-surviving children of Michael and Judith! There can be no doubt that they are real and loved after reading this book. We all have different weaknesses and strengths (sometimes hidden).

Many readers will find new insights into their own special plight from this book.

Thank you, Judith and Michael, for sharing this very personal experience with fellow sufferers and would-be helpers.

Margaret Franklin MBBS (Qld), Dip Ch H (Lond.)

Introduction

Becoming a parent upon the birth of your own biological child can be an awe-inspiring experience, calling for great jubilation and celebration.

For the majority of couples this experience will be one of great excitement and anticipation. From the time the couple decide to have a child, to conception, and then through the long weeks of pregnancy, the only blight on their joy may be physical incidents of little real significance such as morning sickness or varicose veins.

Yet there is a significant number of couples for whom dreams of becoming a parent for the first or subsequent time, will be at worst shattered, at best severely shaken. Some will be unable to conceive easily. Some will lose their child through miscarriage, while others will have their child die before, at, or after birth. Others will have their baby arrive before he/she is fully mature. Still others will have to face the prospect of loving and rearing an ill or handicapped child.

Our society copes easily with the joys of a successful pregnancy. Commercial outlets, the media, friends, and relatives rejoice with the parents and voice society's approval at producing healthy offspring. But our society is not so willing to participate in the sorrow of those for whom bearing a child is more difficult, if not impossible. Infertility, miscarriage, premature delivery, perinatal death, and the birth of an 'abnormal' child become silent subjects. The sooner they can be forgotten, the more comfortable we, as people, will feel. The couple may have to face the pain largely alone, unless they are among the fortunate who find willing, skilled, supportive carers. Unfortunately, many often remain alone, feeling ostracized from society in general by their pain — a slight embarrassment to a society which has lost much of the capacity to cope with situations that do not produce 'good' feelings.

This book is not intended to be a definitive answer to the medical and social problems involved in bearing a child. It is not intended to be a prescription, upon which a 'cure' for the psychological pain of disappointment is based. Further, it is not intended to replace the individual's own search for meaning.

What, then, is this book meant to be?

It is written for those couples who, like ourselves, have faced — or for those who may have yet to face — the disappointment and sorrow when their dreams of bearing a live, healthy child are shattered. In our pain we went looking for answers, for something or somebody to tell us we were not alone. We wanted to know we were understood. This is the first and major purpose of this book.

The book is also written for those who are in contact with such people who are attempting to cope with these crises in their lives. It aims to provide some basic insights into their feelings and their needs. There are also attempts to evaluate many of the common reactions of others to such people, so as to stimulate thought and discussion among professionals and the general population.

We ask you not to view this simply as a piece of research made into book form. Rather, view it as an expression of support and encouragement for you from us — from the authors, professionals, and other individuals who have contributed to this book. We may not know you, but yet we share your pain, for we too have all experienced the heartache and disappointment in our own individual ways.

We make no apologies for the conversational manner in which this book is written. The words and expressions used may not always be scientifically formulated. Yet we have tried diligently to research the issues we discuss. We then attempted to present these issues in language all are able to understand. A scientifically presented work would have prevented us from including our own feelings of concern for couples in crisis, which we have felt with each written word.

Within this book we aim to highlight the problems of those for whom bearing a child does not come easily. In doing so, we will look at the medical and psychological aspects of this painful time, and attempt to demystify the experiences as a whole. Hence this book will combine three aspects: the basic medical knowledge presented in layman's terms, the emotional effects of the situations, and finally, a discussion of some means that others have used to cope with their experiences.

Reactions to child-bearing difficulties are as individual as the persons experiencing them. Some individuals may find their particular crisis relatively easy to deal with. Such persons generally are those who have developed appropriate crisis-coping skills prior to this experience, and who receive appropriate emotional support from those around them. Others, whose life-experiences and support provided are less helpful to them at this time, may experience more extreme reactions. Each person's behaviour and feelings are valid for that person, no matter how these may differ from the behaviour and feelings of others. We have presented here a range of different experiences and an outline of many common reactions which individuals may identify within themselves. This may alleviate fears of being different, 'neurotic', and unable to cope. It is not a yardstick against which persons should attempt to analyse their success or failure in coping with child-bearing difficulties, by comparing their reactions with those of others.

We attempt to look at the person in crisis as a whole, whose being is composed of many overlapping facets. We therefore will address the intellect's thirst for knowledge and the emotions' thirst for understanding, while also considering the philosophical and spiritual facets. Since no one experiences a crisis in an environment completely isolated from others, we have also included attempts to discuss openly the effects on the individual of interactions with other people.

At this point we note that the term 'the couple' will be used throughout this book in an attempt to recognize that these experiences generally affect both parents. However, we certainly do not wish to alienate or insult single parents by this term, and address this issue in Chapter 9.

We must re-emphasize that we do not believe or intend to convey the idea that what is presented here is all that is known about these subjects, or that this book outlines the only acceptable reactions and means of coping with such situations. Some may even disagree with observations made. It is also important to realize that medicine is advancing all the time, and that new treatments are being devised constantly. We ourselves do not have medical qualifications. Our information has been gleaned through research and guidance from medical practitioners. As far as possible, we have tried to present current medical knowledge in a down-to-earth fashion. Yet medicine continues to change, and hence in some places our information may be outdated at the time of reading. We therefore do not want the reader to assume that this book contains all medical possibilities.

Some may believe that providing medical information may only serve to frighten grieving couples further, particularly if they wish to attempt another pregnancy. We do not discount such a possibility. We have weighed this possible fear against the strong desires of most couples to understand their situation. The fear of the unknown is, for many, worse than any knowledge of possible unfavourable outcomes. Hence we encourage the reader *always* to discuss details with his or her doctor. This book may simply provide background knowledge and a foundation for such discussion.

In conclusion, we hope that the individuals who have read this book will be able to feel that they have spent time with people who have shared their pain, and that they have been understood. If this is the case, we will have achieved our aim!

Read on now, remembering you are *not* alone as long as these disappointments continue to plague other couples each day.

1 Our Experience: Judith Tells

We had met and fallen in love while living in a small town in Queensland. Before we were married, we had discussed having children and decided that we would begin a family as soon as possible. We were both in our mid-twenties, and felt emotionally and financially ready for a family. Little did we realize in 1982 that such a simple decision would lead us into the most trying period of our lives so far.

We had read enough about fertility to realize that it could take an average of four to six months to fall pregnant. To our excitement and certain relief, I found I was pregnant in the first month after our wedding. We were elated for a whole week! Then I began to bleed painlessly. This was the first time that the possibility of miscarriage had crossed our minds. The town's general practitioner simply told us to go home and wait. We didn't realize then what a common situation a threatened miscarriage was to him. The bleeding lasted a week, and during this time fear and anxiety became our constant companions.

Although we remained fairly anxious, the next four weeks passed uneventfully. A trip to Brisbane brought a visit to my obstetrician, who suggested an ultrasound scan. We saw our baby for the first time, and were given reassurance as to its security.

On returning home, we were to be put through further uncertainty, as I began to bleed painlessly again during the thirteenth week of my pregnancy. Then, once again the bleeding abated. After these two episodes, fears for the life of our baby destroyed any of the joy we had felt about this pregnancy.

It was only as I approached my seventeenth week that we began to feel a return of some enthusiasm. The doctor and the literature that I had now read indicated that most miscarriages occurred before 14 weeks. We felt heartened. We had made it past the 'magic 14'.

At eighteen weeks pregnant I had gone to bed early, after feeling very tired. At about eleven o'clock I woke, feeling pain in my back. Since this was my first pregnancy, I was quite ignorant and didn't associate backache with my pregnancy. I assumed any trouble would be indicated by abdominal pain. I decided that I must have strained my back. By morning, the pain was severe and regular, yet I still thought it was simply a strained back.

I went to work that morning and taught for half a day, until the contractions — as I now know them to be — became so regular and severe that I was unable to stand without fainting.

Fortunately Michael was home and he rang the doctor, who came immediately. I was contracting, but had no vaginal loss. The foetal heart-beat did not seem to indicate that the baby was in any distress. He gave no diagnosis, and left with instructions to call if any new development occurred. A new development did occur: blood!

By one o'clock that afternoon I was admitted to the small-town hospital, very uncomfortable and emotionally shocked and numb. After he had examined me, the doctor calmly told me I was miscarrying. I had no idea of what was to take place, and no one around enlightened me. A nurse told me to call when I wanted to push. 'How would I know?' I asked naively. But I found that I did know! Without Michael's support and loving presence, I would have found this time even more difficult.

By three o'clock that afternoon, February 15, 1983, it was all over. We had lost our baby, a baby we never saw. The tears flowed freely. Unfortunately, the hospital staff, except for one who had experienced miscarriages herself, found difficulty in coping with the situation. I felt a need to know if the baby had been a boy or girl, and asked the Matron. She said: 'Don't be so morbid! Go home and forget about it!' Those words still ring in my ears. I pressed her. Reluctantly, she told me that we had had an apparently perfectly formed son.

On leaving hospital a day later, I was not told of what might occur. No later check-up was suggested. From reading I had done, I realized that infection was a possibility after a miscarriage. I began taking my temperature in the hope of recognizing just such an eventuality. Four days later it was raised a half degree. I returned to the doctor. Fortunately, the Flying Surgeon was due to visit the following day, and a curette was performed.

The next few days were trying. About a week after the miscarriage we began to wonder about what had happened to our son. With some shock, we discovered that he was disposed of with no ceremony or real dignity. This was a very distressing thought to accept, as to us he had been a person in his own right, from the moment it was confirmed I was pregnant. It didn't seem right, somehow.

The local doctor told us that one miscarriage was common. He found it difficult to understand my fears for future pregnancies. I wanted very much to be pregnant again as soon as possible. The five months spent in trying to achieve this were arduous. Each month when menstruation began I was greatly disappointed. When it failed to appear during the fifth month, we were excited, although we consciously tried to suppress our excitement. A pregnancy test confirmed our hopes.

In my seventh week, I felt a slight backache and began to spot. It was 48 hours before any cramping and heavier bleeding began. Within a couple of hours, I passed a fair-sized clot and the pain subsided considerably. More hopes and dreams were dashed! My confidence had been struck another blow.

I felt more depressed after this second episode than after the first, probably in part because I had never come to terms emotionally with the first loss. I seriously doubted if we would ever have children, and I wanted Michael to leave me and find someone who could bear him a child. Other women around me had children so easily, or so it seemed!

I made a visit to an obstetrician in a larger city, who outlined to me many of the causes of a mid-trimester miscarriage. Which one had applied in my case, he was unable to say. He suggested that cervical incompetence might be my problem, but was not convinced of this.

We began to feel the need to be close to an experienced obstetrician in whom we felt confidence. That need, combined with a drought that forced us to sell out, saw us in Brisbane the Christmas of that year.

By this time I was already two months pregnant again. The news was welcomed by us, but at the same time met with a great deal of apprehension. We hardly discussed it, except in terms of 'if all goes well this time'.

We told only our parents of our news, until a two-day stay in hospital to have a cervical suture inserted at 13 weeks required some explanation. Up until this stage we were anxious lest we experience another early miscarriage. After 13 weeks we were still tense, as we moved toward our 18-week landmark.

From early in the pregnancy, I had believed I could feel the contracting of the uterus, but dismissed this as being impossible. The books spoke only of Braxton-Hicks contractions that began somewhere around 20 weeks. By 16 weeks my tightenings were obvious and quite painful. As they became my constant companions, I decided that if they were going to cause a problem they would have done so by now. I assumed that everyone had them so strongly, and that after two miscarriages I was simply being 'neurotic'.

By 21 weeks I began to experience some periods of happiness not accompanied by anxiety. These times frightened me in some ways, and were ended by thoughts of 'But, what if . . . ?' My obstetrician was able to accept my anxiety, but was pleased to see me becoming more relaxed. At least I didn't burst into tears each time I entered his office!

The evening before my ante-natal check at 23 weeks, a slight backache began. Backache of any type now was accompanied by fear. I entered my obstetrician's office and told him of my concern. He examined me and told me the suture was slightly open. He didn't seem overly concerned, but he may have wished not to frighten me. He decided to admit me to hospital for bed rest and medication.

During the hours after leaving his office and when entering the hospital, my body shook and the tears flowed freely. My old companions, fear and anxiety, rushed back to me, as did those feelings of desolation I had felt after losing our first baby.

The nursing staff were reassuring, although at times I resented them, thinking: 'How do you know it will be all right?' My chart said that I was 'apprehensive', but that the prognosis for my pregnancy reaching term was good. Later, in my grief, I was to resent this prediction. I tried to relax and worry less, until a nursing sister felt one of my assumed normal tightenings and told me she felt that they shouldn't be so strong. After my doctor felt the strength of the tightenings, he told me not to plan to go home. It was at this time that I first heard the term 'irritable uterus'. All anyone could tell me was that some women have a uterus that wants to keep contracting. Why? Well, that was something no one could tell me.

The magic 24 weeks came. This to me marked the day of hope. Every day in the uterus from here on increased our baby's chances of survival. That very evening the pain of the contractions grew in intensity. Next morning the pain and regularity of the contractions heralded my movement to the labour ward. There I was placed on a drip in an attempt to halt labour. The drip was as strong as medically advisable, but the contractions continued.

After I had been on the drip for one day, birth seemed imminent, with contractions about two minutes apart. My memory of the following two days is very blurred, as I was in constant pain and exhausted. I only clearly remember my very wonderful husband, who grabbed catnaps on a beanbag beside me and fed me tomato soup, the only nourishment I could take easily.

Each day my obstetrician visited, and with each visit his face grew more grave. He hurt for us, and his feelings of helplessness were obvious. We felt for him, and now saw him more clearly as a very real person with feelings, rather than an expert who should be able to perform miracles. Because of the constant pain, my inability to eat, and his belief that medical science could do nothing more to stop what now seemed inevitable, he asked us if we would like to have the drip removed. I refused, and promised to try to eat. Each time I found the foetal heart-beat, my resolve was heightened. Where there was life, there was hope!

Finally, after three-and-a-half days in labour, our daughter Kate was born, nearly fifteen-and-a-half weeks premature. It was 12.15 am on Good Friday morning, 1984. We knew her chances were slim, but were heartened to hear she weighed 840 grams, which was a good weight for such a premature baby.

After her birth, I could not contain my fatigue. Before I was taken back to the ward, we were taken to see our daughter in her humidicrib. She was so tiny and so beautiful! My reaction was tears, and many of them.

The paediatrician in charge of the Special-Care Nursery came early the next morning, bearing two photographs of Kate. He told us that X-rays had shown her lungs to be very immature. Kate had a hole in her left lung. He said she was holding her own and that she had a chance as long as the right lung was maintained intact. At about 2 pm we were taken to the nursery to see our daughter. She was covered with monitoring devices, and tubes were inserted into her tiny chest. She was being hand-ventilated to remove air from her chest cavity. The sister explained exactly what was happening, and told us honestly that she didn't feel Kate had much hope of survival. We knew in our hearts that it was only a matter of time.

We spent a time in the chapel, and on returning to the ward were told we were wanted in the Special-Care Nursery. We were told that Kate wasn't going to live, and were asked if we would like to hold her. For half an hour we sat and held her, talked to her and simply loved her. We cried together. The sister cried with us.

As the moment of parting came closer, the sister removed the monitors and tubes and allowed her to die naturally in our arms. She had lived 17 hours. As difficult as those 30 minutes were for us, they were also very special and will always remain so. We were given two other photographs of her as she was, without monitoring equipment or tubes. They remain precious to us.

I was discharged the next morning. The following days were difficult, and we had a feeling of unreality. Feelings of failure, pain, anger, doubt, and hopelessness were all mixed, and appeared without a set pattern. Friends and family were very supportive, but no words would alleviate the hurt. Amid his pain, Michael found strength to support me, and we grew in love those days as never before. The loving support of our families and minister-friend helped us also.

The funeral had to be organized. It provided an important time for saying goodbye to our Kate. We wrote parts of the service ourselves, and were able to say the things we would never be able to say to her again.

At my next visit, my obstetrician answered my barrage of questions honestly. He told us that it seemed I had the problem of an incompetent cervix and an irritable uterus. He could make no promises about the future, but told us not to give up hope. We were determined not to.

In late October, six months after Kate's death, I was pregnant again. In these months we had found much support and caring, and had been able to work through our grief slowly but surely. We had also taken steps to have one more 'really good shot' at a viable pregnancy. We had discussed in depth our feelings, and had tried to build future plans for ourselves without children of our own.

Through much soul-searching, we emerged realizing that we did want a child to love, to nurture, to be a family. It would be nice if we had one child that was biologically our own, but this was not really an obsession. We realized that other children we had loved in our prior dealings with them had been so loved because of the effort we had put into them. We also realized that the rearing of children, even biological ones, was only part of a person's life. There were many years to follow after they left the nest. We looked toward new areas to maintain our closeness as a couple, as individuals who were not parents. Other plans to complete our family through adoption and fostering were put into action.

I also began training in relaxation. Therefore, when our fourth pregnancy was confirmed, although we were anxious, the pressure seemed somehow eased slightly.

In mid-January 1985, 12 weeks pregnant, I entered hospital to have another cervical suture inserted, although this time it was to be positioned closer to the internal os (the inner opening into the uterus). The operation presented no medical problems, and I now looked ahead to a prolonged hospital stay.

By 14 weeks the irritability of the uterus was evident. Admitting that to myself, to Michael, and to medical staff was hard. I didn't want to believe it. The past rushed back to me, and I sobbed that day. The wonderful support of Michael, family, and staff got me over that rough patch and hope returned, although slightly tarnished.

The pregnancy progressed slowly but surely. Some days were better than others. My hospital 'family' were a vital link in my support chain. Michael and my mother, who visited every day, were important sources of courage.

It was a momentus day when we reached 28 weeks, the day that marked hoped for us. At this time I had my first outing from the hospital in 16 weeks. At 30 weeks my obstetrician showed signs of relief. Yet I continued to take it one day at a time, unable to believe it might really work out this time.

Then the day arrived. After an amniocentesis at 37 weeks confirmed that the lungs were mature, an epidural caesarean section was scheduled for the following day. The feelings that we experienced on that day are hard to express adequately. My hospital 'family' and our families and friends were all swept along with us in the wave of expectation.

At 3.11 pm on Friday July 12, 1985, Peter Robert Murray was born. All the effort had been worth it! We thought of Kate and our other children that day, but thought of them lovingly. As much as we would have wished to have them with us, we realized that if they were with us, Peter would not be here. Looking at that precious bundle, we simply felt blessed and eternally grateful.

Peter retained some fluid on his lungs after birth, and so remained under observation in a portable humidicrib for some 36 hours before we had him to hold. It was hard to believe our dreams had come true. In fact, somehow I felt things were too good to be true. The thoughts '. . . but what if something goes wrong?' were still there, tarnishing my joy.

Five days after his birth, I was again emotionally shell-shocked when, on routinely examining our son, the paediatrician calmly announced that Peter had a heart murmur. He didn't seem overly concerned, realizing that this was a reasonably common problem that would most likely correct itself in time and without any medical intervention. I maintained my composure till the paediatrician and a number of visitors left. Then I fell apart! At that moment, I was convinced Peter had a serious problem that would lead to his death. I was unable to hold him or even touch him for a time. I was afraid to love him. I rang Michael in tears, and he came immediately to the hospital. Fortunately, I could lean on his support and calm rationality. I was probably overreacting. Yet those who have shared similar pain to what we had felt over the last three years would probably feel that my reaction was perfectly reasonable. As I write this, Peter is ten months old and a healthy bundle of giggles and mischief, undaunted by a heart murmur.

The reason for telling our story is not to imply that all stories have a happy ending. They haven't! We are among the fortunate ones. Rather, we wish you who read this to know that we understand in some small measure the pain you feel, and thereby offer you our support and that of those other couples who also share your grief. May your life be contented and meaningful.

2 Different but the Same:
Grieving as a Common Bond

Although couples who face difficulties in bearing a child often feel isolated and alone, the statistics indicate that there are many who share such losses.

We hesitate to use statistics, for they, by their very nature, involve generalizations and hence do not consider individual cases. They may cause alarm to pregnant women when alarm is generally unnecessary. More than nine out of ten pregnancies that reach the thirteenth week will end with a couple taking home a live, healthy baby. Secondly, statistics do not comfort a couple who mourn their children, both potential or actual. To know you are a part of a small percentage does not make you feel any more comforted.

We mention these statistics simply to point out that the number of couples who experience some difficulty in bearing a child is not insignificant. They constitute a sizeable minority, yet a minority who are often overlooked by society. This oversight is often caused by self-imposed silence on the part of the couple, or by society-imposed silence.

Approximately one couple in six will experience some problem with their fertility at some stage in their life together. Of those who do conceive, doctors estimate that as many as 20 per cent, or one in five, will lose this confirmed pregnancy through miscarriage. In fact, recent evidence [1,2] suggests that many more pregnancies are miscarried but are not recognized as such because they occur before the woman is even aware she is pregnant. Premature delivery of a child occurs in approximately seven births in every hundred. Of these babes who weigh between 500 and 1,000 grams, some 60 per cent will die, while some 20 per cent of those above this weight will also die![3] A few years ago, the number of stillbirths was estimated to be one to two per cent of all births.[4] The figure may well be a little lower now.

Finally, it is estimated that three babies in every hundred are born with some form of severe congenital abnormality.[5]

If we consider these figures in the light of the Australian population, we note that close to 25 per cent of confirmed pregnancies may develop some problems. This does not even consider those who fail to conceive at all.

However, these statistics fail to show the good news. Most of these affected couples will go on to have a healthy family of their own. Many will achieve this with medical help for an ill infant, or with further successful pregnancies. Others may realize their dream through processes of adoption. But this heartening news does not mean that during their times of difficulty such couples should not be provided with vital and meaningful support. Even the most optimistic couple will experience their own pain in their present difficulties, irrespective of any renewed happiness the future may hold.

Each individual couple will face their particular problem in their own unique way. Each experience will display certain unique characteristics. Yet all of us share one thing in common. We share **grief**.

The Oxford Dictionary defines grief as 'deep and evident sorrow'. Grief is a natural reaction to losing something important. We all grieve because in child-bearing difficulties we have all lost something precious to us. What we have lost may differ, and the intensities of our grief also differ. Yet we all experience the deep sorrow of grief.

The couple faced with infertility will grieve for their unborn children, the loss of their potential to produce a dream. The couple who face an early miscarriage lose a child, for to them it has been theirs to love during those early weeks. Late miscarriage, stillbirth, and neonatal death focus on the loss of a child whose movement heralded its existence. Premature delivery of a child who does survive robs the couple of the end of their pregnancy and the physical contact with their new baby. The parents of an abnormal child also grieve for the loss of their 'perfect' baby. They lose their dreams of this child's brilliant future, and have them replaced by uncertainty.

Each of these couples grieve. Some experiences may produce more intense, prolonged grief. It is pointless to try to compare the grief of one couple with that of another. Suffering is not something to be measured and compared, like the size of a house or the cost of a car.

Suffering hurts, and your suffering hurts you. It doesn't make any difference that another's grief is deeper or more justified in the eyes of others. Grief is a very unique experience. Your grief hurts you more than the grief of others, because it is happening to you. A person may sympathize with another's pain, but to you your pain is greater, simply because you feel it.

Other people's pain is simply happening to them. It won't mean as much to you as your own.

This statement may sound selfish, even cruel, but it is not meant to be. It is meant to help us realize that it is acceptable to feel our pain, even if others around us feel that it is unwarranted. How many times have a couple been told after the loss of a child: 'You can always have another', or 'At least you didn't lose it after a few months like — ', or 'Snap out of it! It was only a miscarriage'. Comments like these only serve to highlight the fact that often a couple who face difficulties in bearing a child are denied the same rights as are afforded to others who are bereaved in our society. They may feel guilty about their feelings and attempt to suppress them, instead of experiencing the pain and coming to terms with it. Such reactions can lead to problems.

Understanding a little about the grief we are experiencing can help us cope with it by removing some of the fear of the unknown. Let us look more closely at grief, our common bond.

Factors affecting grief

The grief we experience through our particular loss is very real. How we cope with that grief will be very individual. We do not enter this difficult period of grieving devoid of a past. Many factors will affect our journey through grief. Some couples will have a relatively smooth, direct journey, while the journey of others will be continually thwarted with delays and detours. Unfortunately, some will even fail to reach their destination, and their unresolved grief may disrupt their lives for many years.

Let us look at some of the factors which vary among couples, and hence may influence their grief in differing ways:

1. Emotional investment in the birth

To assume that the news of pregnancy is a joyous matter for all is misguided, to say the least. Many a woman, because of her marital, family, health, or financial situation at the time, has been troubled by this news. In many cases, the pregnancy is clearly unwanted. In contrast, other couples, particularly those who have faced a period of infertility, may be ecstatic with the news. Similarly, a couple who had doubts about having children at all may feel differently about the blow of infertility than do a couple who desperately want a child. A young couple whose pregnancy was the result of an absence or failure of contraception may deal with an early miscarriage differently from an older couple who have married late and wish to begin a family promptly. A couple who have dreamed of their child taking over a family business may find great difficulty in coping with the news of the birth of a handicapped child. The neonatal death of a child may be a crushing blow to a couple who have already lost a number of other children. Finally, a couple who were eagerly anticipating a 'meaningful natural' childbirth experience may feel at a greater loss during the activity and tension of a premature delivery than another couple to whom the birth process was simply a means to an end.

These examples indicate a vital factor affecting the feelings of grief: the emotional investment of the couple in the event. It is dangerous to generalize, but in most cases, the more important the dream of a live, healthy, mature child, the more intense is the grief caused by a loss. A couple who have seen their future as revolving around their life as a family, may find their grief complicated by a loss of meaning and direction in their life. This is most likely to occur where the couple have no other live children, and hence are not likely to be seen as a family in their own eyes or the eyes of society.

The couple who want a child and have planned for a pregnancy may invest greater emotional and physical energy in the conception and pregnancy. They may carefully cut out habits that may not be advantageous to the developing child, watch their diet carefully, exercise, avoid drugs, and generally treat the mother's body with caution. They may have a loving nickname for the child, and talk about their future as a family. When pregnancy is not achieved or a child is lost, the emotional pain is quite intense.

2. Prior life-experiences

How we deal with any stressful situations in our lives is affected largely by the way we have dealt with stress in the past. From childhood, we have developed our own particular means of coping with stress. As we watch children confronted by a difficult situation, we note different reactions. One child who falls off a horse may get angry and strike the horse. Another may cry and run away, while yet another seeks help and gets right back on to the horse. Adults react to painful situations in similar, yet uniquely individual ways. We all know people who 'run away' from a problem, or who 'explode', or who 'analyse' everything, or who 'go into their shell'.

In our current child-bearing trials we will generally react as we have to previous crises in our lives. Some means of coping are more effective than others in allowing one to work through the problem to a satisfying result. Where an individual has not developed effective coping skills, crises may not be resolved. These experiences may then affect future crises, by making them even more complicated and trying.

3. Preparation for the loss

Relatives of the terminally ill are provided with a period of time during which they can prepare for their loss. If this preparation phase is worked through successfully, some of the stress of the final parting can be alleviated. A sudden death, such as in a car accident, leaves the relatives initially in deep shock and without any psychological readiness to grieve.[6,7]

Such unexpected losses occur in situations of infertility, miscarriage, stillbirth, premature delivery, and the birth of a child with a congenital abnormality. Suddenly one's whole life changes drastically.

Other couples may have time before an event to prepare themselves for the eventual outcome. For example, a woman may begin spotting but not miscarry until after a period of some days, or an ultrasound scan may indicate an abnormality. A woman may have a history of premature deliveries, or a man may suspect a low sperm count after a case of mumps that caused a rare complication in the testes.

Some period of preparatory grief before the actual event may help the couple to cope with the final loss.

4. Life-situation/personality factors

Males and females may differ in their reactions to a loss. Their differing perspectives on life, their hormonal differences, and their conditioning as children may affect their reactions.

Age can be a disadvantage if a couple are attempting to bear a child fairly late in life. Infertility or other loss can see them lose hope that they will have a family, as time seems to be running out on them. Yet age can also be advantageous, in that time may have shown them more disappointments. In coping with these, they may have developed a maturity born out of crisis. The personalities of the partners can affect the process of grief. A person who inhibits feelings or is prone to guilt may cope less effectively than one who is openly expressive and self-confident.

Different cultures and families place varying emphasis on the importance of a couple bearing a child. These differing expectations will either alleviate or increase the tension and grief.

A couple's religious beliefs can also strongly affect their grief. A belief in the goodness and divine reason of God or a Supreme Being may help a couple accept their loss as part of a plan. Hence they are provided with meaning in a seemingly senseless situation.

A couple who must also face other crises — such as financial worries, other bereavements, or unemployment — as well as their child-bearing difficulties, are at a further disadvantage.

Therefore we see that child-bearing difficulties cannot be considered in isolation. The personalities of the couple and their environment have a considerable effect on their grief.

5. The apportioning of blame

As human beings we like to believe that there is a cause for every incident — so that when things go wrong there is something or someone to blame. We find it unacceptable that nature does not follow our rules. We look for something to blame for our troubles, and will even accept the blame ourselves.

If one partner is able to attribute blame, rightly or wrongly, to him- or herself, he/she may feel more intense grief than the partner. For example, a man's low sperm count or a woman's blocked tubes may be the cause of their infertility. A woman who didn't want the child may blame her feelings of rejection for a miscarriage or stillbirth. A partner found to carry a gene for an abnormality or a woman who went into premature labour may find in their bodies something to blame.

Irrespective of whether such blame is justified or not, such persons may experience more intense feelings of grief and depression caused by a turning in of anger on to themselves. In many cases, such anger is difficult to alleviate through rational discussion. Often the loss of confidence and sense of failure that accompany these feelings of guilt are difficult emotions to deal with. Any attempt by a partner to support this person or alleviate his/her guilt may be misinterpreted by the partner who feels guilty. He/she may feel that the partner is 'just being nice' while covering up the anger really felt. In psychological jargon, persons who blame themselves may project their own feelings of anger at themselves on to their partner. In other words, they are angry with themselves and assume that their partner must feel likewise. In some cases there may actually be anger or resentment felt by one partner toward the partner with the physical problem.

6. The support available

Although grieving is essentially a process through which one travels alone, the support available to a couple during their grieving can greatly affect the passage and outcome of the process. The type of support offered varies.

Perhaps the support of greatest significance is that offered by one's partner — the one person in the world who, through a sharing of the loss, experiences similar intense personal feelings. The one's loss is also the other's loss. Even other people who have experienced a similar loss are not able to understand a person's particular loss as acutely as does his/her partner. The couple who cry together, who comfort each other, and who mourn the loss of their perfect child, are one. There may be times when one partner is weak while the other is strong, a complementary situation. But at some darker times, neither will feel the strength to bear the other's pain. It is often at these times that feelings of not being understood can block the communication. We will discuss these times in a relationship in Chapter 9.

Family and friends can also prove vital sources of support. Many couples will be protected under a strong umbrella of loving concern opened about them by family and friends. Unfortunately, others may not encounter this so readily. Distance or death may have separated a couple from their parents and/or closest family members and friends. An inability to understand the feelings of the couple or to cope with any stressful situation may lead some family and friends to avoid these unpleasant situations, and hence also avoid the couple. It is not uncommon, during the time when a couple must face some difficulty in bearing a child, that friendships will be re-evaluated according to the couple's often changed outlook and their experience of the support they receive.

The wider society, involving doctors, nurses, professional counsellors, and support groups, provides another link in the support chain. These people can provide the couple with information, understanding, and friendship. The support groups can further supply a knowledge obtained from other couples' own period of loss. The availability of community support may vary. A large maternity hospital or experienced doctor may have developed specific strategies for supporting a couple who have difficulties bearing a child. This kind of help may not be available for a couple who experience the same problems in a small town or remote area. In addition, many support facilities are dependent on the couple seeking out their assistance. For many people, finding the confidence and courage to do this while depressed is difficult. The realization that many couples face their loss in isolation is of concern to those involved in the task of supporting such couples. Recognizing a couple who are not coping successfully is less likely in our highly mobile, urban society, which is based on the nuclear family. We frequently don't even know the names of the people who live two or three houses from us in the same street.

7. The relationship of the couple prior to the loss

Being faced with the inability to have children, or being able to have them only after some difficulty, places enormous strains on a couple and their relationship. Just as a dry twig will snap under pressure, some relationships — brittle due to a breakdown of communication — do not survive the pain. It is not uncommon for such marriages and relationships to be dissolved at some time following the couple's loss. Other relationships are like a green twig, which bends under pressure but fails to break. When the pressure is eased even slightly, it attempts to return to its previous shape, and usually succeeds, even if that shape is now slightly altered.

A couple who enter into pregnancy in a conscious or unconscious attempt to save a failing relationship may find that once their dream has been shattered, their relationship is at an end also. Others may discover new strengths and qualities in their partners that enhance their partnerships or help them to rediscover the old companionship. Other couples, who have built a strong bond of caring, trusting, and communication, may emerge from their grief changed but intact. In many cases a couple who face such difficulties discover a sense of well-being in the knowledge that their relationship has survived immense pressure. The more trivial pressures of life seem to take on new, less threatening perspectives.

What each couple brings to their experience of grief in terms of individual qualities, communication, and knowledge of one partner by the other, will affect their passage through their present difficulties.

Of course, we must not forget that a growing number of women, through relationship breakdown or choice, may face their parenting disaster without the support of a partner. The grief of such a woman in losing her child is compounded by the grieving for a lost relationship or social disapproval at having become pregnant by choice. A further group, the young unwed mothers who did not plan their pregnancy, must cope with this very difficult situation during a time in their life — that is, adolescence or early adulthood — in which other life-crises are normally present.

Grief is hard work

We hear the statement that grief must be 'worked through'. Psychological textbooks, counsellors, and even the media use the phrase liberally. Yet only one who has faced grief can fully accept how apt that phrase really is. Grief is work, hard work— perhaps the hardest work we may have to face in life. It can't be avoided indefinitely. It stands as a wall between us and our future peace of mind. It is a wall that must eventually be demolished if we are ever to attain some semblance of peace in our lives.

Some people meet the wall well-equipped with bulldozers of support and effective coping skills. They demolish their wall of grief and emerge triumphant, even if a little bruised. Others will attempt to tackle grief less well equipped, armed with only a shovel. They find the going difficult, but, in time, emerge triumphant also. Yet others will attack their grief with their bare hands, emerging bruised, battered, and exhausted. There are still others. They run desperately up and down beside the wall, looking for an easy way around it. Their desperate search will be in vain, and finally they must confront this obstacle.

Even when we confront our grief and attempt to deal with it, the way is never smooth. Just as we may find a brick in the wall that refuses to budge, we may find a time in our grief during which we feel we will never cope. We wonder: 'Will I ever be able to feel joy again?' At other times we may seem to be making encouraging progress, only to be sent reeling back by a significant incident. Our demolition machinery seems to hit a foundation stone.

Let us look, then, at a few points about grief

1. Grief makes no consideration for age, sex, social status, religion, education, wealth, or previous suffering. It does not even overlook those who are in some ways relieved by the loss. Suffering and grief can strike any of us at any time. Your time of grieving just happens to be now, in this situation. But fear not. You will not be alone. It comes to us all.

2. Your reaction to grief has nothing to do with your intellect. You can't simply rationalize it away. It has to be confronted and experienced.

3. Grief has its basis in our humanness. It is common to us all.

4. Grief cannot be denied or ignored indefinitely. You may be able to repress it for a period, but it emerges in some way, such as in later illness.

5. Grief is not pleasant or easy. It is senseless to try to hoodwink ourselves into believing that grief 'isn't really all that bad'. We don't like pain in our society, and prefer to avoid any possible painful experience. Our inability to accept that grief is not pleasant or easy is reflected in the heavy use of tranquillizers prescribed for a person experiencing grief, and in the conspicuous absence of support from some people who are unable to deal with another in pain.

6. Grief is not a rational, logical process. More often it is like groping about in the dark, with no set pattern, looking for a light switch. It's more like two steps forward and one back, with a nudge and a push off to the side. The feelings associated with it may not be constant. Rather, there may be 'up' and 'down' days, the number of each type altering as grief is resolved.

7. Grief is individual. It differs from person to person, couple to couple, family to family, culture to culture, and even pregnancy to pregnancy. It does not have to follow some set pattern.

8. Grief affects the whole person. Reactions to grief can be seen in feelings of sadness, tiredness, hopelessness, anger, and guilt. The body, too, can show the pain the mind is confronting. Loss of muscular strength, stomach upset, shortness of breath, disturbed sleep, and muscle tightness are all common physical sensations of grief. Grief may also be displayed in our general behaviour by absent-mindedness, hyperactivity, irritability, and carelessness.

9. You can emerge from grief a stronger, more capable, and more sensitive human being. Because of this, the pain of grief has actually been good for you, although at the time that is the last thing we want to be assured of! It is a special moment when you come to your own personal realization of this.

10. It is impossible to understand fully another's grief. We can share grief, but there will always be parts of the journey which a person must go through alone. A husband cannot take on to himself his wife's grief. He can share her pain, but ultimately she must come to terms with her unique grief alone. This doesn't mean that the journey cannot be made easier by others. It simply means that ultimately the final resolution is a personal experience.

11. Grieving requires us to confront our loss and to accept it as reality and as being generally irrevocable.

12. Grief can be compounded. Unresolved grief over a prior loss can complicate and deepen the grief of a new crisis.

13. Grief need not be feared. It is a healthy means of coping with an incident in our lives that could otherwise destroy our peace of mind indefinitely. Grief is a form of healing. A broken leg is painful when it is first cracked and as it is set. Eventually it heals, at times even stronger than before. Similarly, grief is a painful experience, but if allowed to proceed will eventually culminate in a new peace of mind.

14. Grief takes time. Grief can't be hurried to an end. Just as healing of the body will proceed at its own pace, so does healing of the mind.

15. You will survive grief, even if at times you doubt it. Don't give up! It will pass!

What is grief-work?

If we are successfully to come to terms with grief, there are certain tasks that must be completed.[8]

A. First, we must accept the facts of our loss. This seems an unnecessary statement to make, but unfortunately this task is often the hardest work of all. A couple may seek out a number of different doctors in a desperate attempt to reverse a diagnosis of untreatable infertility. A grieving mother, who has experienced a caesarean and found the baby stillborn, may accuse others of lying about her dead child. Parents of a congenitally handicapped child may refuse to accept mental retardation in their seemingly healthy, physically attractive child.

B. Once the facts of the loss have been accepted, one must then allow oneself to experience the pain of the loss. This is the period of grief most recognizable to the outside world. Displays of emotion and withdrawal are common. The degree of acceptance by society of outward grief will often depend on the object of that grief. For example, society may more easily accept displays of grief from the mother of a stillborn infant than from a couple who mourn their loss of potential children through infertility.

C. Somewhere among the pain, those who are grieving will move hesitantly toward the next task. In this task they must readjust to a world in which their longed-for dream of a live, healthy baby is not present, at least temporarily. They begin to return to activities that provide for some return to normality in their lives. At times they will re-experience their pain, but eventually their lives focus on new areas.

D. This heralds the final task of grieving. The life energy that was directed toward the dream will finally be diverted to an attainable reality. The person becomes involved in a new dream, or makes another attempt at the old. For many, a new pregnancy will be the focus. In starting to work toward a new goal, those involved begin to make a future for themselves and their loved ones.

Such tasks are generally undertaken in the above order. They appear straight-forward when written down, but the time-span during which these tasks are accomplished can vary from weeks to months to years or even a lifetime. Unfortunately, sometimes life does not give enough time or support for the tasks ever to be completed.

It is easy to outline tasks of grieving on paper. The difficulty arises in trying to convey to a reader just how much emotion and energy is involved in working through them, and just how unclear is the distinction between the end of one and the beginning of another phase.

Common grief experiences

Dr Elizabeth Kübler-Ross, in her work *On Death and Dying*,[9] completed perhaps the most inspirational work on grieving. Although it deals with patients who were terminally ill, her work on what she termed the 'stages of grieving' can be applied to the situation of grieving the loss of being able to produce a live, mature, healthy child.

These stages of grieving do not necessarily follow sequentially. People may drift from one stage to another, or return to a prior stage. They may even experience two stages simultaneously. We shall be looking at varied situations and varying intensities of grief. Therefore we shall concentrate less on the stages of a definite grieving process, and rather view them as common experiences in grief found in couples facing child-bearing difficulties.

Kübler-Ross describes her stages of grief as:
1. Shock and denial
2. Anger
3. Bargaining
4. Depression
5. Acceptance

We shall look at these stages as they apply to the situations we are interested in. We shall also consider them in the above order, but with the recognition that all individual patterns may differ.

1. Shock and denial

Most commonly, the first reaction to news of a loss is shock. The mind and body seem to shut down almost completely. They are numb. Perhaps the body fails to move, thoughts become jumbled, and reactions may appear unusual. It is believed that this may initially be the mind's way of coping with a situation that would otherwise destroy the person. The mind seems to throw up a barrier against the news to try to maintain some equilibrium.

Time may pass in a disorganized sense of unreality. The couple may appear to function normally, but their behaviour is simply a mechanical process devoid of real understanding. It is not a time when a couple can assimilate too much reality, too much information. It is a bit like a 'living death'. Those patients who occupy our mental-health institutions in a catatonic depressive state, divorced from reality, become a little less of an enigma to those of us who have experienced the loss of reality and isolation that can occur during this stage of grieving. The couple may appear devoid of the 'symptoms' of grieving. They may not cry. They may refuse to see their child or sign essential papers. They can't yet accept the reality of the situation.

Denying the existence of a situation as a means of defending the psyche from anxiety was outlined by Anna Freud in her discussion of defence mechanisms.[10] It is perhaps one of the more extreme of these mechanisms, but yet can provide an effective buffer against strong emotional pain. It is important for those close to the grieving person to realize that denial is not necessarily a destructive thing. It is not helpful to try to force the griever to acknowledged the facts before he/she is ready. When the mind is ready to cope, denial will generally fade.

It is not uncommon for a couple faced with test results indicating infertility to desperately seek out the possibility of errors in the test or other opinions that will invalidate the diagnosis. Denial of the pregnancy may follow a miscarriage. Mothers of a stillborn infant have been known to accuse hospital staff by lying to them and of spiriting their child away. Some may go to the nursery in search of their baby. Other women may deny obvious labour pains, rather than admit they may again be facing a premature delivery. Similarly, it is not uncommon for a couple to disbelieve results of tests which indicate that their child suffers from a congenital abnormality.

Generally, over a period of hours or days, people move on to other different grief experiences.

2. Anger

Anger is a very common reaction to loss, and one of the more intense. It is also an emotion complicated by our conditioning. Discouragement of outward displays of this emotion can lead to feelings of guilt in those who feel the anger.

Anger as a feeling is *not* wrong. It is simply a normal human emotion, as are love and sadness. If the feeling leads to violent, destructive, or damaging *behaviour*, then it is the behaviour that is wrong, not the feeling. From childhood, many are not taught how to deal successfully with anger. Hence, it is often unexpressed, suppressed anger, which can linger for years after the situation causing our grief has passed.

Anger can be directed against God, medical personnel, family, one's partner, society, the child that is lost, and — perhaps most commonly — against oneself.

> Why did God let this happen to us? He lets all those who don't look after their children have them, but not us! It's not fair!

Medical malpractice suits, though at times justified, are often instigated by a couple experiencing very strong feelings of anger. Anger at the partner who carried a gene that caused an abnormality, or whose sperm count or failure to ovulate is seen as the cause of infertility, is not uncommon. A child who came too early or who was aborted spontaneousely, may also be the subject of anger.

Yet, perhaps, most commonly anger is directed at oneself, and a feeling of guilt is the result.

> I should never have cleaned the house the day before the baby was born.
>
> If only I hadn't worked through my pregnancy or had taken better care of myself.
>
> If only I had listened to my mother and not fooled around, I wouldn't be sterile now.

The 'if only' game leads to feelings of guilt and anger at oneself. If unresolved, these feelings become a recipe for disaster. In fact, it is believed that prolonged depression often has its roots in such unresolved anger.

3. Bargaining

We often attempt to find someone or something to blame for a problem. We feel that this would provide an explanation for the events, and then we would have a chance of controlling the situation. Control gives us power over a disaster and a means of allowing us to believe that it is not just a chance event. If it were merely chance, we would have to face our human powerlessness and frailty — an unpleasant thought.

We are brought up with the attitude that if we work hard enough in a situation it will be resolved in our favour. This usually appears the case in education, employment, and sport. For many couples encountering problems in bearing a child, this may be the first time in their lives when it is not within their power to change an unpleasant situation. They are out of control!

One means of trying to reinstate our control is to bargain. Often the bargaining is with God.

> God, if you save my baby, I'll start going back to church every Sunday.

This type of bargaining is not new. The First Book of Samuel in the Bible tells of Hannah, the wife of Elkanah. She made a bargain with God. She promised that if he gave her a son after years of infertility, she would dedicate this son to God.

At times, bargaining occurs before the event. For example, a woman who enters premature labour or threatens to miscarry, may attempt to secure a favourable outcome by bargaining with her doctor. The bargain is generally made in silence, but she may, at least unconsciously, agree to do all her doctor instructs and more, in return for the pregnancy continuing.

4. Depression

Just as the setting of a broken leg is followed by a long period of inactivity as the bone knits, grief includes a period of convalescence. This is depression. The mind has finally accepted the news it wanted to avoid, and now must slowly regain its equilibrium.

When we look at grieving practices of the past, we remember that in many cultures mourners were forbidden to take part in gaiety for twelve months. This showed an acceptance of the fact that grieving is a long process. Of course, some situations, such as premature delivery of a child who lives, will be partially resolved by the favourable outcome. Yet there is often some degree of depression involved in even these cases. Other situations, such as prolonged untreatable infertility or the birth of a severely handicapped child, may never be resolved finally, and continuous bouts of depression may result.

Depression is a 'turning in on oneself'. Our minds need to adjust to our loss, and to do this requires most of our energy. Depressed persons may be preoccupied with their thoughts, fears, and even fantasies. They may not be able to find the motivation to carry out normal household or occupational duties. This lethargy of grief is very common. A husband may arrive home to find his wife still in her dressing-gown, weeping. Attempts to force another to 'buck up' usually meet with failure, at least initially. Preoccupation with one's self and the loss is normal.

The griever may express a strong feeling of futility and worthlessness, and display a loss of the will to go on, even to live. This is generally not a feeling to be afraid of. It is part of nature's way of making you slow down so that the healing process can be completed.

We also need to remember that the depression of grief may be further complicated by severe post-natal depression, which affects some ten per cent of women in general.

The symptoms of depression differ, as do people and situations. Some may develop intense fears of pregnancy, menstruation, babies, or death of a partner or other children. Others are discontent to remain at home, and become hyperactive. Others cannot face the outside world. Physical symptoms can include effects on nearly every system of the body. A loss of muscular power, aching or spasming muscles, 'nervous' diarrhoea, stomach cramps, headaches, and nasal congestion are just some of the possible effects on the body. Perhaps one of the most common symptoms of depression is an irregular pattern of sleep, involving continual tiredness or insomnia. Bad dreams may futher hinder the ability to sleep, as the sufferer fears the dreams will recur. Lack of sleep and the use of tranquillizers can create a vicious cycle, leading to a dependence on these prescribed drugs.

The depression may be interrupted by returns to different stages of grief, such as anger. The depression is not generally constant, but varies in intensity. One day you may feel you are ready to face the world again, only to find that this feeling is replaced by deep depression, a day, an hour, or even a minute later. You may sometimes wonder whether you will ever make it back to the land of the living. It may seem a cruel joke — one step forward and three back, two steps forward and one back. Eventually, in time and with support, you will move forward at a faster rate than the rate at which you drop back.

5. Acceptance

Little by little, grieving persons will begin to accept that they have lost something, what that loss meant to them, and that life must go on without their dream of a live, mature, healthy child — at least temporarily. **Acceptance is not happiness**! Acceptance simply occurs when we reach a stage when it doesn't hurt so much any more, and we are able to begin to think about other things and view our loss from a different perspective. The bone has knitted. It is becoming stronger, but there will be times when it will still hurt. Many couples know the renewed pain on the anniversary of a stillborn child's birth, or the news that a relative is pregnant again while they must face infertility. Acceptance does not mean happiness, but it is the foundation upon which new happiness can be built.

Conclusion

Each couple must face their own situation, their own grief. For some it will be short-lived, for others long-term.

It may be necessary to contend with recurring visits from this unwelcome friend called grief. Some will not be able to face this healing process. The bone may be injured again and again, and never knit properly. We are all different. Yet, in losing something — whatever it may be, from the loss of a dream to the loss of a third trimester to the loss of a child's life — we are all the same. We grieve.

References

1. P.G. Whittaker, A. Taylor, and T. Lind, 'Unsuspected Pregnancy Loss in Healthy Women', *The Lancet*, May 21, 1983, 1126, 1127.
2. J.F. Muller, E. Williamson, and J. Glue, 'Foetal Loss after Implantation', *The Lancet*, September 13, 1980, 554-556.
3. David Tudehope, Judith Wintour, Father John Chalmers, and Nursing Sisters in Special-Care Nursery, *Specialized Care for Newborn Babies: An Introduction to Special Care Nursery* (booklet produced for parents by the Special-Care Nurseries of the Mater Misericordiae Mothers Hospital, South Brisbane, Queensland), 5.
4. Peter A. Barr, Julie C. Dunsmore, and Glynis J. Howard, *The Death of Your Baby* (booklet for parents produced by the Department of Neonatology, Royal North Shore Hospital, St Leonards, New South Wales, 1982), 1.
5. D.I. Tudehope and M.J. Thearle, *A Primer of Neonatal Medicine* (Queensland: William Brooks, 1984), 67,68.
6. Colin Murray Parkes, *Bereavement: Studies of Grief in Adult Life* (New York: International Universities Press Inc., 1972), 128,129.
7. Stanford B. Friedman, 'Psychological Aspects of Sudden, Unexpected Death in Infants and Children', *The Pediatric Clinics of North America*, 21 (1) (1974), 103–111.
8. Talk given to Stillbirth and Neonatal Death Support Group Listeners' Course, 1984, by Father John Chalmers, former chaplain of the Mater Misericordiae Hospital, Brisbane.
9. Elizabeth Kübler-Ross, *On Death and Dying* (London: Tavistock, 1969).
10. Anna Freud, *The Ego and the Mechanisms of Defense* (1936) (New York: International Universities Press, 1946).

3 Infertility

'Perhaps the greatest pain is the pain others never see.' This thought could be written as: 'Perhaps the greatest pain is the pain others don't recognize'. Most people can understand and will accept that a couple could be upset by a miscarriage, premature birth, death, or an abnormality. Few seem to realize and accept that perhaps there will be some couples — the infertile — who may even envy the plight of others who lose a child. Nancy had a stillbirth at 26 weeks after eight years of infertility:

> About three months after I lost the baby I thought, 'A year ago if I had heard about someone who had been pregnant and had lost the baby, I'd have been jealous'. At that stage I'd never been pregnant and even had a chance of having a baby.

Infertile couples are often dealt the cruelest blow. They grieve for the loss of the children that they can only imagine. They have no tangible evidence of the object of their grief. Their loss is the loss of their dreams and hopes. Often, others are unable to realize how devastating such losses can be.

It is estimated that between 15 and 20 per cent of couples will experience some period of infertility during their life together. Many of those will go on to have their own children, with or without medical intervention. Others will complete their family through adoption. A number will go on to a change of lifestyle that does not revolve around their being a family. But before any resolution comes, the couple have to face those very difficult months of 'trying', made up of the disappointments and hopes that follow in regular cycles.

The reaction of each couple will depend upon many factors. We must recognize that each species of animal, humanity included, bases much of its society around procreation. Little girls and boys play 'mummies and daddies' at an early age. A woman's monthly cycles, a man's physical make-up, and the emphasis in our society on pregnancy and contraception are very constant, unavoidable reminders of the importance of reproduction in our society. Yet so often we forget the pressure that must then be on the couple who find difficulty in conceiving a child.

Many others, unaffected by the problem, see the infertile couple as not having lost anything! Yet any infertile couple will tell just how much they have lost. They have lost their dreams, their status as a family, and their knowing where they belong in society.

Perhaps of all those whom we consider in this book, we feel that these are the couples who are most sadly affected by nature and society. Yet they continue to live as 'normal' human beings. This chapter, then, is not only about such couples; it is also intended as a tribute to their courage, and as our attempt to help them receive from society some further recognition of their plight.

A couple are considered infertile when they have been unable to conceive within a 12-month period during which no contraceptive measures have been employed.[1] This is because 80 per cent or more of healthy couples who have regular intercourse will conceive within such a period of time.

A note on the term

We hesitate to use the word 'infertile' or discuss the 'infertile couple'. These words may bear some connotation of abnormality. They may insinuate to some that there is something defective about such people. We wish to make it clear that we do not want such couples to view themselves as defective in any way. One part of their bodies is simply not working as it should. Other people have system failures. They have kidney failure, heart disease, or are colour-blind. Unfortunately for the infertile couple, the repercussions of their reproductive system failing to work as it should are more far-reaching than the breakdown of other bodily systems. Such failure strongly involves the self-concept of the person. We wish to stress that we view infertility as a terrible problem, becuase it causes pain to two people who have so much to offer in themselves, irrespective of whether they have children or not.

We shall use the term 'infertile' as it is the word in common usage. It is used in its narrowest context, as meaning 'not fertile' or 'not able to conceive a child'. We stress that although we use this term we reject any connotation of the couple being 'defective'.

The mechanisms of fertilization
The female menstrual cycle

At puberty, the onset of menstruation marks the time for a girl from whence she can become a mother, at least theoretically. Her menstrual cycles usually continue from this time onward until she reaches her middle years.

In considering how fertilization occurs, we shall look more carefully at this cycle. The events occurring during the menstrual cycle are linked with the preparation of a woman's body for accepting a pregnancy.

The whole process is controlled by a part of the brain known as the hypothalamus. The hypothalamus acts like a conductor of an orchestra. The conductor directs certain parts of the orchestra to play in a certain way at a certain time. He blends all the different sections to play in a balanced manner, so as to produce an integrated sound. As different sections of the orchestra finish with their parts, he brings new sections into play. The conductor can make his wishes known by baton movement and by conveying instructions to leaders of particular orchestra sections. The conductor of the menstrual cycle, the hypothalamus, uses chemical substances to relay its messages to its section leader, the pituitary gland.

To continue our analogy further, consider our orchestra. The conductor begins the piece by relaying his directions to the section leaders. These leaders send out messages to their sections through their movement and timing. The section of the moment begins to play its required part until it reaches its climax. Soon its part is finished, and this information is conveyed back to the conductor. He then allows another section to come into play through its section head. This is basically the process involved in the menstrual cycle, although it is more complicated.

During menstruation, the hypothalamus sends a message to the pituitary gland. This message is in the form of FSH-releasing factor (Follicle Stimulating Hormone releasing factor), so called because it allows the pituitary gland, which manufactures FSH, to 'release' this hormone into the bloodstream. A hormone is simply a chemical messenger of the body which is transported in the blood and tells specific parts of the body to act in particular ways.

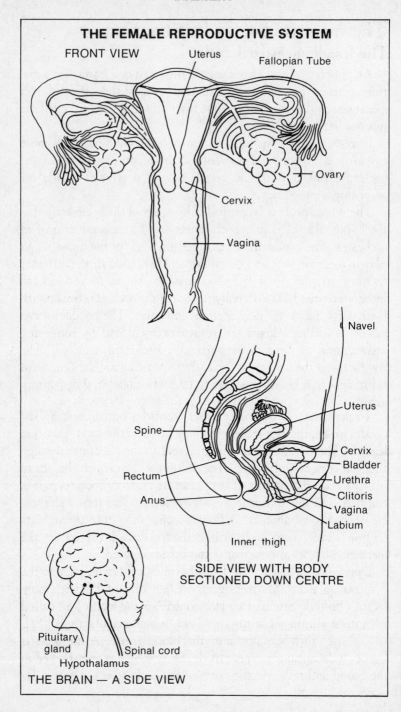

THE FEMALE REPRODUCTIVE SYSTEM

FRONT VIEW

Uterus

Fallopian Tube

Ovary

Cervix

Vagina

Navel

Uterus

Spine

Cervix

Bladder

Urethra

Rectum

Clitoris

Vagina

Anus

Labium

Inner thigh

SIDE VIEW WITH BODY
SECTIONED DOWN CENTRE

Pituitary
gland

Spinal cord

Hypothalamus

THE BRAIN — A SIDE VIEW

As its name suggests, FSH (Follicle Stimulating Hormone) stimulates about 12 to 20 egg follicles (egg chambers) of the ovaries to grow. As they grow, they manufacture more of the special female hormone, oestrogen, thereby increasing its concentration in the blood. The oestrogen, being a hormone, is the messenger to parts of the body telling them to change in some way. For example, it tells the cells of the genital tract to secrete different amounts and types of mucus. It further instructs the cells surrounding the sides of the uterus to secrete material that will build up into a lining inside the uterus that will be capable of nurturing a growing embryo. The pituitary gland continues producing FSH, and so oestrogen continues to build up in the blood.

The conductor of our operation, the hypothalamus, has been monitoring the level of oestrogen in the blood. When it reaches an appropriate level, usually at about 13 days after the first day of the previous menstrual period, the hypothalamus sends out a new direction to the pituitary gland via the LH-releasing factor (Luteinizing Hormone releasing factor). LH-releasing factor tells the pituitary gland to 'release' luteinizing hormone.

This new messenger, LH, is released into the bloodstream and tells one of the growing egg follicles to mature and burst, so releasing its egg and fluid. This is known as ovulation. It then tells the follicle cells to change to a yellow colour. Sometimes more than one follicle will burst to release their eggs. This is uncommon, but it is the reason behind multiple births in which the resulting babes are not identical.

Once released from the ovary, the egg (or ovum) is caught in a current created by the movement of the feather-like ends of the oviduct or Fallopian tube. The egg is guided into the tube, down which it makes its journey. It is generally here that the egg will meet up with the sperm if it is to be fertilized. We shall look at that story later.

Once the follicle has released its egg it collapses, and under the effect of LH, changes its colour to yellow. It now takes on an additional function and a new name, the corpus luteum. It still produces oetstrogen, but now also produces a new hormone, progesterone, the second major female hormone.

This new messenger tells the body to act in new ways. Its most important act is to tell the lining of the uterus to thicken and to produce a fluid that could nourish a fertilized egg.

If the egg is fertilized and burrows into this new lining, the corpus luteum continues producing progesterone while the placenta develops. At about 12 to 14 weeks of pregnancy the placenta then takes over that function.

If the egg is not fertilized, the corpus luteum degenerates, as do the other follicles that had been stimulated but had not been directed to burst. With no corpus luteum, the levels of oestrogen and progesterone in the blood drop. This causes the lining of the uterus to shrink. As it shrinks, the blood-vessels that serve this area break, and bleeding begins. A small amount of blood and the lining are now lost into the uterus. In a matter of hours, the uterus fills with fluid and so contracts to expel this blood and tissue. These contractions, which can vary in intensity among women, are known as 'menstrual cramps'. Menstruation has begun.

The hypothalamus, which monitors this action, notes this drop in oestrogen and progesterone and begins again to produce FSH-releasing factor, so that the process begins all over again. If we think about it, the menstrual cycle is really a lesson in perseverance. From puberty to menopause, a woman's body regularly prepares itself in the hope of attaining a pregnancy.

But this cycle alone is not sufficient to produce a pregnancy. The egg must unite with and be fertilized by a sperm. Hence, we turn now to the male and the part he plays in fertilization.

The production and distribution of sperm

Unlike the female, whose ovaries contain at birth her full complement of eggs, the male begins to produce sperm at puberty, a process which continues throughout his life.

The hypothalamus of the male produces FSH and LH hormones. These controlling hormones stimulate the maturation of sperm and the production of the male sex hormone, testosterone. Sperm production is continuous, and is known as spermatogenesis. It is a delicate business that can be affected by a variety of physical, emotional, and environmental factors. The life of the sperm may be as long as two or three months. They mature continuously, and it is even theorized that their final stage of maturity may not be accomplished until they are actually deposited inside the vagina.

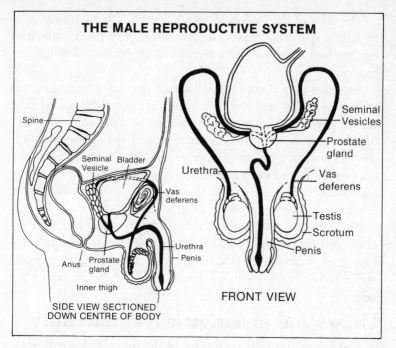

THE MALE REPRODUCTIVE SYSTEM

Spine

Seminal Vesicle Bladder

Seminal
Vesicles

Prostate
gland

Urethra

Vas
deferens

Vas
deferens

Testis

Scrotum

Penis

Anus   Prostate
gland

Urethra

Penis

Inner thigh

SIDE VIEW SECTIONED
DOWN CENTRE OF BODY

FRONT VIEW

For the sperm to enter the vagina, they must move from their storage centre, the epididymis, via the vas deferens, to the seminal vesicle. It is here in the seminal vesicle that the seminal fluid is produced, which, combined with prostate gland fluid, will transport the swimming sperm down through the urethra, out of the penis and into the vagina.

For this movement to occur, rhythmic contractions of the muscles of the male genitalia are needed. This is known as ejaculation, and occurs in conjunction with orgasm. Once ejaculated into the vagina of the female, the sperm must make their way up the cervical canal. It is believed that a selection process occurs here, and deformed, unhealthy, or injured sperm are rejected and destroyed by the immune system of the female. Once the selected sperm have negotiated the cervical canal, they must then swim toward the Fallopian tube openings in the upper part of the uterus. Many will not survive the journey. In fact, it is estimated that, of the 20 million to 250 million sperm contained in an ejaculation, only about one to two thousand of the healthiest sperm actually make it to the ends of the Fallopian tube. Of these, only one will finally succeed in fertilizing the egg.

The cells of the Fallopian tube secrete a nutritious mucus, in which the sperm can survive for an average of 48 to 72 hours. If an egg has been released when live sperm are present, fertilization may occur.

Although only one sperm will finally penetrate the egg's outer membrane, it is believed that many others are needed to help achieve this aim. The sperm carry an enzyme called hyaluronidase, which turns the jelly-like material around the egg into liquid, through which a sperm may enter the egg. It is probably the combined effect of many sperm releasing this enzyme that actually allows for final penetration. Once an egg has been entered, its membrane prevents the entry of other sperm.

The fertilized cell begins to divide. Approximately seven days after fertilization, the fertilized egg or embryo, now called a blastocyst, burrows into the lining of the uterus. If this process of implantation is accomplished successfully, a new pregnancy has begun.

Causes and investigations of infertility

If we consider the complexity of the process of fertilization outlined in the previous section, we will probably regard it as more awe-inspiring that the majority of couples fall pregnant so easily, rather than that some have trouble in conceiving. So many different aspects must come into play, and if any of these fail to function correctly, then difficulties in conceiving arise. Let us work through these aspects, as we consider the causes and investigation of infertility.

One point before we begin this section must be strongly emphasized: Medical science, particularly in the treatment of infertility, is advancing at a tremendous rate. New techniques and treatments are being devised and refined all the time. New knowledge of causes is also being accumulated. Therefore it is vital that the reader does not assume that the following information is the most up to date available. Couples must consult their doctors, who may wish to use new and different techniques from those discussed here.

The hypothalamus and pituitary gland

As we have seen, these structures deep within the brain play important roles in the control of the menstrual cycle.

a) Some rare diseases, congenital abnormalities, or developmental mishaps can cause disruption to the functioning of these structures. The symptoms of such dysfunctions are usually noticeable at an early age. Fortunately, such problems are very rare. It is suspected that there may be fertility problems if a girl has not begun to menstruate by her very late teens to early twenties, or if secondary sexual characteristics have failed to appear. Specialized tests and treatments, which we shall not discuss here, are carried out.

b) Some doctors have considered the possible role that anxiety and stress may play in infertility. They cite cases where some women's menstruation has ceased when they have been under stress, such as when they begin a new job or during a marriage breakdown. Other instances involve couples who have been infertile for a number of years, yet who fall pregnant after they have taken steps to adopt a child. However, more recent thought suggests that such couples may have fallen pregnant anyway at this time! In yet other instances, women who had previously had normal periods can experience cessation or irregularity when they are to undergo artificial insemination.

These incidents are possible indications of the effect of anxiety on fertility. Unfortunately, the story is not so clear-cut. Many doctors view anxiety as an effect of infertility, rather than its cause. Yet, anxiety may work against conception in indirect ways. For example, it may place a strain on the sexual relationship that can lead to ineffective intercourse. Some theorize that the anxiety can cause muscular contractions of the Fallopian tubes that prevent the movements of the egg toward the sperm.[2] Other evidence suggests that anxiety alone cannot cause infertility. Many doctors believe that anxiety may be a factor to be considered in some women, but not in others.

Where no other problem can be found, it is easier to attribute the infertility of a couple to anxiety and hence to prescribe relaxation. Unfortunately, such a diagnosis fails to help many couples. A diagnosis that the problem is 'all in your head' can lead to feelings of guilt and a loss of self-confidence. You can see that, when these feelings are combined with the depression caused by not being able to conceive, this diagnosis — rather than helping — can actually make matters worse.

We must realize and accept that we still know very little of the mechanism of the working of the brain and its effect on our bodies. We are beginning to accept that the influence may be profound. There is no conclusive proof that anxiety may be the cause of infertility. It is still only a suspicion, even if a convincing one.

Perhaps telling a couple that it is believed that as many as 15 to 20 per cent of couples cannot conceive at will, and that medical science does not have all the answers as to why this occurs, may at least relieve the feelings of being 'the only ones' or 'a freak'. As couples who have wanted to fall pregnant will tell you, being told to relax, and actually achieving that aim, are two different things. Encouragement to take steps to heighten health and self-esteem may be of more use. We discuss this in greater detail in the section on coping with infertility, presented later in this chapter.

Hormones and ovulation

Obviously, if no egg is released, fertilization cannot occur. There are various means of checking for the occurrence of ovulation.

You will remember that after ovulation the corpus luteum begins to produce progesterone. One effect of this hormone is to cause the body temperature to rise by up to 0.5°C. This rise of body temperature can occur up to three days after ovulation. The body temperature generally maintains its new raised level until the onset of menstruation. A woman can check this rise herself. On first waking in the morning the woman takes her temperature with a medical thermometer placed under the tongue, leaving it in place for about four minutes. Alternatively, the vaginal temperature can be taken. The woman then graphs this temperature during her whole cycle. If a constant rise is not noted in the second half of the cycle, failure to ovulate is suspected. However, it is important to note that many women who do ovulate normally have temperature charts that are difficult to interpret clearly. Therefore your doctor should be responsible for interpreting these charts.

Another means of checking that ovulation is occurring involves noting changes in the mucus secreted by the cervix. This is achieved by testing vaginal smears taken by the doctor during both the first and then the second half of the cycle. Women themselves can use cervical mucus patterns to detect ovulation.

The Billings Method of conception and contraception[3] is based on recognizing fertile mucus that is produced around the time of ovulation.

Blood tests can also be taken in the second half of the cycle to measure the level of progesterone in the blood. A further method, not commonly employed and used only for specific reasons, is the endometrial biopsy. Here a smear is taken of the uterine lining. Ovulation can be confirmed or denied from these samples.

If it is found that a woman is not ovulating, drug therapy is often attempted. Drugs such as Clomiphene (Clomid) and gonadotrophins can assist in bringing about ovulation. At times, more than one egg will be released under the effect of such drugs, and a multiple pregnancy may result. These drugs are commonly known as 'fertility' drugs.

In some cases, the hypothalamus may be affected by extreme weight loss caused by heavy exercise or anorexia nervosa.

The hormone prolactin, which is responsible for the production of breast milk, has been linked in some instances to cases of infertility. Often a nursing mother under the influence of prolactin does not ovulate until the child has begun to be weaned. It is therefore believed that infertile women who in the non-pregnant state have high levels of prolactin in their bloodstream, may be blocking fertility. Blood tests can determine the levels of prolactin, and if they are high, drugs such as bromocriptine can be administered to lower this level.

A small group of women actually suffer from premature menopause, and hence a cessation of ovulation. This situation may be caused by chromosomal problems, chemotherapy and radiotherapy used in cancer treatment, pituitary tumours, or unknown factors.

The physical aspects of the process
The female

If ovulation is occurring, the egg and sperm must successfully make their respective journeys through the female reproductive system for fertilization to occur. Let us consider first the journey of the egg (or ovum) to the uterus.

Once released from the ovary at ovulation, the egg makes its way into the Fallopian tubes. Problems with these tubes can exist. A very small number of women are born without tubes or with abnormal tubes. More commonly there are tube losses, blockages, or scarring of the tubes due to other problems. Some causes of such problems are: the presence of adhesions following previous surgery or infection; a mucus plug; previous infection and pelvic inflammatory disease; a previous ectopic pregnancy; prior advanced venereal disease; ovarian cysts; endometriosis; appendicitis; and bowel inflammation. At the end of a menstrual period the doctor may carry out specific tests to identify how healthy or 'potent' these tubes are.

The hysterosalpingogram (HSG) or uterosalpingogram is carried out by injecting into the uterus an opaque dye that can be picked up by an X-ray or ultrasound scan. Information about the uterus, the cervical canal, and the Fallopian tubes can be gleaned from these procedures. As the dye is injected and the uterus and tubes fill with fluid, there may be some slight discomfort similar to menstrual cramping. This cramping is least when the woman is as relaxed as possible.

The laparoscopy is performed under a general anaesthetic. Two small incisions are made in the abdomen. Forceps and a narrow telescope-like instrument, which has its own light-source, are introduced into the abdomen, allowing the doctor to view the reproductive organs directly. Dye may also be injected into the uterus and tubes to highlight these structures.

If a blockage or obstruction is found in the tubes, attempts may be made to correct the problem with microsurgery. Australian microsurgeons have favourable success rates with these procedures, which are also used for the reversal of tubal ligations. Other methods of unblocking tubes are also used.

The last decade has seen the beginnings of an exciting new hope for couples with tubal and other problems. This hope is in the In Vitro Fertilization (IVF) programs, in which Australian doctors display skills recognized by the rest of the world. In vitro means 'in glass'. A woman is stimulated through the use of drugs to produce mature eggs. Just prior to ovulation, a number of mature eggs and their surrounding fluid are removed during a laparoscopy. Recently supplied male sperm are then added to the eggs in a small dish or test-tube. If fertilized by the sperm, the resulting embryos are allowed to divide to a two, four, or eight cell stage. At this time, where possible, approximately three embryos are returned to the woman's uterus. It is hoped that at least one will implant and go on to produce a live baby. At present, techniques are available that allow for any excess embryos to be frozen and thawed for later use if an implantation fails or is miscarried, or if a couple desire further children. In 1983, Australia saw the birth of its first frozen-embryo child.

Attaining a successful pregnancy on entering the program is not guaranteed. Figures show that a very limited percentage will achieve a viable pregnancy on one attempt. These figures will improve as techniques are refined and more IVF units are established.

Once the egg has made its way through the Fallopian tube and has been fertilized, it must then implant successfully in the lining of the uterus. Little is known of the problems that may be encountered here. There are theories that suggest that antibodies in the lining, or the condition of the lining itself, may make implantation difficult. In fact, it is believed that some women classified as infertile may not have a strictly correct diagnosis. Fertilization may occur, but problems at the time of implantation may cause the fertilized egg to be lost before a pregnancy is even suspected. Scientists have now discovered a substance secreted after fertilization that prevents the body rejecting the embryo. This tiny new life is half composed of foreign matter, the father's genetic material, to which, the body would normally be hostile. Detection of this substance in the blood would show that an egg has been fertilized, thus indicating that conception is not the actual problem for some women.[4]

The theory behind the use of the Intra-Uterine Device (IUD) as a contraceptive is that it may irritate the uterus sufficiently to prevent implantation. Similarly, perhaps naturally occurring irritation may contribute to infertility.

Some infertile women have been rendered such by the need to remove ovaries, both tubes, and/or their uterus by surgery. Disease, such as cancer, or repeated ectopic pregnancies can bring about such losses in the reproductive system. Where the uterus is intact but ovaries and/or tubes have been removed, the use of donated ova and the available IVF procedures may hold hope for some women. Women who have suffered the loss of the uterus may be tempted to look for help to the controversial area of surrogate motherhood and future research into substitute wombs.

Endometriosis is a condition in which the tissue that normally lines the uterus and changes under the effects of the hormones of the menstrual cycle, grows outside the uterus, often affecting the tubes and ovaries. Menstruation then occurs at these abnormal sites. Infertility may result, due to blockages or biochemical dysfunctions. Drugs, such as the synthetic steroid Danazol (Danol), or progestogens such as Duphaston and the contraceptive pill, have been used to treat this condition. Some treatments cause the troublesome reproductive cells to shrink and gradually disappear. Menstruation will also stop, as the tissue of the uterus is affected, but normal cycles return when the drug therapy ceases. IVF procedures have been used to help some sufferers achieve a pregnancy. In severe cases of endometriosis, and where cysts have developed, conservative surgery may be required. A treatment known as diathermy has also been employed.

In some women, benign cysts known as Fibroids block tubes or restrict the walls of the uterus, thereby preventing implantation. Yet, some women have large fibroids and still have no difficulty conceiving. Hence, these cysts may be a factor in the infertility of some women and not others.

Let us now consider the journey of the sperm through the female reproduction system.

Once released into the vagina, the sperm must make their way through the cervix. Just prior to, and at the time of ovulation, the cervix produces a clear, slippery, viscous mucus that assists the sperm to swim up into the uterus. If the cervix fails to produce the mucus, if its production is damaged through treatment such as in a cone biopsy of the cervix, or if infection is present, the sperm's movement is hindered.

The mucus can also be 'hostile' to the sperm. The sperm, as foreign matter in the female body, are subject to attack by the immune system, but they are most likely protected by the fertile cervical mucus and by their swimming action. It is believed that the mucus of some women contains antibodies that kill the sperm before they have successfully negotiated the cervix. This is known as 'hostile' mucus. To diagnose this, a post-coital test is carried out. At a time close to ovulation, the woman usually presents herself at her doctor's surgery, two to 24 hours after intercourse. A small amount of mucus is collected by syringe or forceps, and this is then placed on a slide ready to be viewed under a microscope. If the mucus is not hostile, there should be a large number of active sperm to be seen under the microscope. If few live sperm are found, the mucus is suspected of being hostile. Unfortunately, even if hostile mucus is found, the results are not conclusive, because many women with such mucus still conceive easily. Once again, we see that this factor may be significant in the infertility of some couples only.

However, here too the pressure and anxiety involved in having to perform sexually immediately prior to the post-coital test may itself have a possible effect on the male ejaculate and the female mucus secretion.

Procedures may be used to withdraw the hostile mucus and to introduce the husband's sperm artificially in an attempt to prevent their destruction.

The male

Sperm are produced in the testicles and then stored in the epididymis. Disruption in this production can lead to an absence of sperm or a reduction in their number. There are varied causes of such problems.

a) In comparatively rare cases of mumps in childhood or in the adult human, the infection can invade the reproductive organs, causing inflammation. It is important to remember that this will occur in only a small number of men (about ten per cent) who contract mumps. Other infections, such as gonorrhea, can also cause such a lowering or cessation of sperm production.

b) Other factors which can lower male fertility are under the control of the man himself. Excessive smoking, alcohol, and poor general physical health have been suspected. Physical problems, such as maldevelopment of the testes or uncorrected undescended testes in a male newborn are more uncommon causes of later male infertility. Prior injury to the testes may also be involved.

c) As in the female, the pituitary gland is responsible for maintaining adequate production of the male sex hormones. These hormones are required for the production of sperm. If levels of the hormones are insufficient, injections of them may be considered.

d) It has been found that some men's bodies produce too high levels of the hormone prolactin, which is suspected to lower fertility. As in women, such levels can be reduced through the use of drugs. The excess production of the hormone FSH in some men is also believed to affect fertility.

e) Cancer or other growths in the male reproduction system, and the resulting treatment of such conditions, can also affect sperm production.

f) Infection or inflammation of the prostate gland or seminal vesicles can give rise to abnormal, damaged sperm, and the appearance of pus in the semen. Clearing of such infections may then boost male fertility, as long as the infection was not severe enough to cause permanent damage.

g) The nestling of the testes in the scrotal sac allows them freedom to move up and down to assist in regulating temperature. Sperm production requires a constant regulated temperature. In cool conditions, the testes move up closer toward the warmth of the body, while they descend to regulate for excess warmth caused by external forces such as weather, or internal forces such as fever. Inappropriate temperature control may occur if the testes are unable to overcome body temperature or are restricted. Such problems may occur as the result of excessively hot baths, too hot electric blankets, the wearing of close-fitting underwear, and obesity.

h) The male semen also contains sperm antibodies, whose job it is to destroy unhealthy sperm. At times, these antibodies can also destroy the healthy sperm, lowering their numbers in the ejaculate considerably. If this is the case, the semen can be 'washed' and the concentration of antibodies reduced. The treated semen can then be artificially inseminated into the female.

Compared to many of the tests that are involved in investigating the internal female reproductive system, those concerned with the male system are relatively simple to perform, mechanically at least. A male is required to provide a sample of semen through masturbation. It sounds simple, but the emotional pressure involved in going into the strange surroundings of a doctor's office or of an unnatural situation at home devoid of a partner's sexual stimulation, can lead to temporary difficulties of impotence or lowered levels of ejaculate. The whole situation can be very embarrassing for a man. At times he can feel a bit like a stud bull to be purchased or discarded according to its potency. Many men in our Australian culture, consciously or unconsciously tend to see this procedure as an attack on their manhood. Masturbation has been frowned upon, and over time it has been erroneously linked with physical and mental disorders caused by such a 'dirty' practice. In some cases, these feelings about masturbation and potency can be so strong that the male will refuse to be tested.

> When my wife started going to the doctor to be tested, I never thought it would have to involve me. I never considered the problem could be in me. After all, I was a man, and like many men had never questioned my virility. I wasn't going to be tested. I thought, 'It wouldn't be me. That's a woman's problem.'

Many doctors refuse to carry out any but the simplest tests on the female until the male is tested. This is because procedures such as laparoscopies and drug therapy require some element of risk. Ethically, they cannot and will not subject a woman to such risk if there is any chance at all that the male might hold the answer to the fertility problem. Many women are willing to undergo all tests, and feel upset when the doctor refuses to proceed with further testing for them.

> My husband wouldn't agree to be tested. I kept changing doctors, hoping they'd finally test me fully. I kept getting the same answer. I'd come to a full stop. I was prepared to go through anything. I couldn't understand their reluctance.

Perhaps there are also other factors, besides the medical, that are valid in this situation. Pregnancy, if achieved, is a time in a couple's life during which the male must play a supportive role. This role is played out more easily if he is also committed to the idea of having a child. Reluctance to undergo testing may mean that the male needs more time and understanding in coming to terms with his perspective on infertility and his commitment to becoming a father.

However, it may be that the main problem is embarrassment. Difficulties with doctors' appointment schedules often mean that the sample must be obtained at a specific time. Perhaps some flexibility needs to be allowed, so that the couple is encouraged to obtain the sample and bring it to the office some time over a period of days. Even a doctor who is able to recognize and discuss these difficulties with the couple, and reassure the male that he is not alone in his feelings, may help considerably.

When the specimen is obtained, it will be examined for a number of characteristics. The semen should be a runny, jelly-like, white or off-white liquid that is not transparent. There are usually two to five millilitres of the fluid, and in general this should contain about 20 to 250 million sperm per millilitre. Such a number seems almost unbelievable when we consider that only a few hundred will ever reach the Fallopian tubes of the female. Of these millions of sperm, at least 75 per cent must still be alive and moving after one hour. No more than 40 per cent must be abnormal. These investigations provide a sperm count, which, if low, could indicate the cause of infertility. The semen is also scanned for pus cells. If a number are found, an infection is suspected.

Semen analyses may be followed by blood samples to detect hormone levels or identify some other physical illness. In some cases a needle biopsy is performed, in which a sample of the sperm-producing cells is taken for examination.

If sperm being produced are few or abnormal, the amount of seminal fluid small, or the male impotent, the couple can consider AIH (Artificial Insemination by Husband). This procedure is also used when intercourse is not possible, due to such factors as physical handicap. Semen is collected at intervals and frozen until a sufficient concentration is obtained. The semen is then deposited into the female's system at ovulation. The woman may even be able to do this herself or with her husband's assistance, by using a special cervical applicator.

If no sperm are being produced, a man has been unsuccessful in achieving a reversal of a vasectomy, or there is a chance of a genetic abnormality carried by the father being inherited, AID (Artificial Insemination by Donor) is an option. However, this option requires some careful consideration.

AID would allow the woman to experience a pregnancy. The child would also be genetically hers. The physical characteristics of the donor can be matched closely to those of the male partner, but the child will not be genetically his. This is the same situation for the male as would occur in adoption. The male partner may need some understanding in coming to terms with his feelings, so that no one suffers in the future. Will he resent his partner, who really is the mother of this child while he is not the biological father? Will he feel less responsibility for, and involvement with, the child? Will he feel uneasy when questions are asked as to how a pregnancy was achieved after years of infertility? We will discuss these feelings in greater depth in the section on considering adoption. We make the point here that the female, so relieved at knowing she may have a child by this method, must give careful, loving consideration to her partner. He must not only cope with the prospect of not being the biological father to the child, but must also deal with the blow to his confidence caused by being labelled 'sterile'. She may have to consider giving her husband time to work through his grief before embarking on an AID pregnancy.

In many cases, both husband and wife will be thrilled at the prospect of having their longed-for child. The male may believe strongly that it is the care, not the biology, that makes him this child's father. How the pregnancy has been achieved may be unimportant to them both. On the other hand, some women may feel that they are being self-centred in wanting to become pregnant without their husband's participation, and they must weigh this against their overwhelming desire to have a child. The husband may perhaps take part in the AID process to help both partners feel more involved in the actual conception. Unfortunately, the stark, clinical, mechanical side of the insemination can often prevent such participation.

The recent successful use of donated ova in IVF programs has placed women in a similar position, although at least she feels part of the child she will carry through pregnancy.

Both partners may share the normal fears of other pregnant couples about the possibility of an abnormality in the child. AID couples may feel more concern, due to fear of inappropriate donor selection. They may share with AIH couples fear that the procedures involved may have damaged the sperm in some way. These fears are generally unfounded, and the couple share the same risk as any other of abnormality — a very small one. However, the AIDS (Acquired Immune Deficiency Syndrome) crisis has caused the closure of some AID programs until reliable screening of donated sperm can be assured.

It must be remembered that AID is not a cure for infertility. It is an option the couple may consider after accepting the fact that they are infertile. That is, as a couple they will never produce a child genetically linked to both of them. Therefore, like adoption, AID is something that must be considered carefully, and where possible worked through by the couple in conjunction with some form of counselling.

Because AID and IVF with donor ova involve a biological parent outside the marriage, some people consider these procedures morally unacceptable.

IVF programs are now offering some hope for male infertility. The figures suggest that in about half the cases of male infertility, the problem can be overcome by IVF procedures.[5] In fact, males whose sperm are blocked in the testicles may be able to have such sperm aspirated, treated, and then used in IVF procedures to attain a pregnancy.

In other cases of male infertility, there may be blockages in the vas deferens that prevent the sperm stored in the epididymis being deposited in the vagina. Infection or other causes may have blocked these hairlike tubes. Microsurgical techniques have been used to unblock the tubes, but the procedure does not carry a guarantee of success. Varicose veins surrounding and constricting the vas deferens can also reduce their efficiency.

Some men who have had a vasectomy seek a later reversal of the procedure. Where the vasectomy has been carried out skilfully and the division made well away from the epididymis, chances of reversal through microsurgery are good.

Problems in the sexual act can also lead to infertility. Impotence in the male needs to be handled with loving care. Any possible physical causes, such as a thyroid problem, must be first ruled out through medical examination. Where impotence is linked to stress, emotional, or relationship problems, the couple need to work these out together, perhaps with the support of a trained counsellor.

The 'normal' infertile couple or idiopathic infertility

It is generally believed that about 40 to 50 per cent of fertility problems can be related to the female, 30 to 40 per cent to the male, and 20 to 30 per cent to both partners. For some, the cause of their infertility will remain unknown.

Those in this latter group, consisting of about five to ten per cent of infertile couples, are termed 'normal' infertile couples. No direct cause of infertility can be ascertained, even after exhaustive testing. Obviously, there must be something amiss, but as yet we don't know what. Medical knowledge is still limited. Such couples are left with no diagnosis and generally no prognosis.

When a problem is discovered, an infertile couple can either hope for treatment that can overcome the problem, or begin to work their way through their grief. On the other hand, the 'normal' infertile couple may alternate monthly from hope to despair for many years. They never really have a chance to grieve, for while there is no definite problem, there may be hope.

Since medical science seems limited in its ability to help them, such couples may seek out other forms of healing. Unfortunately, some grasp at 'wonder cures'. They may go from doctor to doctor, desperately hoping that an initial diagnosis is wrong. We do not suggest that couples should not seek a second opinion. Even among specialists, there are differences in expertise. Generally, most doctors are willing to refer their patients to colleagues specializing in infertility. Today there is also more acceptance of alternative medicine. For many couples, a firm belief in a therapy, together with the therapy itself, may help in the problem. Such forms of treatment can't simply be discounted. But there is a difference between healthy investigation and desperate searching as a result of an inability to accept the situation.

Many 'normal' infertile couples will conceive in time without assistance. Others may enter IVF programs to achieve a successful pregnancy. IVF programs cater for many 'normal' infertile couples, as well as those suffering from tubal blockages and other problems. A small number will never conceive. Because there is no cause to which they can attribute their problem, their confusion and sense of loss is heightened.

Factors that may, or may not, affect fertility

Some general factors are believed to have possible effects on fertility.

There seems to be a fairly rapid decrease in fertility in females from the age of 35 years onwards. In males, the decline is more gradual, becoming noticeable at about age 60. Therefore, the older the couple, the greater difficulty they may have in conceiving. But this is far from always the case.

Unless adequate safety precautions are taken, the occupation of either partner can have an adverse effect on fertility, particularly if he/she is dealing with radioactivity or some chemical substances. A job fraught with a great deal of stress can also affect fertility if it leads to difficulties in, or infrequency of, intercourse. Stresses within the couple's relationship (including infertility) can also cause such problems. The less frequent or effective intercourse is, the easier it is for the appropriate days of the woman's cycle to be missed.

The health and medical history of the couple are also important. Certain chronic diseases, such as diabetes or kidney problems, can lower fertility. Even common illnesses can affect fertility temporarily. Other health factors are also emerging. For example, it is suspected that a link may exist between the drug DES (diethylstilbestrol) given to pregnant women in the 1940s and 1950s and infertility problems in the daughters — and perhaps even sons — of such mothers.

Certain factors believed at one time to be associated with infertility have been found to be innocent. Painful or irregular periods are generally not linked with infertility, and nor are infrequent periods. Infrequent period sufferers generally have the same level of fertility as others, but their number of chances of achieving a pregnancy is fewer. If intercourse is timed to coincide with ovulation, such women have just as much chance as any other of falling pregnant. Predicting ovulation is the difficult aspect, but here doctors can provide some assistance. Even the woman can predict this event through observation of her mucus.[6]

Most commonly, the uterus tilts toward the front of the body. In some women it tilts toward the backbone. Opinion is divided as to whether or not this retroversion is significant in infertility. Many doctors believe that unless the uterus is attached in this retroverted position and unable to move, it is about as significant as being right or left handed. It is simply a variation of normal.

A parent or other relative who suffered from a period of infertility does not predispose a person to this same problem.

Many couples fear that the form of contraception they used prior to trying to conceive may be to blame for their infertility. Generally, if the contraception is used correctly and properly managed, this should present no problem.

The barrier methods, such as the diaphragm and condom, are considered safe. The spermicidal creams used with such devices are deposited only in the vagina. The vagina is a self-cleaning part of the body, and soon disposes of these creams.

The IUD (Intra-Uterine Device) is a small plastic or metal device that is fitted into the uterus. It is believed to discourage implantation of the fertilized egg. In some rare instances the IUD can cause infection, usually introduced when bacteria enters the uterus via the string attached to the IUD. The IUD may also perforate the walls of the uterus. Problems can then result. If there is any pain or discharge associated with having an IUD inserted, see your doctor immediately. Many doctors will discourage the use of IUDs in women who have not had children or have had an ectopic pregnancy. This is because they appear to have more risks associated with them than other methods of contraception.

The contraceptive pill is probably the most researched drug ever used. Yet opinion is still divided on its possible effects. Generally, doctors believe that the pill is safe and is not linked to infertility. Some women do experience some delays in the return of ovulation (anovulation) on ceasing the pill. But in time the cycle returns to normal. Only a very small number of women, such as one in a thousand, fails to ovulate in time. Doctors often believe that such women may have suffered from infertility problems anyway. Treatment with drugs will generally stimulate ovulation. There is some evidence that the pill may cause raised levels of prolactin in some women. But the fact remains that the vast majority of women who have used the pill will conceive without difficulty after discontinuing its use.

In recent years, medicine has made spectacular progress toward assisting the infertile couple. At present, at least half of all infertility can be diagnosed and treated. With new techniques and refinements of old treatments, these figures are liable to rise.

Therefore there is cause for hope and expectation among infertile couples who are willing to accept medical intervention.

Emotional reactions to infertility

Unlike the grief that surrounds events such as miscarriage, premature labour, or perinatal death, the grief of infertility is often insidious and gradual. In some cases, such as situations involving hysterectomy or the absence of the reproductive system, infertility is expected. But in most cases the suspicions grow each month as menstruation appears. Few couples worry for the first few months, but as a year passes the nagging fears become pressing. They feel disappointed with each period, yet try to hope with each new month that 'maybe this month'. These continual cycles of hope and disappointment can be extremely difficult times for a couple who want a child.

Often couples have worked hard to achieve financial and emotional security before deciding to have a child. They may have arranged to buy a home and meet their commitments on one wage. They assume the female will be pregnant in a few months, and that she will leave work as the day of delivery draws near. They see themselves as a happy family. Mum and baby will wave to Dad in the morning as he leaves for work. Other children will join this happy scene at planned intervals. Their lives will contain family outings, involvements in pre-school and school activities. They will see their children into a rewarding occupation and enjoy their grandchildren in their twilight years. This dream of the future may not be one shared by all couples who desire children, but it is a common one. As the months crawl by and pregnancy is not attained, the doubts and fears arise that their dreams will not come true. For the couple in their mid to late thirties, we must add to these fears the knowledge that 'time may be running out'.

Some couples react differently. In the present age, when there is an emphasis on career and alternate lifestyles, there is a growing number of couples for whom children do not play a central role in their future dreams. Some of these couples decide to have a child when their careers are established. They worry that if they don't have a child they may regret this later in life. They may be ambivalent about this decision. For some, infertility may even be a relief, for it seems that the decision concerning whether or not to have children is made for them. The lives of such couples will continue, and infertility, though a disappointment and a slight shadow on their self-concept, does not mean devastation.

> The feeling wasn't that we had to have children to make our lives complete. We decided we'd never go through IVF or anything. We felt that if we weren't meant to have children, then we didn't want to 'fiddle' too much with things that just weren't meant to happen. Ross's work took a lot of time, and the dogs kept us busy. We were happy to just be the two of us.

We can see, then, that the emotional reactions of a couple to infertility will depend to a large degree on the strength of the desire of that couple to have a child, and on the part that child will play in their future as they see it.

In present-day Australian society, the traditional structure of the nuclear family is still recognized as the norm. Because of this, it is common for infertility to be a huge burden a couple must bear. Debate still rages as to whether the source of the desire for a child is due to an innate maternal (or paternal) instinct, or whether social conditioning plays a more important role. Perhaps another factor to consider is that infertility removes a couple's options in deciding their own future.

It seems farcical to many couples during these difficult waiting months that prior to this time they had always been so careful with contraception. It seems a cruel joke! Through the use of contraceptive measures they felt they were exerting control over their lives. Suddenly, they are no longer in control. They cannot command events, no matter how hard they try.

Each appearance of menstruation means a loss of hope for that month, and so there is often some grieving. It may be displayed in tears, a period of depression, irritability, or other negative feelings. This plainly is grief, even though it may pass in a few hours or days, as hopes for another try next month take over. A month is a long time when you're trying to have a child! As time goes on, the depression can beome more constant. Hope becomes more difficult to muster. At times, the depression can become excessive, and may affect functioning in everyday life. If this is the case, professional help should be sought. In general, though, the depression is more a feeling of deep disappointment and unhappiness. After years of infertility, these feelings are almost like old friends. The couple may wonder if they will ever feel excited and frivolous again, not weighed down by these empty feelings.

In an attempt to exert some control, many couples will begin to seek out information on methods of increasing their chances of attaining a pregnancy. The fertile days of the cycle are calculated carefully, and intercourse planned for these days. For some couples, such planning may help them relax, as they now feel that they have a better chance of achieving their aim. For many others, preoccupation with charts, mucus, and 'required' intercourse can destroy the spontaneity and enjoyment of sex.

A male may resent his being called on for 'stud' purposes. One partner may not be able to understand his/her partner's preoccupation with becoming pregnant. Doubts about sexuality and potency may begin to haunt both partners.

The mechanical nature of 'required' sex can interrupt the normal sexual act. Climax and ejaculation become of foremost importance in love-making, and the security of foreplay is often lost or severely limited. These emotional and physical deficits can severely affect the progress of intercourse and ultimately the climax. In some instances, males can face impotence or great difficulty in ejaculating, which can further lower self-confidence as well as reduce the chances of conception occurring. He may become concerned that his partner views him as a breeding machine, rather than the man she loves.

> My wife and I never had any sex problems until 'those days'. I just couldn't relax. We were comfortable with sex two or three times a week. But 'those days' it was every 36 hours or so. Sometimes I really had to work at a climax. Neither of us really enjoyed it.

In this tense atmosphere, the woman may also be left feeling drained and unfulfilled. She may feel under pressure and anxious, concerned only that her partner ejaculate. Tension and lack of foreplay may lead to less natural lubrication of the vagina, and intercourse may cause discomfort. She is less likely to reach orgasm. For both partners, the whole sexual act becomes 'something that must be done', rather than an act of love.

If the couple are unable to discuss these feelings of dissatisfaction with 'required' intercourse, difficulties may spread into their relationship as a whole. Sexual difficulties, which can naturally occur in any relationship, are more damaging when the importance of intercourse is out of perspective, as is the case when there is an intense desire to conceive. Even for a couple who are both committed to having a child, the loss of spontaneity and the loss of their dreams can be real passion-killers! The loss can even lead to lasting sexual problems.

> I grew up in a 'Puritan' environment, where sex was never discussed. My mother died when I was 19. I was led to believe sex was only for the procreation of children. After my hysterectomy I was so bitter and resentful, and turned away from my husband. I could not meet his demands, even though he was not over powering. I was ashamed, and could not even discuss with him how I was feeling. Sex was, and still is, bad for us.

The couple who have made known to others their intentions to have a child may encounter increased pressure, due to others enquiring: 'Are you pregnant yet?' Even if couples have not announced their intentions, the social enquiries may begin after a year or two of marriage. The general societal assumption that children follow soon after marriage can make the couple who have difficulty conceiving feel that their relationship or marriage is somehow less valid than one that produces children. Being regularly confronted in social situations with questions such as 'And how many children do you have?' or 'When are you going to have some children?' cause many couples embarrassment. They can be found fumbling for answers, such as 'We're not ready for children yet' or 'When we're financially secure'. The real truth is not commonly offered as an explanation. Their shaken self-esteem is too closely involved with such a topic to discuss it openly.

> I can remember I was angry toward my mother because as a teenager I can remember her saying that people who didn't have children were just selfish, wanting to go out to the pictures and have holidays. When we couldn't have any children, I was too proud to say this to Mum. I deliberately encouraged people to think that if I didn't have children that was because that was the way I really wanted it.

Some couples will seek out medical opinion before 12 months have passed. Most commonly, doctors will suggest that they wait until the 12 months have elapsed, reassuring them that many couples can require such time to achieve a pregnancy. The belief in 'do no harm' seems to suggest that it is better, within reason, to let nature take its course. Some of the tests of infertility performed on the female require general anaesthesia, and hence some risk. Doctors do not take such risks lightly.

A reassuring visit to the doctor may be all that is necessary to relax some couples. It may help them further to feel that they are doing something to clarify the problem and to contribute to its solution. Tests of infertility that involve no risk or money, such as the charting of the basal body temperature, may provide some concrete means for the couple to feel in some control. Discussion with the couple about methods of predicting ovulation, combined with an open discussion of optimum intercourse and the problems of anxiety, may provide more hope for anxious couples than simply telling them to go home, relax, and keep trying until the 12-month period has passed. On the other hand, some may feel threatened by the mechanical aspects of the process.

> That first visit I got all the temperature forms, and he told me to do it for three months. I thought 'Hell!' I think I went along to that first appointment thinking we were going to find out for me straight away what was wrong, rather than this continued thing that seemed like it would go on for ever, changing our sex-life.

The doctor will need to use his/her knowledge of different couples when deciding which approach to use. In some cases, particularly those involving older couples, the doctor may decide to begin testing before the end of the 12-month period.

The period during which a couple undergo testing can be very taxing. The tests themselves, unless handled discretely, may add to the embarrassment and cause a further erosion of self-esteem. We have already discussed this embarrassment in terms of the reactions of the male to providing a semen sample. The woman may have to undergo internal examinations, injections, and drug therapy, which may leave her feeling embarrassed, uncomfortable, and even ill. She may forget that there is any part of her body other than her reproductive organs!

Couples may have varying reactions to testing. Many are relieved that at last they may have their suspicions confirmed or denied. If no problem is detected, there may be relief, and the tension involved in the situation may be diffused. Others feel that they would prefer to find a rectifiable problem, which, once overcome, will lead to their dream of pregnancy.

Some may initially deny the existence of the problem, while others experience anger toward themselves, their partner, the doctor, their bodies, God, those who 'breed like rabbits', pro-abortionists, child abusers, pregnant women, and a multitude of others. They may become depressed and withdraw from others, particularly children, families, and pregnant women. To put it simply, these couples are grieving their loss.

The loss of their dreams, their potential, meaning in their lives, and the experience of pregnancy are shattering to these people. Yet generally this is not recognized by the rest of society.

> I was actually mourning the children I'd never have. I was often very very sad, but I couldn't actually tell people I was feeling sad because of this, because there was nothing concrete to mourn.

These couples may be denied the right to grieve in a very grievous situation. As we saw in Chapter Two, one of the tasks of resolving grief involves the experiencing and the discussion of the loss. If these needs are frustrated through being unacceptable to others, the couple are unable to move toward acceptance of their loss.

There are varying reasons why the chance to grieve may be denied these couples. Firstly, infertility strikes close to the very heart of a man's and a woman's identity. Their most obvious characteristic, their gender, is 'tainted'. They may feel a failure as a man or woman. There may be a mixture of feelings of confusion, embarrassment, and shame. Hence, they may prefer to keep the problem a secret from others. This may be more pronounced when the male is the source of infertility. Male sterility, rather than being confined to an inability to have children, is often erroneously seen as a slur on a male's masculinity in general. Little wonder, then, that in our culture men don't discuss it very often!

> Often I've wished it were me with the problem. At least then society would be on my side. An infertile man is too often made to feel his masculinity is on the line.

Many couples, when they find a problem, are unable to grieve because they are not sure if they have anything to grieve about. Many problems can be rectified. The couples still have hope, unless the situation involves such problems as a hysterectomy, premature menopause, or azoospermia (complete lack of sperm). Couples don't feel that they should grieve when there is hope. Yet they have lost their innocence about child bearing, and each month they have lost those particular hopes of attaining their dream. They have also lost the ability to control their fertility, a fact others take for granted. They have sufficient reason to grieve.

When a problem is diagnosed to involve only one partner, this partner must deal with an added dimension to his/her grief, that of guilt feelings. The feeling of guilt is a very strong, destructive emotion. The 'guilty' partner may try to punish him- or herself, or seek some means of undoing this 'punishment'. Guilt feelings are difficult to deal with at any time. When your problem affects someone you dearly love and also prevents him/her from being fulfilled, its pangs tear deeper. It is often easier when it is you alone who must face pain and disappointment, rather than when your problem hurts one who is trying to be supportive and caring. The 'guilty' partner, whose self-image is so badly affected, may feel that he/she doesn't deserve consideration from the other. The 'guilty' partner may then accept negative behaviour toward him/her as being justified. He/she doesn't deserve any better, according to these feelings. This low opinion of his/her worth can go beyond the relationship with a partner, into outside activities.

> When my wife found out I was sterile, she became more and more distant. Our marriage finally broke up. I don't blame her, though. She tried, but she wanted a child so much. She was better off finding someone who could give her that. I couldn't. It wasn't her fault.

The time spent waiting for test results can be filled with tension, adding further difficulties to the situation.

> Every time I went to get the results, my hands used to tremble as I opened the letter or picked up the phone. Sometimes I was crying before the doctor even came on the line.

With IVF procedures and other medical advances, the probability of success in attaining a pregnancy for many infertile couples continues to increase. Unfortunately, there will continue to be couples who are unable to achieve a pregnancy with such intervention. IVF success-rates are not high, and even AIH and AID are not successful in every case. Medical intervention may not be possible for others in cases of severe chronic maternal disease, a hysterectomy, or severe reproductive-system abnormalities. There will continue to be those couples who will never have their own biological child.

The publicity that has occurred in the last few years surrounding IVF, has opened up the subject of infertility for discussion. Unfortunately, it has also created a belief in some sections of the community that such procedures are the answer for all infertile couples. Comments such as 'O well, you can go on IVF' exemplify a failure to understand the true situation and success rates. The couple's problem is almost dismissed as insignificant. Other misunderstandings have arisen through the public awareness of the role of venereal disease in some cases of infertility. Many people in society are therefore suspicious of such couples, believing them to have been promiscuous. Hence, such couples are put under further pressure through the withdrawal of some social support and compassion.

A couple's reaction to their fertility problems can fluctuate widely and often. At some times they are optimistic, and begin to believe that it will happen. They may even succeed in forgetting the problem for a while. They may struggle to keep this positive attitude, only to find it replaced in time, varying from minutes to weeks, by a dark depression and a feeling of 'What's the use? It will never happen.' They may just want to give up or run far away! These mood swings are normal, and they may occur without a precipitating event. They may also be triggered by simple events, such as the sight of a baby or pregnant woman or a television program on children. Good intentions to relax and remain positive are difficult to fulfil!

Some couples seek to forget their pain through 'consolation prizes'. Feeling that their years of waiting and saving have been wasted, they may spend a substantial amount of money on other things, such as a trip, stereo equipment, or clothing. The infertile woman who has put off buying clothes in case she gets pregnant, may rebel against her situation and go on a spending spree for new fashionable clothes. The anger of grief is then satisfied in a splurge of healthy rebelliousness. The fight is not lost, only delayed!

In very rare instances the desire to have a child can lead to an emotional disorder known as a pseudocyesis, or phantom pregnancy. Menstruation ceases, the abdomen enlarges, and other symptoms of pregnancy seem to appear. Yet there is no pregnancy causing these changes. The mind has taken over the body to play out a role it desperately wants to fulfil, that of being pregnant. A pregnancy test will show negative results, and no pregnancy sac is to be found. This situation shows a person in deep distress, and requires a great deal of tender loving care and professional support if further emotional damage is to be avoided.

During the months of trying and testing there may be disruptions in the woman's menstrual cycle, which can lead to a belief that she is pregnant. If menstruation is simply delayed, the let-down can be crushing.

> The month before I fell pregnant with Brenton, I'd gone nine weeks and convinced myself I was pregnant. I'd felt all the things I thought you should feel when you are pregnant. After I started to bleed, I couldn't go to work the next day. I was so upset.

Some infertile people fantasize about longed-for children, and then feel guilty for 'being so silly'. It often remains their secret. When baby-sitting other people's children, they imagine them to be their own.

> I went through a stage of imagining children, not babies, but those of about three or four. It was my secret vice. They were quite real. They had names — Sophie and Daniel.

A pregnancy that is attained after years of infertility can be a joyful, yet fearful, experience. These prospective parents have lost their innocence about child-bearing. They may become extremely concerned about miscarriage or other pregnancy losses. The loss of this cherished pregnancy would be a blow from which many feel they would never recover. Once again, understanding and acceptance of their fears by doctors and others is vital, even if some fears seem irrational.

Over time, many couples resolve their grief and come to an acceptance of their infertility. It still has the power to hurt them, but it is now seen from a new perspective. The couple are able to focus on their relationship and other areas of their lives. At this stage, couples who continue with treatment find some of the pressure and tension alleviated by this change of attitude.

Other couples discontinue infertility treatment at this time. To them this is preferable to coping with the gruelling cycles of hope and despair. They are no longer prepared to have their lives ruled by one desire, and seek out new experiences for themselves. This is a very difficult decision for a couple to make. Such a decision means surrendering their dreams of the future. It is a decision that can also involve some feelings of guilt. They may feel guilty for 'copping out', for giving up 'without a fight'. They may feel guilt for giving up on something they spent so long trying to achieve.

The feeling of guilt is made more intense when only one partner wishes to discontinue treatment. He/she then must experience the added feelings of disappointing his/her partner, as well as possible feelings of resentment on the partner's part. A decision to discontinue treatment then requires a great deal of courage and soul-searching, and hence is not a decision to be denigrated by others.

Coping with infertility

In discussing coping with infertility, we make the point that what follows is not meant as a prescription to magically relieve the pain of couples facing the problem. There is only one sure cure, and that is a conception eventuating in a live, healthy child! What are presented here are suggestions that may provide support to couples in developing their own individual means of dealing with the problem. In the end, it is vital to remember that books and others cannot tell you how to cope. Ultimately, coping is the domain purely of each individual. The thoughts presented here may simply help to provide a move in the right direction.

1. Prepare yourself for a pregnancy!

It may seem ironic to suggest that a couple should prepare for a pregnancy that may never eventuate. Yet we feel that it is no more strange than the suggestion that a couple relax and forget about pregnancy!

Let us acknowledge the fact that for a couple who do want a child, it is virtually impossible to forget about it. Therefore they shouldn't be made to feel guilty about it, and hence become anxious that their thoughts are somehow blocking conception. Instead, face it! They want a child!

Prepare the body in the best way possible for a pregnancy, so that when it does occur the baby has the best possible chance in life. When one feels like giving up, it shows in one's body and the lack of care for it. The best body for pregnancy is a healthy one! Therefore, by being healthy and having fulfilling intercourse, a couple are doing the very best they can to achieve a pregnancy.

The couple need to consider their diet, and alter it if it is inadequate or inappropriate (see Chapter 11 for suggestions). Even when they don't feel like eating properly, they can tell themselves: 'I am doing this for a reason. A healthy body has the best chance of pregnancy.' There is no need to be too self-critical. A splurge on a huge piece of cake when you're feeling very low does not make you a failure!

Combine good eating with exercise. The body during pregnancy is under strain, and a healthy body bears this strain more efficiently. A healthy body also produces healthy sperm, usually two or three months before they are actually used. If they have the time and opportunity, the couple may join an exercise class or a sporting club, or devise an exercise program in consultation with their doctor for their combined home use. It's hard keeping up an exercise program, but the wish to promote pregnancy can be a strong motivator.

Besides preparing the body for pregnancy, the pursuit of health has other advantages. Firstly, it gives one a feeling of being able to do something to help oneself. It makes the individual a participant, along with his or her doctor, in helping to achieve a pregnancy. Such a role is more encouraging than that of passive recipient of treatment.

Secondly, good health seems to actually have an effect on feelings of well-being. The body works more efficiently and suffers from less illness. People who are fit not only feel good, they also look good. There may be a loss of some excess weight. The body is more attractive to others. In fact, research shows that the physique can affect the way in which others treat a person.

In going to exercise classes or joining a sporting team, the couple may have a chance to meet people who know them only as they are now, not as a depressed infertile couple. When others react to them as more positive people, they begin to realize that they are more than, as one woman put it, 'a defective breeding machine'. They may even find other infertile couples among their new-found friends!

2. Seek satisfaction in your medical advice

When a couple decide to consult a doctor about their fears, it is important to seek eventual referral to a specialist in gynaecology or infertility. Some specialists actually develop further expertise in the area of infertility, and may be attached to IVF programs or infertility clinics of major hospitals. The specialist should be able to provide the couple with the most recent information on, and treatment of, infertility.

Perhaps as important as the doctor's knowledge, is the relationship of the couple with him/her. The testing and treatment periods are often lengthy. It is during these difficult times that a couple need to feel comfortable with their doctor. They are then more willing to ask questions, and will feel less embarrassment during the procedures. Communication and support from one's doctor is vital in overcoming the tension.

It may take time to find the doctor with whom one feels comfortable. Different personalities require different interactions. There is no crime in seeking out the doctor with whom your personality is suited.

3. Relaxation

Simply making a decision to relax is often insufficient. There are techniques that can be learnt and employed quite easily by a couple to facilitate relaxation. With practice, these may help them attain greater tranquillity (see Chapter 11 for more details).

4. Expend time and effort on your partner

Infertility can be a great strain on a couple, so great in fact that some relationships do not survive it. Couples who have experienced long periods of infertility will attest to the fact that it can permeate their sexual relationships, social contacts, and communication. Problems in a relationship only serve to make this difficult time even worse. Anxiety and difficulties in intercourse may arise, which further decrease the chances of attaining a pregnancy.

The couple need to try to turn their thoughts away from pregnancy for at least a part of the month. What better time than those non-fertile days! During these days, they should concentrate on each other, thinking of ways to please the other. It might be making a special meal or having a candlelight dinner, writing a poem or a song for a partner, or dancing to favourite music. They might even enjoy an intimate evening and intercourse, but *only* when pregnancy is *not* the aim. Let the aim be simply to enjoy each other's company. Make a determined effort to spoil the other.

It is very sad if, for the want of a child, the most important relationship is neglected. Make the effort to thank your partner for his/her support and love. Remember that you were interested in each other first as a man or woman. The wish is not simply to have a child, but to have one by the person you love!

Unfortunately, for a few the want of a child can overpower feelings for their partner, and a breakdown occurs. Such a break is devastating to the partner who is deserted, particularly if his/her self-esteem has already been shaken by the effects of infertility. Fortunately, most couples are able to face their disappointment united. To keep their unity strong under such pressure, it must be nurtured and treated with care. We discuss this further in Chapter 9.

5. If necessary, unashamedly seek professional help

Unfortunately, people in our society are less willing to accept assistance in maintaining their mental health than they are for their physical health. Just as there is no shame in seeking help if our body is unwell, so there is no shame in seeking support for our mental health before it becomes seriously affected.

At times, the pressures of infertility can be so intense that they begin to interfere with a couple's normal daily functioning. There are trained counsellors who may be able to help guide them through this emotional maze in which they seem to be wandering. Such professionals are often attached to support groups in your state, or attached to hospital units. For the sake of both partners, the future, and the chances of attaining a pregnancy, help needs to be sought if one feels that it is 'all becoming a bit much'. One can usually recognize when that time comes. If you are in that situation, you needn't feel a 'freak' or inadequate. You aren't! Many people lack the support of family and friends through distance or other circumstances. There may have been other pressures, financial or emotional, which are significant in themselves. Little wonder that there comes a time when it becomes too much! Professional help is simply providing the support one may have missed elsewhere. Rather than feel ashamed, the couple should feel proud that they have the courage to do something about a problem before it becomes unmanageable. The importance of preventive medicine applies in mental health also.

6. Develop your other unique talents

When a couple face difficulties in bearing a child, the effort and time required in dealing with this problem can blind them to the other aspects of their lives. The constant timing of ovulation, doctors' visits, and treatments serve to focus their attention on one aspect of themselves — their ability to reproduce. When they seem to be failing in this area, they can begin to see themselves as worthless people as a whole. Nothing can be further from the truth.

Each individual has unique talents to contribute. While they are trying to conceive a child, the couple need to look for their unique talents, if such aren't already obvious. Such a pursuit may at least occupy some of the time which may be spent in depression. At best, it may open up a whole new world and future for them.

Look into further study or adult education groups. Write a children's story or a novel. Make all your Christmas presents. Take up part-time, full-time, or voluntary work. Help out with remedial reading or mathematics at the local school. Bake biscuits for a restaurant. The list goes on!

The couple experiencing depression may not feel the urge to get out and develop new talents. Perhaps they could join a club or do a course *together*! They may need to think to themselves: 'Depression, even if it doesn't prevent my conceiving, is not helping me. Maybe if I can get more involved, it might help. If not, it's still better than spending my time like this. It can't hurt!' Activities may serve simply to fill those long days of the month. On the other hand, they may become so absorbing that pregnancy becomes something only in the back, not the forefront, of the mind — for a while at least.

7. Think through carefully why you want children

This may seem an unusual suggestion, but is probably of vital significance in coming to terms with our fears. Most people, if asked why they wanted children, are stumped for an answer. The following are some reasons people have children:

a) It's the 'done thing'.
b) All their friends are having children.
c) That is the future as they see it.
d) Their parents want grandchildren.
e) They like children or babies.
f) They want to be 'a family' or a mother or a father.
g) Their partner wants children.
h) They want someone to care about them in their old age.
i) They want to leave something of themselves when they die or someone to carry on the family name.
j) They don't want to be lonely.
k) They want someone who will love them and whom they can love.
l) They want someone else who is like their partner or themselves.
m) They want some meaning in their lives and a position in society.
n) They may regret it later if they don't.
o) Time is running out on their fertility.
p) Their children can become the kind of people they wanted to be.
q) They have never had contact with, or considered, any other lifestyle.

The list goes on. Generally, though, most couples have a child without even considering why. Couples facing infertility often know that they desperately want a child, but actually why they want this is difficult to put into words. Yet perhaps this is vitally important.

If we look at the reasons listed above, we see that many people have children to fulfil their own needs. This is perfectly valid if the child's needs are also fulfilled. Parents and children are then mutually rewarded. Unfortunately, at times, the parent's needs that urged them to have a child blind them to the individual needs of that child. Children are frustrated and parents disappointed. As the children grow, some parents begin to wonder whether it is all worth it, and what it will be like to be 'free' again.

Perhaps the strongest motivation for having a family is that it is the 'accepted thing'. We are conditioned as children in a nuclear family to see marriage and children as the natural progression, the way of nature. When a couple are confronted with the possibility of not producing children of their own, their world is thrown into confusion.

The status of 'parents' gives one a position or niche in society. One is a mother or a father. With these titles come duties, responsibilities, ways of behaving, something to occupy one's time, a conversation point, and an entrance ticket to all those institutions that are served by, and serve, parents. The position in society of those who are not parents is not so clear. They become part of a minority. They are faced with non-inclusion in their peer group. It's a painful adult version of being the new kid at school, who didn't really fit into any particular 'crowd'. Human beings are communal creatures. We want and need to belong, to identify with the majority. Infertility robs couples of their belonging. They are on the outside looking in. It hurts! A child would make them part of the group. But is it legitimate to place such a fulfilment of one's needs on a child?

The couple need to ask themselves some of the following questions:

1. What do we see ourselves doing in 30 years?
2. What do we want to get out of life?
3. In the people we admire most, what are the qualities we admire? Is it their children?
4. Do we want children because we can't imagine a life without them?
5. Do we feel pressured to have children by anyone?
6. Why do we want children?

When a couple begin to think seriously about such questions, they may see a little more clearly through the haze that surrounds them. Children will not live parents' lives for them. They will go their own ways one day. Their needs may be in conflict with those of their parents.

Children are a wonderful source of joy; if we weren't convinced of that, none of us would try to have them. But they can't be one's whole life, even if there is no trouble in producing them.

Children provide a way of allowing parents to live on after death. They are parts of them. Is it the genetic make-up of a child that makes parents love them, or is it the effort they put into them? This is an important issue to consider if couples are thinking about adoption or artificial insemination by donor.

Couples cannot rationalize their wishes for a child. Perhaps some of this urge is innate, to ensure continuation of the species. When they can't produce a child at will, a couple must be prepared to look at alternatives for their future, rather than spend a life of depression and bitterness lamenting over something they cannot change. Facing the unfavourable prospect may actually help to destroy its sting.

If, after consideration, the couple come to the conclusion that children are an important part of their life, they may decide on adoption, fostering, or an occupation dealing with children. If not, they may look to a cause or a career. The couple shouldn't be afraid to think about what they will do if they can't have children. But this needn't be rushed. Some are not able to cope with such thoughts while deep in grief.

What could their future hold for them? They may make moves toward a future that would at least be satisfactory, even if not their hearts' desire. If the worst then happens, and they have no children, they have a position, some plans. If they do have children, they can only be pleasantly surprised. Thinking through these issues, even in this instance, can only help the couple and their later children. They will know clearly in their own minds why they had this child, something many parents have not thought about.

When their future takes on a clearer dimension, and does not centre solely on having a child, the couple may find some of their fears slightly relieved, and the difficult months may be a little easier. Of course, reaching a point at which they can think through these issues may not come immediately; for in such thinking couples are often beginning to resolve their grief.

8. Talk selectively about your infertility

Support for infertile couples comes from words and actions of others who try to understand and who accept the couple's right to be upset. Not everyone will feel comfortable about discussing the problem. If the subject is broached, some will try to change the conversation's direction. Unfortunately, others may want to discuss the issue as a curiosity, a piece of gossip. Therefore, when a couple feel the need to discuss their difficulties, it is important that they seek out those persons who can provide genuine concern for their feelings.

Often this type of concern will come from close family members. However, at times families are also unable to understand the depth of emotions involved. The infertile couple may feel jealous of brothers and sisters who have a child. They are torn by their feelings of jealousy and disappointment, and yet feel guilty about such feelings. Family births, christenings, and celebrations can be a trial for the infertile couple. Brothers and sisters, feeling deeply for the affected couple, may be embarrassed about their pregnancies and families. They don't quite know how to react. Do they involve the couple in family gatherings and act naturally, or do they try to protect them from such situations? If feelings are not discussed within families, then a rift may occur.

There is one group of people who can often provide the greatest understanding — other infertile couples, or couples who at one time faced the problem. Support groups provide contact with other couples who know only too well the trials and pain of infertility.

If he/she feels the need to talk, the infertile person should seek out a listener. The listener is often the person who has been there before in the good and bad times. They are the ones with whom the sufferer feels free to be himself/herself. The couple have a right to feel pain, and a right to be soothed and coddled. No one ever outgrows that need!

Of course, one's partner is the person from whom the greatest support usually comes. Honesty between husband and wife is vital. If one partner feels hurt when a friend excitedly announces her own pregnancy, he/she should tell his/her partner. One's pain and anger should not be directed toward one's partner because of his/her untidiness, cooking, or manners. A partner can't help ease the other's pain when he/she is not aware of it.

The suggestions we have presented here are based on the assumption that when a couple encounter infertility it can become a focal point of their life during that time. Instead of suggesting that they try to forget it and relax, we suggest that they do everything humanly possible to achieve a pregnancy and prepare their lives to accept a child. The advantage of this approach is that the couple no longer need to feel guilty for thinking about a pregnancy. They have the best motivation for carrying out the suggestions. Some of the activities may even enrich their lives as individuals or a couple.

Considering adoption?

Adoption in Australia is handled by State government departments concerned with Child Welfare, and, in some States, by private institutions. In most developed countries where there is widespread use of contraception and the practice of abortion, the numbers of children available for adoption have been greatly reduced. Waiting lists and waiting periods are long. The adoption agency will investigate a couple fully before approval. For information on the procedures carried out in your State, contact the local child-welfare agency. The State government pages of local telephone directories generally list the necessary contact numbers.

Here we wish to look more closely at adoption as an alternative to infertility. As we mentioned earlier, both adoption and artificial insemination by donor have within them an inherent danger for the future outcome of such a situation. In both cases, the child will not be biologically linked to one or both parents. The child may look like the parent, but he/she has got those characteristics from another. This child cannot ever be genetically yours. This is a fact which must be faced.

This fact may be obvious intellectually. However, accepting it can be emotionally more difficult. As we noted in the previous section, a biological child can fulfil a parent's need to reproduce his/her own genetic patterns. An adopted child can never do this. A child who is adopted as a second-rate replacement for a much-wanted biological child can never make the grade.

> I have never really accepted my infertility, but my husband did agree to adopting a child. She was ten weeks old when she came to us. But subconsciously, she was never my own, though I loved her dearly. Although my husband agreed to the adoption, she was never his. Sometimes he would become angry with me and about

our child, and would say 'People who can't have children of their own should not adopt other people's children!'

In some rare cases, child-welfare departments find adopted children being returned to their care in later years. These children usually didn't fill the gap in their parents' life adequately.

An adopted child must be loved as a child for his/her own sake. It must be the effort that is put into bringing up that child, rather than the biological act, that makes a child part of these parents. We hesitate to use the words 'that makes these children yours'. Commonly, we use terms like 'Bob and Jane's children', as if they were owned by their parents. But children are not chattels; no one 'owns' a child, even if it is biologically determined by their union.

Children, whether adopted or biological, are given in trust to parents to be nurtured to maturity, at which time they must decide their own future. Perhaps there is one advantage adoptive parents have over natural parents. They may not try to force the child to be like a parent or relative. In some ways, dealing with an adopted child is dealing with a mystery. What talents that child may possess are largely unknown, unless there is in-depth knowledge of the biological parents.

It is likely that an adopted child may one day wish to seek out his/her natural family. This is a possibility that must be accepted before the adoption occurs. Such a search is not a denigration of adoptive parents. It is a part of the adopted person's understanding of who he/she is and where he/she fits in the world. Unfortunately, accepting such a search can be difficult for adoptive parents, whose self-confidence may never have fully recovered from the pain of their infertility; or, if they have recovered, the pain may be reawakened by this search.

If the parents accept that an adopted child has rights as an individual and if they maintain their position in society in other ways than through children, the joy and security of adoption for both parents and child will usually be undisturbed. If a couple want children because they honestly believe it is the way of life for them, and they feel that it is the child who matters, then adoption may be for them. If adoption is a 'poor second' to their own children, with the adopted child being 'better than nothing', then for the sake of both that child and themselves, the couple should think seriously about other alternatives to infertility.

Conclusion

Infertility or difficulties in conceiving a child affect about one couple in six at some stage during their reproductive lives. At least half of these couples will be diagnosed as having problems that can be treated or overcome through medical intervention. Many of the remaining half will eventually fall pregnant as time passes without any such intervention.

A small proportion will have problems that cannot be overcome, or will simply never conceive. These couples must then consider alternatives to having their own children. This sentence is so inadequate, since it fails to suggest the pain and agonizing that goes into such decisions. We do not profess even to be able to convey the hurt these couples experience. We simply salute them for their incredible courage.

In many cases of protracted infertility, the couple look closely at the factors for and against parenthood. Some even go close to convincing themselves that they don't want children after all. Some won't have them. But most others will continue to strive toward that aim. For some, it will become an obsession.

In today's world, the infertile couple have reason to be hopeful. For some, achieving a pregnancy may take a great deal of patience and perseverance. However, most are prepared to spend the time, and somehow they muster the courage. None of these couples enter parenthood as blithely as do many others, or even as they themselves may have done before this time. Many make fine concerned parents, a bonus outcome for all their effort.

References

1. Derek Llewellyn-Jones, *Everywoman*, 3rd ed. (London: Faber and Faber, 1982), 97.
2. J.P. Greenhill, 'Emotional Factors in Female Infertility', *Journal of the American Academy of Obstetrics and Gynecology*, 7(6) (1956), 602–606.
3. Evelyn Billings and Ann Westmore, *The Billings Method* (Victoria: Ann O'Donovan, 1980).
4. Glenn D. Braunstein, William G. Karow, William D. Gentry, and Maclyn E. Wade, 'Subclinical Spontaneous Abortion', Obstetrics and Gynaecology, 50(1) (1977 Supplement), 41s–44s.
5. Talk by Professor John Leeton to IVF Friends, Melbourne, March 26, 1985, and printed in the Newsletter of IVF Friends, June 1985, 13,14.
6. Billings, *op. cit.*

4 Miscarriage

'I had a miscarriage.' Those words are said by many women, but they fail to convey the depth of feelings that accompany the event.

'O well, it was probably for the best.' 'You will have lots of other children.' We have all heard these comments. It makes no difference that in most cases they are true. The couple who lose their child through miscarriage, particularly one that occurs before 14 weeks, are at times denied the right to grieve for that child, a child who has been a part of their lives. For many, this child was not just a mass of cells that bore little resemblance to a human being. It was a child who had lived and perhaps gone on to become the Prime Minister — at least in their minds.

No — perhaps they never held him/her. Yes — perhaps the child may have been born with an abnormality. Yes — they may have been fortunate not to have felt its movements. But, no — you can't deny a child that was yours by producing logical explanations.

Some will be relieved that an unwanted pregnancy resolved itself. Others may have fallen pregnant unexpectedly, and are optimistic about their next planned attempt. But to deny a couple the right to grieve a miscarriage is to deny the importance of this child, to deny a life. From the moment a pregnancy is confirmed, a woman is aware that her body sustains another life. For a couple who want this child a great deal, it is a time of great rejoicing.

Unfortunately, many women who miscarry a first pregnancy are unprepared for this event, and hence the blow is shattering. Unless they have encountered others who have lost in this way, their chances of being naive about such losses are high. Society is generally quite silent on this subject.

We are not by any means advocating that women should be encouraged to brood about this possibility, and hence rob themselves of the enjoyment of a most wonderful time of their lives. The majority of women will go on to carry their babies to term. We simply suggest that the silence and ignorance surrounding miscarriage only serve to heighten a couple's sense of isolation.

In many medical circles, miscarriage is viewed as a normal divergence of pregnancy. Unfortunately, the feelings that accompany it are far from so easily accepted. We realize that doctors and others may simply be trying to keep the couple feeling optimistic. Couples appreciate these intentions and human thoughtfulness. Unfortunately, by failing to acknowledge that it is a terrible blow and that couples do have a right to feel sad, others can leave the couple feeling that they may be overreacting to the situation. The couple may little realize that similar events have caused major traumas in the lives of others, simply due to the shattering nature of the situation.

The medical terms
Miscarriage and spontaneous abortion: some confusion

Within this book we shall use the term **miscarriage**, for it is the word in common use. The word, though, does hold the possibility of being misconstrued.

When a pregnancy is lost through miscarriage, this does not insinuate that there is anything 'miscarried', in the sense of 'badly carried'.[1] The woman has not done something wrong in the way she 'carried' the child. Therefore she is not at fault, and need feel no guilt. Except in cases of severe physical abuse of her body or the use of substances poisonous to the foetus, the mother is in general powerless to instigate or prevent a miscarriage. Miscarriages are natural processes. As with many aspects of nature, they occur irrespective of how human beings feel about it, and are unaffected by their attempts to change the situation. If nature deems it, the child will be lost.

Your body has for some reason followed a dictate of nature, and you can be sure that you are not at fault. To relieve feelings of possible guilt and give a pregnancy its best chance, doctors often prescribe bed rest and a good diet when a miscarriage looms. Unfortunately, it is not proven that these have any effect in preventing such an occurrence. If the woman has done her best to ensure a healthy child and yet nature deems that this child is to be lost, irrespective of any medical intervention, then no one is to be blamed.

Doctors do not use the term 'miscarriage', but rather call such a loss a **spontaneous abortion**. A spontaneous abortion is the ending or termination of a pregnancy prior to the time at which a baby or foetus could live on its own, and which involves no outside agent. Approximately 15 to 20 per cent of confirmed pregnancies will be lost in this way, with about three quarters of this number being lost before 14 weeks' gestation.

Our society popularly uses the term 'abortion' in a more controversial manner, referring to a voluntary ending of a pregnancy by physical intervention. This is an **induced abortion**. Some States of Australia have passed legislation to legalize some induced abortions, which are then termed **legal terminations**. The availability of such terminations in different States varies.

It is important that couples who abort spontaneously, or miscarry, are aware of this difference. Some hear their doctor say that they have aborted, and are confused, somehow feeling that they have voluntarily caused their child's death.

The miscarriage itself

The onset of vaginal bleeding in a pregnant woman is a frightening experience. A proportion of women do bleed during pregnancy with no damage to the child. At times this is due to the process called nidation, whereby the fertilized ovum burrows into the uterine lining. Some small amounts of blood may be released at this time. Other amounts may be lost later, as the placental attachment grows in size. Other women experience some bleeding during the times when menstruation would have occurred if they were not pregnant. Blood loss may also be associated with a urinary tract infection, a polyp, or an erosion, or be linked to a drop in progesterone as the placenta takes over its function.

Fortunately, most cases of bleeding in early pregnancy are not related to the health of the foetus, and hence will not lead to miscarriage.

Although not all vaginal bleeding indicates that a miscarriage is in progress, doctors err on the side of conservatism and consider such bleeding as a **threatened miscarriage**. A threatened miscarriage is heralded by vaginal bleeding and may also be accompanied by some cramping, although this is not always the case. There may be other ambiguous symptoms, such as gas pains or diarrhoea associated with it. The distinguishing feature of such a threatened miscarriage is that, on examination, the cervix is closed. At this stage it is difficult to predict whether or not the pregnancy will continue. An ultrasound scan may be used to check on the health of the foetus. This, combined with a test measuring the levels of HCG (Human Chorionic Gonadotrophin) in the blood, gives an indication of the inevitability of the miscarriage. Unfortunately, it is often a case of a very anxious waiting game.

Bleeding can continue for varied amounts of time before a definite outcome becomes obvious. This period of limbo, during which the couple try to prepare for the worst while hoping for the best, can last from hours, to days, or even to a couple of weeks. At some time, though, all becomes settled, and the pregnancy continues or the miscarriage becomes inevitable.

Few doctors would like to try to predict when a threatened loss becomes an **inevitable miscarriage**. Bleeding generally becomes heavier, and is often accompanied by contractions or cramping. With these contractions, the cervix is opening in preparation for the loss of the pregnancy. Lower back pains of a periodic rhythmic nature are often felt as the cervix opens.

The severity and duration of the symptoms of a miscarriage can vary greatly from woman to woman, and even from miscarriage to miscarriage in the same woman. Some women experience very little bleeding and cramping, while others experience pains similar to normal birth contractions. Why this is the case is unknown. It is believed that in many women the physical pain of miscarriage is heightened by the anxiety and mental pain the woman is experiencing at the loss of her child. Generally, the pain is influenced by the duration of the pregnancy. Miscarriages that occur before 12 or 13 weeks are termed **early miscarriages**. It is important to realize that this is only a tendency, and there exists no general rule governing pain during miscarriage. This is understandable, since in general there are large variations in people's ability to withstand pain of any type.

At some stage, the actual miscarriage or spontaneous abortion will occur. The foetus, pregnancy sac, and placenta, together known as the **products of conception**, will be passed from the uterus. In very early miscarriage this may take the form of a clot of a few centimetres in diameter. For pregnancies of greater gestation, the pregnancy sac may be visible and the small foetus and umbilicus are able to be seen. It can be frightening and upsetting for a woman to look into the toilet bowl or on to the bed and see a formed foetus and cord, particularly as she is generally unprepared for such a sight. In late miscarriage it is even possible that the foetus will actually live for a very short period of time.

Although difficult, it is very important that, if she is not in a hospital, the woman keep all clots and tissue for the doctor to examine. There are two important reasons for this. By examination of the tissue, the doctor can determine whether or not all the products of conception have been expelled. Secondly, after examination of the foetus, the doctor may in some cases determine if the foetus was normally developed or suffered from some abnormality.

If all the products of conception have been expelled, the miscarriage is termed a **complete abortion**. Bleeding will ease and change colour from red through pink to a brown discharge. The cervix closes, and the woman's system begins the mending process.

If all or parts of the foetus or placenta are not expelled, the placenta may continue to function. The uterus will be unable to return to its normal size. The cervix will not close, and bleeding will continue to some extent. This is termed an **incomplete abortion**.

If this is the case, a procedure called a D and C (dilation and curettage) is performed. The procedure is commonly known as a curette. The D and C requires hospitalization, as it is performed under general anaesthetic. An instrument called a dilator is inserted to open up, or dilate, the cervix. Once this is accomplished, other probes are used to gently scrape the walls of the uterus to remove the troublesome tissue. This removal then prevents any risk of haemorrhaging or infection. Infection may be indicated by a rise in body temperature. If you have any doubts or concerns after a miscarriage, such as a fever or feelings of ill-health, seek out medical advice. Don't feel you are being 'neurotic'. A doctor who is worth your patronage will be only too willing to examine you to ease your concern.

Sometimes the foetus dies while in the uterus, but is not naturally aborted by the body. The foetus begins to degenerate. The signs of such an occurrence in the mother's body are that the symptoms of pregnancy, such as tender breasts and nausea, are reduced in their intensity and then disappear. Some discharge may occur, but this is not always the case. This occurrence is known as a **missed abortion**. Usually the dead foetus will abort spontaneously. If not, the doctor may perform an examination. He or she may note that, rather than show an increase in size for the increase in gestational age, the uterus has actually become smaller. A negative pregnancy test is the final indicator that no further pregnancy hormone is being produced. An ultrasound scan will also be used in most cases. Some doctors will wait for a period of time to see if the body will expel the foetus naturally. If not, a D and C will be performed, or labor induced if the pregnancy is well-advanced.

Fortunately, a miscarriage is usually a unique event. Some women will miscarry a second time, and doctors accept this as within the range of possibility. The chances of such women carrying a next child to term is just slightly below that of the general population.

Unfortunately, there is a small group of women who miscarry three or more consecutive times. This sentence is easy to write on paper, but it does not convey the anxiety and pain experienced by such women, who are medically labelled **habitual aborters**. We shall not discuss this problem here, as it will be discussed in detail in Chapter 8.

A problem of definition and dignity

When does a miscarriage become recognized as the death of a prematurely delivered child? In years past, the age of viability was 28 weeks; foetuses born at that age or higher were classified as premature births. At that stage the child, if born, might have survived.

With more recent advances in the care of premature babies, survival from 24 weeks onward is possible, although less likely between 24 and 27 weeks. In 1983, we heard of the survival of a baby girl born in America at 22 weeks' gestation.

It is often difficult for a couple who have felt the movements of their child to think of their loss as a miscarriage. To experience labour and the delivery of a small, fully formed baby is difficult to integrate with the attitude that this was 'simply a miscarriage'.

The law in Queensland recognizes the child at 20 weeks, for after this time a dead child must be buried or cremated. Yet how difficult it is for a couple whose child is lost at 18 or 19 weeks, as they later wonder about what became of that child! We do not advocate full rites of passage for miscarried foetuses before 20 weeks. But we are advocating the rights of the couple to know that the remains of their child, the foetus, is disposed of with dignity. Such consideration for these couples and their children would in many cases assist the couple in their grieving.

Some hospitals have considered this question carefully. One Brisbane maternity hospital has made arrangements with a local funeral director to have constructed a set of 'Angel' boxes. Into such a box is placed each aborted foetus, after being wrapped lovingly and carefully in white cloth. The funeral director then arranges for burial of the box. Such actions are often extremely comforting to parents of the lost child.

Many couples may not be concerned about these issues. But it is thoughtless to assume that others aren't. This child, even if spontaneously aborted before 20 weeks, is a lost life, and may have been the focus of the dreams of a grieving couple.

Rowena had already lost six pregnancies when her membranes ruptured at 18 weeks. She felt the need to have this child recognized:

> When my membranes ruptured with Shaun, the first thing I wanted to do was to get him to 20 weeks so that I could bury him, so that he would be recognized as a baby. I think I was affected here by having had miscarriages before, and feeling the end was not really right for these babies.

The physical after-effects

The physical after-effects of a miscarriage will differ, depending on what stage of pregnancy had been reached. In early miscarriage, the body will generally return to normal quite quickly. Menstruation will generally recommence within four to six weeks. In late miscarriage, the body has been in a pregnant state for much longer, and hence will take longer to return to normal. As after the birth of a live child, the breasts will fill with milk about three days after the loss. Many doctors prescribe a drug for women who experience late miscarriage. This drug suppresses lactation, so that breast milk is then not produced. If this drug is not prescribed, the breasts will 'dry up' naturally if the milk is not used. However, this process can cause some discomfort. Milk painkillers and warm showers can often relieve such discomfort. Within a week of 'filling up', the breasts will return to normal. Unfortunately, this action of the breasts and the vaginal discharge that may occur for up to three weeks are difficult reminders of a child who is no longer there.

Menstruation will generally have returned within ten weeks after a late miscarriage, although it can take longer to re-establish due to the intense stress of the situation itself. Stress itself can affect the onset of ovulation and hence menstruation. If you are concerned that menstruation has not returned, seek your doctor's opinion, even if only to relieve any unnecessary worries that this may indicate a problem.

The development of the child

Before we look at specific causes of miscarriage, it is important for us to look at the development of a child from the moment the sperm meets the ovum within the Fallopian tube.

The ovum and the sperm carry within them all the necessary genetic information to make a new human being. A few hours after fertilization, the first cell-division will occur. Each new cell contains the same maternal and paternal chromosomal information. During the next 72 hours, each new cell continues to divide, so that the number of cells increases from four to eight to 16 to 32 and then 64 seperate cells. At this stage the group of cells is known as a morula.

By seven or eight days after fertilization (about day 21 of a 28-day menstrual cycle), the morula has developed a space in its centre and is known as a blastocyst. Projections known as the chorionic villi have formed on the outside of the blastocyst, and these will embed the blastocyst into any local tissue. By this time the blastocyst has moved down the Fallopian tubes to the uterus, and it is here in the rich lining that the blastocyst embeds. This is known as implantation. Very occasionally, this implantation is accompanied by a slight blood-stained mucus discharge known as an 'implantation bleed'.

In some instances, the blastocyst's journey down the Fallopian tube is hindered by some obstruction. Seven days after fertilization it may still implant in local tissue, this time in the walls of the Fallopian tube. This is known as an ectopic pregnancy, and will be discussed later.

The blastocyst generally implants in the upper rear part of the uterus, at which site the placenta will develop. Occasionally it will implant in the lower part of the uterus, leading to a condition known as placenta praevia.

The blastocyst will burrow into the rich uterine lining, and cell division will continue. As yet, the woman has not missed her first menstrual period and will not generally realize that she is indeed pregnant.

The hormone progesterone maintains the pregnancy. If the blastocyst has implanted successfully, the corpus luteum will continue to secrete this hormone. One effect of the hormone is to suppress menstruation. This is usually the first sign of pregnancy noted by the woman. Some women do note other symptoms, such as nausea, breast tenderness, or frequency of urination, before this event.

Pregnancy is determined from the date of the first day of the last menstrual period. Fertilization then occurs at approximately the end of the second week of a common 28-day cycle, implantation at the end of the third week, and the suppression of menstruation at the end of the fourth week of pregnancy. Over the next nine weeks, the foetus will develop, so that by the end of the thirteenth week of pregnancy, the foetus is properly formed with all its body systems. The remainder of the pregnancy is devoted to an increase in size and the maturation of these systems.

We see that the first 13 weeks of pregnancy are therefore extremely important, and it is during these weeks that adverse conditions and stimuli can severely affect the foetus. During the fifth week of pregnancy, the spine is beginning to form. This is followed in the sixth week by the formation of a head, chest, and abdominal cavity. The heart and circulation are beginning to function, as are other abdominal organs. During the seventh and eighth weeks, the limbs and senses are forming. Development continues rapidly, as body organs and sense organs grow and develop more completely.[2]

Once organs are fully formed, it is difficult for any adverse conditions to affect them. Therefore, considering the immense development occurring in the first 13 weeks of pregnancy, it is no surprise that most deformities occur within these first months. Similarly, it is not surprising that most miscarriages occur during this time.

The causes, treatment, and investigations of miscarriage

An important note

Before we go on to discuss causes of miscarriage, we wish to state clearly that in most cases of miscarriage a cause will not be found, and that a subsequent pregnancy will have a greater than 80 per cent chance of success. This is almost the same chance of success as exists for a woman who has not previously miscarried.

The causes presented here are only possibilities. We do not want to make a woman excessively fearful of a recurrence, or provide some basis upon which she can blame herself for the loss. In general, the cause of a miscarriage is unknown. But it is known that it has not been caused by some action on the part of the woman.

1. Chromosomal/Genetic

As we noted, a new life begins with the uniting of the female ovum and the male sperm. The sperm and the ovum each contain 23 long strands of material known as chromosomes. Contained on these chromosomes are the genes. Genes are minute structures that carry within them the vital information about the new individual to be formed. Every detail, from eye colour to height to blood-vessel structure, is carried on these genes.

At fertilization, the 23 chromosomes of each of the ovum and sperm combine to produce a new cell. This is the beginning of a new being, one having 46 chromosomes. The number 46 is no accident. Each cell of the human body, except the ova and sperm, contains 46 chromosomes. Other animal species have cells which contain other specific numbers of chromosomes. This ensures their continuing common characteristics.

The 46 chromosomes form into 23 pairs as each cell is about to divide. Any extra chromosome, or the loss of a chromosome or its parts, will lead to a genetic abnormality. For example, an extra chromosome on the twenty-first pair produces Down's syndrome.

Once the fertilized ovum, now of 46 chromosomes, has been formed, the cell begins to make an exact copy of itself by a process known as mitosis. Each new cell will then continue making such exact copies. If exact copies are to be made of the original fertilized ovum, and a mistake in the chromosomes is present in this original cell, we can see that this mistake will be repeated in every cell of the body. Hence, if the mistake is present in either the ovum or sperm, or occurs at fertilization, it will involve every cell of the body. Such abnormalities are more likely to lead to the spontaneous abortion of the foetus early in the first trimester. In contrast, cells that develop some abnormality only after fertilization are more likely to affect one body organ or system, rather than the entire being. It is believed that at least half of the miscarriages that occur in the first 13 weeks may be linked to some chromosomal abnormality.[3]

These chromosomal mistakes are generally simple chance events, unlikely to recur. Many doctors will begin to look for some possible chromosomal problem only after three miscarriages, accepting even three as possible chance events. We will discuss the types of genetic problems in more detail in Chapter 7. Even if a problem is found, the prospects of an eventual healthy pregnancy are not bleak, although sound genetic counselling is vital.

2. Developmental

From fertilization through the next three months, the foetus develops all the organs and senses of the body. At times, this development will fail or be interrupted.

A. Faulty implantation

If implantation is not successfully achieved, the pregnancy will generally be lost. Often this occurs without the woman being aware that she is pregnant. These miscarriages before about six weeks' gestation are referred to as preclinical pregnancies. Women may simply recognize them as a 'late period'. If such losses are considered in addition to miscarriages of confirmed pregnancies, some researchers theorize that the rate of miscarriage of a fertilized ovum could be as high as three in four. Some couples classified as infertile may actually be able to conceive, but may be suffering from repeated preclinical miscarriages.

B. Blighted ovum

In some cases the ovum is fertilized, but fails to develop. The pregnancy consists of a placenta and pregnancy sac, but no foetus. The pregnancy may be able to continue for up to 12 weeks. This is because, in the initial stages of pregnancy, it is the corpus luteum, not the foetus or placenta, that maintains the hormones of pregnancy. At approximately 12 to 13 weeks the corpus luteum breaks down, and the pregnancy becomes dependent upon the foetus and placenta. If no foetus is present, the pregnancy is lost. It is not known conclusively what causes a blighted ovum, but present thought suspects that an abnormal sperm or ovum may lie at the root of the problem.[4]

Blighted ova are not likely to recur in subsequent pregnancies.

C. Hydatidiform mole or molar pregnancy

In very rare instances the foetus is not present, and the placenta develops abnormally. It grows into a mass of small fluid-filled sacs. The condition is characterized by extremely high levels of hormones, severe nausea and vomiting, and a uterus that enlarges at a much faster rate than normal. Most molar pregnancies spontaneously abort. If not, they must be removed. In very *rare* cases, a form of cancer can develop after such a pregnancy. This particular cancer is completely curable if detected early. Therefore, a woman is advised not to fall pregnant for at least one year after a molar pregnancy, to make absolutely sure any potential problem is detected early.

D. Ectopic pregnancy

In about one per cent of pregnancies, a tissue or mucus blockage or a dysfunction in the Fallopian tube prevents the movement of the fertilized ovum to the uterus, and it implants in the tube. The tube is not able to accommodate the growing pregnancy. At or before eight weeks' gestation, the pregnancy must be removed, or it may rupture the tube and then haemorrhaging can occur into the abdominal cavity. This is a life-threatening situation. Any severe abdominal pain that occurs in early pregnancy should be immediately reported to your doctor. The pregnancy and damaged tube will have to be removed. It must be remembered that one damaged tube does not mean that a couple will then face infertility. Only one functioning ovary and Fallopian tube are required for successful conception. Women who have had one ectopic pregnancy are watched carefully during later pregnancies, as there is a slight possibility that another ectopic pregnancy may occur. An ultrasound scan performed very early in pregnancy can determine if a pregnancy sac is visible within the uterus, thereby indicating that implantation in the uterus has been successful.

E. Foetal malformations

A proportion of foetuses that are miscarried are found to have had major malformations of important organs. Severe defects of the neural tube or of the heart would mean that the child would not have lived.

F. Placental position and insufficiency

In some cases, the placenta implants lower down in the uterus than usual, and the risk of miscarriage is slightly increased. At other times, the placenta may not develop sufficiently to be able to supply the needs of the growing foetus. Many babies will still survive some insufficiency, but will grow at a slower rate. Unfortunately, if the insufficiency is severe enough, the foetus may be lost.

3. Hormonal

A. Corpus luteum insufficiency

The corpus luteum secretes progesterone, and is hence responsible for maintaining the pregnancy in the early weeks. In the past, a threatened miscarriage accompanied by lowered levels of progesterone was treated with administration of this hormone. The rationale behind such treatment was that a malfunction in the corpus luteum was causing the threatened miscarriage. Present-day thinking is now that the reverse may be the case. That is, a malfunction of the pregnancy itself may be reflected in the corpus luteum breakdown. Hence, most doctors now allow nature to take its course. Concern is that administration of progesterone may simply cause a missed abortion.

B. Other body hormone systems

Chronic malfunctioning within the body's hormonal systems that are not specifically related to pregnancy, may also predispose the woman's body toward miscarriage. An over-active or under-active thyroid gland, or an abnormal adrenal gland, may result in miscarriage. Uncontrolled diabetes may also be involved. Generally, such conditions are diagnosed before pregnancy. In fact, in some cases such conditions have been linked to infertility. These conditions can be controlled by medication and other treatments. If this is done, the risk of miscarriage is significantly reduced.

C. Reproductive hormones

In some cases of early miscarriage, it is suspected that inappropriate levels of the hormones oestrogen and HCG (Human Chorionic Gonadotrophin) may lead to inappropriate feedback to the brain. The brain may not recognize the pregnancy and the body may shed the uterine lining, and hence the pregnancy is lost. Injections of these hormones may be required if an inappropriate balance of hormones is found in the bloodstream of a woman prone to early miscarriage.

4. Anatomical abnormalities

During the formation of the reproductive system of the female foetus, abnormalities may result that can predispose toward miscarriage. Other abnormalities may occur after previous reproductive difficulties, or gynaecological problems.

A. Uterine malformations

The uterus and vagina of the foetus are formed when two Müllerian ducts join. This development can be incomplete, leading to a variety of malformations. Approximately three per cent of women have some such malformations.

There may be a wall of tissue, a septum, running down the middle of the uterus (septate uterus or subseptate [heart shaped]); a double uterus; bicornate uterus; a uterus with one horn (unicornate uterus); or other combinations.

UTERINE MALFORMATIONS

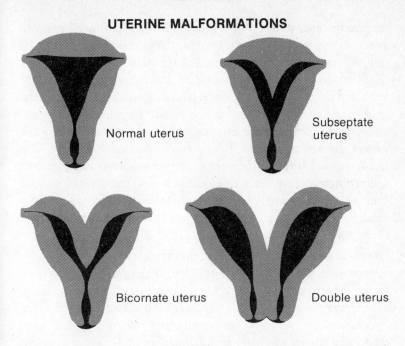

Normal uterus

Subseptate uterus

Bicornate uterus

Double uterus

Many women who have these malformations fall pregnant and carry to a normal full-term delivery without problems. Other women with such malformations may suffer from second-trimester miscarriages or premature delivery.

To diagnose a malformation, a test known as a hysterosalpingogram (HSG) is carried out. We discussed this test in Chapter 3. If a malformation is detected, treatment may vary, depending on the severity of the malformation. In less severe cases, it is found that further pregnancies may 'stretch' the uterus sufficiently to accommodate a full-term pregnancy. In other severe cases, surgery may be indicated, which may then allow for a full-term delivery.

B. Cervical incompetence

A proportion of women who miscarry within the second trimester are found to have an incompetent cervix. It is difficult to diagnose such a problem prior to a first loss. Symptoms are generally vague. There may be excessive vaginal discharge, with some lower abdominal discomfort or backache. The woman may have the sensation of a lump in the vagina. An incompetent cervix is not able to withstand the weight of the developing baby and begins to open painlessly, thereby allowing the membranes to bulge. If the condition is not treated, the membranes will rupture and the foetus will be miscarried or the baby born prematurely. The loss is generally heralded by leaking amniotic fluid or ruptured membranes. Little or no pain may be associated with the opening of the cervix. Such is the classic incompetent cervix.

Diagnosis can be made by ultrasound or by examination of the cervix through the vagina. If a probe of a certain diameter can be easily passed through the cervix, it is considered incompetent. Unfortunately, few cases produce such clear-cut symptoms, and true incompetence may be rare. A definite diagnosis may not be made. More commonly, incompetence is simply suspected.

There are three basic causes of cervical incompetence:[5]

(i) Traumatic. Any procedure that involves the dilation of the cervix, such as D and C, therapeutic abortion, induced abortion, or a difficult forceps delivery, has the potential to cause damage to the cervix, rendering it incompetent at a later date. Where procedures are skilfully performed, this risk is minimal. It is important to inform your obstetrician of any such procedures performed in the past. Some women may not inform doctors of previous pregnancy terminations through embarrassment, but such information is vital. Medical ethics assure you of complete confidentiality.

(ii) Congenital. In some cases, an incompetent cervix is found in conjunction with other malformations of the uterus we discussed above. In others, cervical incompetence cannot be linked to any prior trauma. It is then assumed to be a congenital condition.

(iii) Functional. It is believed that in some cases a normal cervix is forced open by premature and uncommonly strong, yet relatively painless, non-labour uterine contractions. In this way, although the cervix is not incompetent in itself, the outcome is the same.

The treatment of incompetence is relatively simple and highly effective, with success rates approximated at 75 to 80 per cent. A stitch or cervical suture is placed around the cervix, and this serves to hold it securely closed until just prior to delivery. The most common sutures employed are the Shirodka and McDonald, named after the doctors who developed them. The suture may be inserted between pregnancies, early in the second trimester of a pregnancy, or, in cases of early detection, after the cervix has already begun to open. Most commonly, the suture is inserted at approximately the fourteenth week of pregnancy, after the risk of early miscarriage has passed.

The procedure, requiring a stay of a few days in hospital, is performed under general anaesthetic through the vaginal opening. The suture may be of a soft non-dissolving silk or nylon thread, which is passed around the cervix and pulled tight like a purse string. The position of the suture in the cervix will depend on the doctor and the patient's obstetric history. Commonly, it is placed around the external os, the outer opening of the cervix into the vagina. It may be positioned closer to the internal os (the inner opening into the uterus), if this is indicated from a patient's obstetric history.

After this procedure the woman may generally lead a relatively normal pregnant life, although she must ensure sufficient rest each day. If labour commences prior to 37 weeks, the suture must be removed immediately. Otherwise it is usually removed at approximately 37 weeks. The removal requires a simple dividing of the suture, which then allows for a normal vaginal delivery.

Today, suturing of the cervix is carried out in some cases of mid-trimester miscarriage and threatened premature labours, even though cervical incompetence has not been conclusively diagnosed.

C. Uterine growths and other problems

(i) Fibroids. A fibroid or myoma is a non-cancerous growth in the uterus. The fertilized ovum may implant on to this fibroid, which is unable to maintain the necessary blood supply to allow the pregnancy to grow. At times, the fibroid grows large enough to interfere with the growing pregnancy, and so a miscarriage may occur. However, the presence of a fibroid in the uterus does not indicate that it caused a miscarriage, since in most cases the position and size of the fibroid has no effect on the pregnancy.

(ii) Adhesions of the uterus (Asherman's Syndrome). At times, due to disease or medical procedures, the walls of the uterus can become scarred and develop fibrous tissue known as adhesions. Some believe that such adhesions may lead to the loss of a pregnancy by preventing implantation. Evidence is inconclusive, since many women with adhesions have carried pregnancies to term.

(iii) Polyps. Non-cancerous growths in the walls of the uterus, known as polyps, are suspected by some of being involved in the loss of pregnancy through miscarriage. Once again, evidence is inconclusive; polyps may be a factor in the losses of only some women.

5. Environmental factors

A. Drugs

Most research into the effects of drugs on the foetus has involved their possible link to abnormalities. The abuse of drugs, both illegal and prescription types, are suspected of causing damage to the developing foetus. No evidence has been found that drugs available over the counter from chemists, and those prescribed by doctors, such as aspirin, antibiotics or paracetemol, are in any way linked to miscarriage. A good rule of thumb is to take no drug unless it is prescribed or sanctioned by a doctor who is aware of a woman's pregnant state.

One drug that has been linked with pregnancy difficulties, including miscarriage, is Diethylstilbestrol (DES). This was prescribed by doctors during the 1940s and 1950s for women with a history of miscarriages, threatened miscarriages, or diabetes. No obvious dangers were associated with the drugs until the generation of babies born to mothers who had taken DES began themselves to reproduce. These offspring experienced a higher than normal rate of a cancer known as clear-cell adenocarcinoma, abnormalities of the reproductive system, premature deliveries, malpresentations, infertility, and miscarriages. It may be a good idea for a woman who suffers repeated unexplained miscarriages to seek information from her mother concerning any difficulties she experienced or medications she took during her pregnancy. Any evidence of possible DES administration should then be reported to one's doctor.

B. X-rays

Although the evidence is debatable and inconclusive, there is believed to be a possible link between X-rays and miscarriage. Therefore, for safety's sake, it is best to avoid X-rays, particularly in early pregnancy. If a woman is attempting to conceive, or if there is any chance at all that she may be already pregnant, it is best to avoid any X-rays during the second half of the menstrual cycle. It is also advisable for women who work with X-rays, such as radiologists, radiographers, and metal industry and airport workers, to adopt careful protection measures during pregnancy.

C. Radiation

Evidence from Hiroshima, nuclear accidents, and leakages from nuclear waste dumps seems to suggest links between radioactivity, chromosomal damage, and increased rates of miscarriage. Research into this hazard of the modern world is continuing.

D. Chemicals

A variety of chemicals has been suspected of having effects on foetal development. These include some petroleum products, such as insecticides, some plastics, solvents, and lead. Household chemicals are generally safe. If in doubt about the advisability of using such products during pregnancy, seek advice from your doctor or the Poisons Information Centre in your capital city. Women working within the chemical industry are best advised, prior to pregnancy, to seek their doctor's guidance on safeguards. Evidence of danger from anaesthetic gases during early pregnancy is inconclusive, but it is generally accepted that such should only be administered to pregnant women in emergency situations. Women who work in hospitals should also take adequate safety measures to relieve any fear of loss due to contacts there.

Most research on smoking and pregnancy has linked smoking and 'small-for-date' babies. Tendencies toward higher rates of stillbirth have been noted in women who smoke heavily. There also appears to be an increased rate of miscarriage among heavy smokers. Damage due to the heat generated by the cigarette, or the drugs in it, is considered possible. If a woman finds herself unable to give up smoking prior to pregnancy, it is vital, if she is a heavy smoker, that she lower her daily consumption.

E. Alcohol

Once again, most recent research involving alcohol and the foetus has revolved around the identification of babies suffering from what has become known as Foetal Alcohol Syndrome. Most babies with this syndrome are born to mothers who consumed large amounts of alcohol throughout pregnancy or 'binged' during early pregnancy. Further evidence suggests a possible link between alcohol — particularly heavy use — and miscarriage rates.[6] As with smoking, women contemplating pregnancy or already pregnant should stop drinking. At the very least, they should cut down considerably on the amount consumed.

6. Viruses and infections

The effects of a viral or bacterial infection on the foetus depend generally on the type of infection, the severity of the attack, and whether or not the virulent is able to cross the placenta and enter the bloodstream of the foetus. With vaccination procedures and the development of antibiotics, most serious bacterial infections such as tuberculosis, typhoid fever, and diphtheria have been controlled. Viral infections are more difficult to control. Most common infections and childhood illnesses such as the common cold, mild influenza, and gastroenteritis need cause little concern. These are believed not to harm the foetus unless they are accompanied by high fever or severe dehydration. Rubella (German measles) is the exception to this.

Some infections are known to be able to cause damage to the foetus, and hence raise the risk of miscarriage. These are toxoplasmosis, syphilis, rubella, cytomegalovirus, and herpes. We shall discuss these in greater detail in Chapter 7.

Some infections, such as the T-strain mycoplasma, are believed to be associated with miscarriage, although, as with many other supposed causes, evidence is inconclusive. Once again, these infections may be factors in the miscarriages of some women but not others.

7. Immunological dysfunctions

Incompatibility of rhesus factors of the blood of mother and baby were in years past a cause of some miscarriages. Today, injections of gammaglobulin (Anti-D) after a previous birth or miscarriage have made such problems rare.

Recent research has been looking at the possibility of a blocking factor being produced during pregnancy. The embryo, being composed of genetic material from both mother and father, contains material foreign to that of the mother's system. In theory, the mother's immune system should therefore develop antibodies to fight this intruder. A blocking factor appears to be produced to protect the developing foetus against attack. Some suggest the mother's body must recognize the foreign cells to produce this blocking factor. In genetically similar people, this recognition may not occur. A breakdown in production of this blocking factor may lead to miscarriage. Some attempts to overcome these immune problems, such as injecting the woman with white blood cells from the father of the child and others have been used.[7] Research on such possibilities is still in its infancy, but may hold hope in the future for some facing repeated early miscarriages.

8. Accident

The uterus provides an amazingly safe, secure, shock-proof environment for the developing foetus. Minor accidents or injuries are not generally accepted as causes of miscarriage. Yet a woman is more likely to remember such an accident after having a miscarriage, and hence link it to the loss. Serious injury or abdominal surgery may present some risk to the foetus, depending on its position and severity.

9. Intercourse

Many couples fear that intercourse may have been the cause of their miscarriage. It is now generally accepted that intercourse will not cause miscarriage. If there is any vaginal bleeding, it is best to avoid any activity that may irritate the uterus. This includes intercourse. At times, women who have suffered a number of miscarriages, particularly those in the mid trimester, may be advised to avoid intercourse. In such cases, this abstinence will be discussed by their doctor.

10. Occupation

There is no evidence that a woman's occupation will cause miscarriage. There may be exceptions in occupations dealing with the manufacture of certain chemicals where adequate safeguards are not maintained. If a miscarriage threatens, work involving heavy lifting should be curtailed until a doctor advises that normal duties may be resumed.

11. Age

Maternal age has been linked to higher rates of miscarriage. The older the mother, the more likely is a miscarriage. It must be remembered and stressed that the great majority of older women who fall pregnant will go on to term pregnancies. Increased paternal age in combination with higher maternal age has also been suggested as being a factor.

In stark contrast, there is also some suggestion that very young teen mothers also experience an increased risk of miscarriage.[8]

12. Prior contraceptive measures

Many women are concerned that the method of contraception they used prior to conception, or were using when conception occurred, may have been responsible for their loss. The contraceptive pill has no link with increased risk of miscarriage if the woman ceases taking it prior to conception. There is no evidence to support the fear of some women that their loss was due to falling pregnant 'too soon' after coming off the pill. It is suspected that there is a very slight increase in the risk of miscarriage if conception occurs while the woman is still using the pill. The intra-uterine contraceptive device (IUD) has a stronger link to miscarriage, but only when pregnancy occurs while the IUD is in place. If the IUD is removed prior to conception, it is not linked with any increase in miscarriage. If the IUD is not removed, the risk of miscarriage is heightened. Even if the pregnancy is not wanted, the IUD must be removed to rule out any risk of infection.

Condoms, diaphragms, and spermicidal creams have not been linked with miscarriage.

A previous induced abortion has not been linked with increased rates of miscarriage, unless the procedure used caused damage to the cervix, rendering it incompetent. The most common methods of induced abortion used today involve suction and the use of prostaglandin gels which reduce this risk. The effect of a number of induced abortions on miscarriage rates is unknown.

13. Heat

In recent years, doctors have suspected a link between excessive body heat and damage to the foetus, miscarriage, and premature labour. This body heat may be associated with high fever, excessively hot baths, spas, or excessively strenuous exercise.

14. Stress and anxiety

Throughout history, emotional stress or sudden shocks have been blamed for miscarriages. Many women who have experienced miscarriage seek a reason, and have identified a particular stress as the 'cause' of their miscarriage. Others have noted the obvious anxiety of a woman suffering repeated miscarriages and associated this anxiety with her losses. Doctors believe her anxiety is more likely to be the effect of her losses, not the cause of them. To suggest that anxiety alone is the cause of miscarriage may only help to aggravate the situation. Adding feelings of guilt to the woman's anxiety, when such guilt is not justified, may only serve to increase her tension.

15. Unexplained

We have outlined many possible reasons for miscarriage. Yet in 50 per cent or more cases of miscarriage no one particular cause can be identified. Nature still keeps many secrets from medical science in this area. It is a terrible frustration to be told, particularly after repeated miscarriages, that no cause can be identified. Yet, this is commonly the case. The best that doctors can do is to examine the woman for any of the above causes.

A woman often fears that she may have to face another miscarriage. These fears are generally increased when the doctor is unable to specify a cause for a previous miscarriage. She may feel powerless. Some of these feelings can be alleviated if the woman feels she is doing something to prevent in some small measure a recurrence of the couple's loss.

There are a limited number of actions a woman can take to try to prevent miscarriage in later pregnancies.

1. Ensure a nutritious, balanced diet, containing all the major food groups during pregnancy (see Chapter 11).

2. For a period of months prior to conception, the woman should follow a routine of diet and exercise that will ensure a healthy body.

3. The male should also follow a similar health regime for at least three months before conception to ensure the production of healthy sperm. Avoidance of tight underwear or trousers and excessively hot baths or showers that may impede sperm production may also be advisable.

4. Ensure that any chronic maternal disease, such as diabetes, renal and heart problems, thyroid disorders, and hypertension, are under control.

5. Avoid contact with X-rays and industrial chemicals.

6. Cease the intake of alcohol and tobacco. At the very least, curtail their use.

7. Within reasonable limits, avoid contact with persons suffering severe acute viral infections. One cannot and should not become withdrawn from society for fear of contracting a virus, as most common varieties will not harm the foetus.

8. Avoid any activities that encourage excessive body heat.

9. Develop personal means of relaxing under stress through activities that have been able to relax you in the past. Otherwise, seek out professional assistance to develop new relaxation techniques.

Aside from measures such as these that the couple can control, there is little else one can do to prevent miscarriage. In looking at the causes of such losses, we can see that most are mistakes of nature over which the individual has no control. This is a difficult fact to accept, but the truth nonetheless. If a couple have done all that is humanly possible to ensure a healthy pregnancy and still miscarry, they should feel no guilt.

Emotional reactions to miscarriage

Reactions to miscarriage are as individual as the couples who experience the loss. Some feel saddened, but soon recover. Others are shocked by the severity of their feelings. There are a number of factors that can affect reactions to miscarriage.

1. The importance of the pregnancy

Perhaps of greatest significance is the importance of the pregnancy to the couple. A pregnancy that resulted from a contraceptive failure may not be grieved as intensely as that which was planned and awaited expectantly. This may not be the case if the woman, though initially ambivalent about the pregnancy, later accepted it and grew to enjoy it. She too, may then grieve intensely.

A miscarriage that follows a period of infertility, or is one of a series of losses, may produce quite intense feelings of anger and depression. A first child lost due to miscarriage may also be more intensely grieved than one lost through miscarriage to a family in which children are already a part.

These are general tendencies, but reactions must never be assumed for any particular couple on the basis of such tendencies.

2. The stage at which the pregnancy is lost

Generally, the longer the period of pregnancy, the more intense are the reactions after miscarriage. Miscarriages before 12 weeks are painful and difficult, but later miscarriages may also be complicated by other factors. The foetus may live for a very short time after delivery, and the physical reminders of the baby may persist for longer. The couple may have also begun to prepare for their baby as its movements made it seem more real to them.

3. Previous obstetric history

It is often reassuring for a couple at the time of their first miscarriage to realize that the chances of a recurrence are minimal. They may be able to deal with their pain, buoyed by some feelings of optimism about their future.

This may not be the case for the unfortunate few couples for whom this miscarriage marks a second or even later loss. Fear and anxiety concerning their future, particularly if the couple have no living children, can heighten their feelings of grief over this present loss.

A miscarriage threatens

Unfortunately, it is more common for a first pregnancy, rather than a later one, to be lost through miscarriage. It is unfortunate because the majority of couples enter child-bearing blissfully ignorant of what can go wrong. The announcement of a pregnancy is often greeted with great anticipation. For some who greet the news of a pregnancy with trepidation, the acceptance of it may have been part of the first weeks. During the first weeks, most couples have begun to sink comfortably into their roles of prospective parents. Then the bleeding begins!

For many, bleeding makes them consider for the first time that all may not be well. Although more than half will go on to a normal pregnancy, the fear and anxiety that accompanies bleeding is intense. Panic, and all its physical symptoms such as shaking and crying, may emerge as they do during any traumatic event. If the woman is alone at the time, these feelings may be more intense.

> I got such a shock when I went to the toilet and there was blood. I really panicked, yet I was shocked. I couldn't think straight. I started to shake and cry, and went to ring the doctor. He had a patient with him, so I couldn't talk to him right away. I waited on the line for him. They were the longest two minutes of my life! By the time he answered I was in such a state that I just sobbed into the phone: 'I'm bleeding!'.

Most women will, quite correctly, visit or phone their doctor. This may be where the first breakdown in communication occurs. The woman, unaware of how common such occurrences are to her doctor, may be mystified at her doctor's sometimes seemingly offhand manner. To the woman threatening to miscarry, this is an emergency situation! To her, the doctor is the expert, and he seems to be taking it so calmly. The doctor's advice may well be to go to bed and contact him/her if the bleeding continues. This may not be very reassuring to the woman who is in a state of panic. If the doctor can explain what may be occurring and why a waiting game must be played, the woman may understand the advice more easily. To further facilitate communication and peace of mind in the woman, a doctor may suggest that the woman or her partner keep the doctor informed of progress at reasonable intervals. In this way, the couple may feel that the doctor is concerned and is 'keeping a close eye' on the situation. A suggestion that she be visited by her doctor as soon as possible may be even more reassuring.

A woman with a young family or other commitments may be unable to follow the bed-rest suggestion. As we mentioned earlier, she may then feel guilty if she goes on to miscarry. The benefit of bed rest in preventing early miscarriage is still controversial. For a later threatened miscarriage, bed rest may be of greater value, and therefore it is advisable for the woman to follow this course of action.

This waiting game may last only a matter of hours if the miscarriage is already inevitable. Yet it may go on for up to a period of a couple of weeks, until the situation resolves itself one way or the other. This period can be a cycle of highs and lows, with the couple's feelings alternating between hope and despair.

Each visit to the toilet is a major emotional strain for the woman who is haunted by the fear of what might be found. At times, a woman is prescribed sedatives to help relieve this tension and relax the body.

> The bleeding went on for about a week. Sometimes it would change to a pinky brown colour, and I'd start to feel some hope. No sooner had I got that hope back than the red blood would return. I felt as if I was on a roller-coaster ride. By the end of the week I was wrung out. I'd given up. I told myself I didn't care. I was sick of it.

Even if the bleeding abates and pregnancy continues, there is still a loss of innocence. Future hopes are viewed more cautiously.

The miscarriage

Unfortunately, in about one pregnancy in five, the bleeding will not abate and cramping may begin. Very early miscarriages may be allowed to occur at home under a doctor's supervision. At times, they happen quickly before hospitalization can be sought. It can be frightening for a woman or a couple to see blood and clots of tissue. This can be such a shock that they do not retain clots or tissue for examination by the doctor. Even to be instructed to 'keep any clots or tissue' can be abhorrent to the couple. These are not clots! These are their *baby*!

> I'll never forget. I felt crampy and felt this urge to open my bowels. Yet when I got to the toilet, I felt something come out of the vagina. When I looked, there was a tiny foetus with the cord from it surrounded by blood. I was absolutely shocked. Without thinking and in panic, I flushed the toilet! I was hysterical. I don't think I'll ever get over that thought of what I had done. It just happened! I didn't mean to do it! It was done before I realized what I was doing. I have this fear of meeting this baby in heaven or something, and he/she asking me: 'Why did you flush me down the toilet?'

Hospitalization can be a fearful and depressing experience for the couple facing miscarriage. Women are generally admitted to the obstetric section of a hospital. The couple may then be confronted with pregnant women and babies at a time when they must face the possible loss of their own baby. The waiting game played out in hospital surrounded by babies' cries can be even more difficult.

Pain relief is generally offered once the miscarriage becomes inevitable. To be examined and told calmly that one is miscarrying, when the couple are desperately hoping it will 'work out all right', can be difficult to accept. This may be realized by the staff through the woman's reactions.

> As the cramps got worse, the nurse came in and asked me if I wanted an injection to relieve the pain. I remember saying that I would have it as long as it wouldn't harm the baby. The nurse looked at me strangely. I realize now that she must have thought I was a bit balmy. I knew I was losing the baby and at 16 weeks it had no chance of life. Yet somehow I couldn't accept that it would soon all be over. I was hanging on to that baby I'd protected all those weeks.

Women are often surprised at just how painful a miscarriage can be. Yet, particularly with late miscarriages, labour contractions occur. The first stage will be basically the same. The second stage is generally easier than normal, due to the size of the foetus. However, fear and emotional pain often increase the physical pain beyond the expected level. The presence of a woman's partner can provide her with reassurance.

> My husband and I lost our son at four-and-a-half months pregnant. As I went into labour he was there to comfort the pain, while he held into himself his pain at the loss of our child. I could feel his presence and meet his loving eyes whenever I needed it. He sang to me once while the cramping was strongest and I cried, but they were tears of relief and security in his love.

Whether or not the couple see the foetus, and how it is shown to them, is a delicate but important issue.

> When I had the urge to push they came back in and made me sit on a bedpan. I delivered into this. I can't tell you how much it upset me that they expected me to deliver my baby into a bedpan as if it was a waste product! I said nothing, but that really hurt me. Obviously my baby meant nothing to them, but it did to me!

The couple should be asked if they wish to see the foetus. Some are helped by the sight, as it allows them to accept that the loss has really occurred. In case of early miscarriage, where the woman's body-shape has not altered, accepting that a pregnancy has been lost can be difficult. If the couple decide to see the foetus, they should be prepared for what they will see. Rather than being presented in a metal dish surrounded by clots and tissue, the foetus may be cleaned and presented to them on a clean cloth. Many couples will not wish to see the foetus, and this desire should also be respected.

If the products of conception are not fully removed during the miscarriage, the ordeal continues as a D and C is carried out. Some see this as a continuation of the event, while others see the D and C as helping them put an end to the event, a certain relief. Some women see the D and C as cutting off the last link with this child they don't really wish to lose so prematurely.

For many, a miscarriage may be the first time they are faced with a gynaecological operation. To encounter the procedures accompanying a general anaesthetic for the first time can be stressful in itself, without the added complications of the loss. The woman may be unsure of the procedures and of any after-effects. The procedures and the reasons for the operation must be explained carefully.

Over but just beginning

Once the physical side of a miscarriage is resolved, the difficult emotional reactions begin to take precedence.

The woman who has been hospitalized may remain there for a day or so to ensure that there are no complications. Being in an obstetric unit can be very difficult. Rooms and routines are set up for live births. Nurseries, feeding routines, baby-linen containers, and baby cries are often grim reminders of a lost child. Couples should be provided with privacy, away from the nursery or newly-delivered mothers. A private single room provides the couple with the opportunity to express their intense disappointment and pain without fear of embarrassment. If they desire it, couples need time to be together, to cry, to talk, to console. For couples who can spend such time together, this is often the beginning of healing. Unfortunately for some couples, the shock and anger and disappointment will prevent them from helping each other at this stage. If desired, husbands should be allowed unlimited visiting privileges, including a cot for an overnight stay where feasible. Staff may wish the woman to sleep, and may feel that a husband's presence would prevent this. However, they must realize that the woman's first priority at this time may not be sleep, but to have the security of the one who may be the only other person able truly to share her pain. The male, if separated from his partner, may also have his feelings of helplessness and isolation increased.

While the woman is hospitalized, it is vital that a lack of communication does not increase difficulties. The security and comfort of a few caretakers who know the situation can be reassuring. To be confronted with questions or statements such as 'Why aren't you feeding, dear?' or 'How's the little mother today?' or 'You're not very big yet, are you?' can be devastating. A problem exists in determining how to communicate the loss to those having contact with the couple without invading their privacy.

The couple have lost a child, and they must grieve this loss. The process continues long after the couple leave hospital. Shock and disbelief may render the first days an emotional blur.

For some, for whom the pregnancy was unwanted or unplanned, the miscarriage may bring some feelings of relief which are seldom voiced. There is guilt about feelings such as these. The woman wonders: 'What kind of person am I? Did I want my baby dead?'

Guilt is a common feeling, experienced by many women who miscarry. In trying to make some sense of the situation, many women will try to pinpoint some activity in which they participated prior to the miscarriage, which was 'responsible' for it. Housework, exercise, shopping, or intercourse may be blamed.

> My mother told me not to work while I was pregnant. She said it wasn't good for the baby. The doctor said it was OK, but maybe Mum was right. I should have given up.

Some of the guilt may be translated into anger and blame. A woman may decide that intercourse caused her miscarriage, and blame herself or her partner for initiating it. If her anger toward herself is not resolved, it can lead to severe depression. The woman may feel a failure as a wife, a mother, and a woman.

> I really felt like a failure. Other women got pregnant, and that's all there was to it. But me, I can't do it properly. There were three

girls at work who were all pregnant when I was. They all had healthy babies, but not me! I couldn't give Bob a baby, while their husbands were over the moon. I just wanted to fall off the face of the earth.

If the foetus is found to have an abnormality, one or both partners may feel that there is something freakish about them, as they can't produce a normal child. It is important for the couple to be able to discuss fully with their doctor the causes of this miscarriage, if it is known. If it is unknown, they need to be reassured that no one is to blame for their loss, and that in the great majority of cases nature, not humanity, is fully in charge of the situation. Being out of control, perhaps for the first time in their lives, can lead to feelings of powerlessness and helplessness.

There are often differences between the reactions of the man and those of the woman in cases of miscarriage, particularly early in pregnancy. This is due to the woman's more intimate knowledge of the baby. Bonding with her baby often begins even before conception, as she anticipates pregnancy. She may begin to prepare emotionally and physically for her new role of motherhood. Even before her pregnancy is confirmed by a doctor, it is anticipated from the day menstruation fails to begin. Early pregnancy often displays itself quite dramatically to the woman. Her breasts become swollen and sore, and she may experience degrees of nausea and fatigue. For the male, the baby is at this stage an intellectual phenomenon. Unlike the woman, he has not been able to begin bonding with this child. Therefore, if a miscarriage occurs at this stage, his reactions may not be as intense as those of his partner. He may be disappointed, but may not understand her intense feelings of loss. On the other hand, she may see him as unfeeling. Neither is wrong in their reactions, for each is reacting to his/her own experiences of the child.

If miscarriage occurs later in pregnancy, there may be less obvious differences in partners' reactions. The woman has shown obvious signs of her pregnancy, and movements allow both male and female to become keenly aware of the existence of their baby as a separate entity. Society is now aware of the pregnancy, and the enthusiasm of friends and family can further strengthen the man's identification with the child. Both now look forward to the birth of their child.

Late miscarriage, being less common than earlier losses, can be a terrible shock. The reactions of both the man and woman may be more intense, for the period of their bonding with the child has been longer. Their confidence of delivery, which had grown with each passing week, is also now shattered.

The woman's reactions can be further complicated by the hormonal changes that occur in her body as it returns to a non-pregnant state. In cases of late miscarriage, these hormonal changes, the swollen breasts and vaginal discharge, are stark reminders of the lost child. For many women who miscarry, it seems like a never-ending nightmare!

> First there was the miscarriage and all that. I just thought it would all be over then, but then came the curette. I got home from hospital wanting to just forget, and then a couple of days later up came my breasts. They ached and leaked. I was miserable. The discharge kept on and on. I felt as if it was going to go on for ever and I was never going to be allowed to forget it. I was fed up!

The question 'Why us?' haunts many. It may be asked with feelings of anger at oneself, at society, at those who have induced abortions, at those who don't 'deserve' a child, at fate, or at God. For others, it will be asked in deep depression as the couple search for some sanity in a seemingly insane situation. The couple, particularly after a number of miscarriages, may share with infertile couples the pain of a loss of their dreams and a fear for the future. They may experience feelings of jealousy toward others who fall pregnant and deliver a live child. These feelings may be particularly strong toward those whose babies are due at the time when their lost child was due to be born.

One further difficulty the couple saddened by miscarriage must face is that generally they have no tangible memories of their child to mourn. They were generally unable to hold the child or remember its features. Often a lot of blood and tissue are their only reminders. As we discussed in Chapter 2, preoccupation with memories can be an important part of grieving. With so few memories of their child, it is not unusual for the couple, particularly the woman, to relive and repeat the circumstances surrounding the loss a great number of times.

A lack of tangible evidence of a baby can also lead to a lack of understanding from others. In the case of an early miscarriage, many people are not even aware that there had been a pregnancy. Therefore, it is difficult for many people to understand the intense reactions of the couple. If the woman still seems to be depressed after a couple of weeks, many begin to feel she is 'putting it on' or 'looking for sympathy' or 'being dramatic'. Even husbands may begin to feel this way. In an atmosphere where others don't understand the intensity of reactions to miscarriage that can occur, the couple can feel very alone and may withdraw into themselves, while putting on a brave front for others.

> After a while people didn't want to know about my miscarriage. At parties everyone, particularly the women, would stop talking when I came. I know I wasn't full of life, but they made me feel guilty, as if I was making everyone else feel uncomfortable. Even David couldn't stand me crying. So during the day I'd cry, but when he came home I'd stop. If I had to cry when he was home I'd make the excuse of going to have a shower. I was so clean those days!

To others it may be 'only a miscarriage', but to the couple it is a major event over which they have a right and need to grieve.

Try again

There is often a very strong need among women who have miscarried to become pregnant again as soon as possible. Often the birth of a healthy child provides the ultimate resolution of grief over the miscarriage.

For some, the difficulties and misunderstandings of grief may strain a couple's relationship in such a way that another attempt at pregnancy is delayed. For example, a man, fearing more pain for his partner, may try to convince her, sometimes against her wishes, to wait. Intercourse may revive memories of the miscarriage, and so is avoided. In most cases, though, the couple often agree to try again as soon as possible. But how long do they wait?

Most will seek the advice of their doctor concerning this, and here opinion is divided. Physical evidence suggests that after the return of menstruation the lining of the uterus is fully renewed, ready for another pregnancy. Some evidence suggests that there may be a slight increase in miscarriage if ovulation and fertilization occurs very quickly (within a couple of weeks of a previous miscarriage). This is a fairly rare event, as ovulation usually occurs within four to six weeks after the event.

Intuitively, many doctors suggest a waiting period of three to six months after an early miscarriage, and six to nine months after a later one. The belief is that such a period of time will allow the couple to grieve their loss and also allow the woman to recover physically from the effects of pregnancy. Discussion with one's doctor about his/her reasons for particular advice is vital. The couple may then be guided by the doctor's thoughts and their discussion with him/her.

Once the couple begin to contemplate a new pregnancy, they are often faced with a few months of waiting. For many, there is a fear that they will not be able to conceive again. Fortunately, for the great majority of couples, this fear will be dispelled by a new pregnancy within a few months. Perhaps those who require special understanding are those whose miscarriage follows a period of infertility. Their already damaged self-confidence is further disrupted. They must again find the courage to face the possibility of further periods of infertility. For some, the miscarriage may be seen as being good news. They know that they are able to conceive.

Of course, the couple are very concerned about the possibilty of another miscarriage. For the majority of cases, the statistics are heartening. The general population has about a 20 per cent chance of miscarriage. After one miscarriage, the risk of a second is only slightly above the general population, at between 22 and 24 per cent. After two miscarriages, there is still a 75 per cent chance of a normal pregnancy. Even after three miscarriages, the chance of a fourth is just over 30 per cent.[9]

There is some evidence to suggest that if all a couple's miscarriages have occurred before 14 weeks, the chances of another loss may be slightly lower than the figures above. If previous miscarriages have been later in pregnancy, the figures may be slightly raised.[10] Still, the figures are heartening! There is good reason to be optimistic. Most couples who experience miscarriage will go on to have children of their own if they persevere.

Coping With Miscarriage

Coping with a miscarriage is a very individual matter. The process can be aided or hindered by the reactions of others. Below are some suggestions that may aid in the resolution of this loss.

1. Accept that miscarriage is a substantial loss

The loss of a child through miscarriage is a terrible experience. The couple have a right to grieve for this child and the lost hopes and dreams of their future. Even if others are unable to accept a couple's pain, and hence try to force them to forget it and get on with living before they are ready, they should feel no guilt about their grief. The miscarriage of this particular couple has happened to them *now*. Its pain is new and raw, and has a right to be expressed.

2. Express your feelings openly

Feelings after a miscarriage may be raw, intense, and confusing. One may be angry, sad, disappointed, relieved, guilty, or numb. If the person wants to cry, he/she should! If the griever wants to talk or pound a fist or strangle a pillow, he/she should! Yet the feelings and security of others, particularly children, must be considered, and extreme behaviour avoided or coped with professionally. The vast majority of couples will find that talking and crying without fear of embarrassment allows them to express their intense feelings. In time, the need for such expression eases as grief is resolved.

Other people may be unable to cope with a couple's feelings. It is common therefore for couples to 'put on an act' for those unable to cope. This allows them to rejoin society slowly, as long as they still have those with whom they can express themselves honestly.

3. Find someone with a willingness to be a constant listener

There is a wonderful security for grieving persons if they have at least one person whom they know they can rely on for continued patience and a listening ear at any time. This person may be one's partner, a close family member, or a friend. Such a person can help to make those grieving feel confident and cared for, even when they feel they are losing touch with reality. The listener can provide a different perspective, while allowing the grieving person to express his/her concerns and confusion. If there are difficulties in the male's and female's reactions, this third party may provide some balance. Support groups, being composed of people who are familiar with the feelings, can fill such a role.

It is important that the male, too, is provided with such support. Miscarriage is too often viewed as the woman's sorrow. It is a shared sorrow, and the male must also be provided with the security of being able to confide his grief to another.

4. Ask questions

At times, the explanation given by doctors is incomplete or confusing to the couple. Often all that is required to remedy this is that the couple ask the doctor what they want to know. In the hours and days immediately following a miscarriage, the couple may be confused and unable to assimilate information. Later, unanswered questions may plague them, causing unnecessary concern in a later pregnancy. If a couple have questions, they should make an appointment to see their doctor. At this time they can ask these questions. The majority of doctors will be happy to discuss with them what information is available.

5. Be reassured about the future

As we have already seen, couples experiencing miscarriage generally have a great deal to be hopeful about. Even habitual aborters, who 20 years ago were believed to have about one chance in three of a normal pregnancy, have today been found to have approximately a 70 per cent chance of eventual success. Unlike many things in life, miscarriage appears to be one area where persistence generally pays off. At least, couples generally are fertile. Armed with this knowledge and that of their high chance of eventual success, they can look to the future with hope.

6. Be honest. Ask for what you need

Many people around the couple are unsure of how to help. Because of such uncertainty, they often fumble and end up saying or doing the wrong thing. Many would be relieved to be asked by the couple to fulfil a specific request. It is important that the grieving couple are honest about their needs. If a conversation is increasing the pain, they should gently inform the other person that they'd prefer to discuss something else. If one feels a need for company or for solitude, he/she should ask for it. If a woman can't face the shopping or a doctor's appointment alone, she should ask for another's support.

It is important that one doesn't expect others to read his/her mind, and then resent it when they can't. Feelings need to be expressed, and requests for support should be made openly.

7. Be gentle with yourself

Some couples try to return to 'normal' life before they have allowed themselves time to be sad. Normal activities can be helpful, as long as the couple accept that there will be times when feelings or situations bring the pain bubbling back to the surface. The couple need to give themselves time, and should refuse to berate themselves when their timetable for grief or one imposed on them by others is not followed.

Conclusion

Miscarriage is a common event, with one in five pregnancies being ended in this manner. In fact, many doctors view miscarriage as a normal variation in the process of pregnancy. When we look at the complexities involved in the processes of fertilization and the development of a baby, it is even more surprising that more foetuses are not lost in this way.

In the majority of cases, there is little, if anything, that can be done to prevent a miscarriage occurring. No one is to blame. Yet, though common, miscarriage is still a major event in the lives of the couple who experience it. Reactions can vary widely, depending on many factors. Each individual and each couple may experience differing degrees of emotional pain.

Incidents surrounding the miscarriage can be painful and confusing, and require careful handling by doctors and hospital staff.

The couple are grieving a substantial loss, and so may easily suffer in the same ways as couples bereaved by other means. They require care and understanding.

Although miscarriage is a traumatic event, there is great hope for the future. The great majority of couples will go on to have another child at a later time, following a normal healthy pregnancy.

References

1. Hank Pizer and Christine O'Brien Palinski, *Coping with a Miscarriage* (London: Jill Norman, 1980), 11.
2. Gordan Bourne, *Pregnancy* (London: Pan Books, 1979), 66–70.
3. Derek Llewellyn-Jones, *Fundamentals of Obstetrics and Gynaecology*, Vol. 1: Obstetrics, 3rd ed. (London: Faber and Faber, 1982), 184.
4. Bourne, *op. cit.*, 274.
5. The Staff of the Mt Sinai Hospital, New York City (J.J. Ravensky and A.F. Guttmacher, eds.), *Medical, Surgical and Gynecologic Complications of Pregnancy*, 2nd ed. (Baltimore: Williams and Williams, 1965).
6. Jennie Kline, Zena Stein, Patrick Shrout, Mervyn Susser, and Dorothy Warburton, 'Drinking during Pregnancy and Spontaneous Abortion', *The Lancet*, July 26, 1980, 176–180.
7. Colin Taylor and W. Page Faulk, 'Prevention of Recurrent Abortion with Leucocyte Transfusions', *The Lancet*, July 11, 1981, 68–69.
8. A.K. Awan, 'Some Biologic Correlates of Pregnancy Wastage, *American Journal of Obstetrics and Gynecology*, 119 (1974), 525–532, 528.
9. Llewellyn-Jones, *op. cit.*, 191.
10. S.J. Funderbuck, D. Guthrie, and D. Meldrum, 'Outcome of Pregnancies Complicated by Early Vaginal Bleeding, *British Journal of Obstetrics and Gynaecology*, 87 (1980), 100–105. Also Ann Oakley, Ann McPherson, and Helen Roberts, *Miscarriage* (Glasgow: Fontana, 1984), 166.

5 Premature Labour and Premature Babies

Approximately seven babies in every hundred (seven per cent) will be born at between 20 and 37 weeks' gestation. Such babies are classified as premature. What causes labour to begin prematurely is in many cases a mystery to the medical profession.

The premature baby, born before it is really ready to cope with life outside the womb, has a battle to fight against the many factors that threaten its well-being, even its very life. Prematurity is the major cause of death of infants in the first week of life. Of course, the more premature the babe, the greater the risks. Ten years ago, it was unlikely for a child born before 34 weeks' gestation to survive. Today the prospects are much brighter.

For the parents of a premature infant, the birth and following weeks can be a frightening experience, in which hope and despair may follow in quick succession as the condition of their baby changes. The beautiful birth experience they may have looked forward to, and the closeness that was expected after the birth, are taken from them. These positive experiences are replaced by uncertainty, confusion, and fear. If their child does not survive, the couple must then experience the intense grief of those whose children die. Even for those parents whose babies survive, there is loss. There is the loss of the expected birth experience, the loss of the physical contact with the child, the loss of control, and the loss of the third trimester of pregnancy, during which they were to adjust to the new life that was to be theirs. Accompanying their loss are painful feelings of grief. Yet, if their child survives, they may be denied the right to experience these emotions.

The causes and investigations of premature labour

In looking at why labour begins prematurely it may be best to look at labour itself. For labour to begin, two events must occur. Firstly, the cervix must 'ripen'. The collagen tissue that normally composes the cervix changes in structure, so that thinning and dilation are possible. Secondly, the contractions of the muscular walls of the uterus must become regular and coordinated in such a manner that descending motion is produced. To this day, medical science is unable to specify exactly what initiates labour. More and more is being learnt, and many likely theories are put forward.

The hormone progesterone is responsible for the maintenance of pregnancy. It is believed that this hormone, in combination with other hormones, inhibits labour; the progesterone may become blocked by other hormones, such as oestrogen. Simultaneously, substances known as oxytocins and prostaglandins increase within the uterus. Such substances are believed to stimulate the uterus toward labour. Therefore, in this way there is a reduction in the effects that inhibit labour, and an increase in those conditions that stimulate it.[1] It is believed labour may be instigated through this. What may cause these changes in concentrations of the hormones to occur is unknown. Herein lies the dilemma in trying to determine the reasons for the onset of premature labour!

Although we may be uncertain of how conditions cause labour, we can outline the more common conditions that can result in premature labour.

1. Premature rupture of the membranes

In some pregnancies, the membranes containing the baby and surrounding amniotic fluid may rupture before labour begins. In some cases the membrane rupture may be due to bacterial infection that weakens the membranes. How the pregnancy will be managed after this occurs depends on the period of gestation. The decision will be made after all the possible risks to the baby are considered. Once the membranes have ruptured, there is a risk of infection developing within the uterus and affecting the baby. Such a risk must be weighed against the risks to the baby associated with prematurity.

If the pregnancy is of less than 34 weeks' gestation, it is often felt that the dangers to the baby of prematurity outweigh those of infection. Most often, labour will occur within 48 hours of the rupturing of the membranes. If this has not occurred, the woman may be allowed to get out of bed and may even go home, as long as she rests sufficiently and is supervised carefully. Any rise in temperature must be reported to the doctor, as it may indicate infection.

If the pregnancy is further advanced than 34 weeks, labour may be induced, since the risks due to prematurity are significantly decreased. Unfortunately, the reasons behind premature rupture of the membranes are generally unknown. Hearteningly, though, it is found that the condition is unlikely to recur.

2. Pre-eclampsia (PE)

This condition is characterized by high blood pressure, severe swelling of the extremities, and protein in the urine. Severe pre-eclampsia is an important cause of premature labour, being involved in approximately 20 to 30 per cent of such instances. In some cases, labour is initiated by this condition. In other cases labour has to be induced, as the baby must be rescued from the hostile environment the uterus becomes under the effect of severe pre-eclampsia. The mother's life, too, can be in jeopardy unless delivery occurs. Appropriate antenatal care is important in recognizing the symptoms of pre-eclampsia, monitoring it, and making attempts to alleviate it.

3. Overdistention of the uterus

The most common cause of overdistention is a multiple pregnancy. Multiple pregnancies show a higher incidence of anaemia, pre-eclampsia, and hydramnios (an excess of amniotic fluid). Hydramnios in itself is believed to be a cause of premature labour, yet the reason for it is generally unknown. In rare cases, the condition may be linked to foetal abnormality, such as Trisomy 18. A rarer cause of overdistention is linked to infection in the membranes of the uterus or in the foetus.

4. Maternal disease

Chronic severe hypertension, heart disease, kidney inflammation (nephritis), diabetes, and severe acute infections such as urinary tract infections and pneumonia are all believed to be involved in cases of premature labour. Any chronic conditions should be controlled prior to pregnancy, where possible. In some cases, labour may be induced prematurely to protect the child from the hostile intra-uterine environment. Maternal disease may be involved in approximately ten per cent of premature labours.

5. Placental haemorrhage (abruptio placentae)

In approximately five per cent of cases of premature labour, there is an accidental haemorrhage of the placenta. If the haemorrhage is moderate or severe, it is important that the child is delivered as soon as possible, since such severe haemorrhaging can be a life-threatening situation for both mother and child. In severe cases of haemorrhage or clotting, it is almost impossible to stop the progress of labour.

6. Placenta praevia

In a small number of cases, premature labour occurs when the placenta is found in the lower part of the uterus between the baby and cervix. Any bleeding in the second half of pregnancy suggests placenta praevia. An ultrasound scan can confirm the diagnosis. As pregnancy progresses, the mother is carefully watched. Often bed rest is suggested in more severe cases, and this is generally undertaken in hospital. Haemorrhaging is possible in cases of placenta praevia. Delivery is usually by caesarean section, unless the praevia is only partial.

7. Foetal malformations

In the rare occurrence of a foetus being severely malformed, there is a tendency for such babies to be delivered prematurely.

8. Uterine malformations and cervical incompetence

As we noted in Chapter 4, malformations of the uterus can in some women initiate miscarriage or premature labour. In some cases of cervical incompetence, the cervix does not begin to open until late in the second trimester, or early in the third. If this is undetected, premature labour may follow rupture of the membranes. However, if the problem is diagnosed before rupture, a cervical suture may be inserted, or the woman confined to bed. The bed-end is raised to position the hips above the abdomen. Such a position, known as the Trendelenburg position, relieves the pressure on the cervix, and in this way seeks to prevent further dilation.

9. Heat

Excessive body heat is believed to be a factor in some premature labours. Acute infections producing high fevers, excessively hot baths and showers, or strenuous continuous physical exercise, may produce such body heat and are best avoided.

10. Uterine activity

It has been suggested that high levels of uterine activity in the form of strong tightenings may indicate that the pregnancy will end in premature labour. Unfortunately, evidence is inconclusive, and uterine activity is believed to be a factor in the premature labours of only some women.

11. Orgasm and breast massage

In general, doctors advise that it is perfectly safe to continue intercourse throughout pregnancy. Irrespective of this, most couples abstain as delivery draws near. It is believed that in a very small number of women, orgasm may actually contribute to initiating labour. Orgasm is associated with increased levels of oxytocin, prolactin, and prostaglandins in the mother, as well as increased uterine blood flow and contractions.[2] Some doctors therefore believe that if the uterus is 'ready' — that is, quite reactive prematurely — labour may be initiated. Intercourse without orgasm does not increase maternal levels of the above instances, and is therefore not considered a problem.

Breast massage is also believed associated with increased levels of oxytocin.[3] Therefore women who have a history of premature labour, placenta praevia or late miscarriage and who exhibit a strong orgasmic response accompanied by painful uterine contractions, may be best advised to avoid orgasm during intercourse and leave breast massage until late in pregnancy.

12. Unknown

In at least 40 to 50 per cent of cases of premature labour, the cause cannot be precisely determined. Doctors may only be able to make an educated judgment as to the cause. Therefore, prevention of premature labour at a later time may involve only careful antenatal supervision and early recognition of symptoms.

Who is at risk?[4]

For those attempting to prevent premature labour, it is vital to be able to recognize women who may suffer from the problem. It is important to remember that even a high-risk mother is not *destined* to have another premature labour. It simply means that her chances of doing so are higher than the general population.

a) High-risk patients

High-risk patients are generally monitored carefully by their doctor for any signs of premature labour. Many will go on to normal term deliveries, but others will begin to labour prematurely. The sooner this is discovered and treatment begun, the greater is the chance of halting the process. Hence the careful monitoring. High-risk mothers include those who have had a previous premature delivery, those who have experienced a number of second trimester miscarriages, and those who are carrying a multiple pregnancy.

b) Moderate-risk patients

A number of factors working within a pregnancy indicate that the mother needs to be considered a moderate-risk candidate for premature labour. In some, but not all, women with uterine malformations, premature labour occurs. Evidence of placenta praevia, excessive amniotic fluid, maternal disease, second-trimester bleeding, a second-trimester miscarriage, or a thinning or dilating cervix indicates that supervision or treatment is required to ward off premature labour. Women aged less than 18 also tend to be moderately at risk of premature labour.

c) Mild-risk patients

Some factors appear to be related to a small degree with premature labour, but generally would not produce it by themselves. These factors include a number of first-trimester miscarriages, an abnormally low weight gain in pregnancy, fever, smoking, fibroids, high blood pressure in pregnancy, and heavy, tiring work. A very short or very light woman, such as one weighing below 45 kilograms before pregnancy, may also be more inclined to deliver prematurely than the general population. First-time mothers, those over 40, and mothers who have had many pregnancies also have a small risk of delivering prematurely.

What are the symptoms of premature labour?

Unfortunately, only about a half of all premature labours will be predicted. The very early symptoms of premature labour are mild and quite nonspecific. They include a dull, low backache, an increase or change in vaginal mucus or discharge, and a dragging sensation and pressure in the lower abdomen, spreading into the back and thighs. These symptoms may also be accompanied by intestinal disturbances, such as nausea and diarrhoea. Gradually strengthening contractions or tightenings occurring at less than ten-minute intervals for an hour or more must be considered seriously. In other cases, such as premature rupture of the membranes and placenta haemorrhage, symptoms are more dramatic and obvious. It is important that women report to their doctor any consistent changes in their pregnancy that are similar to those mentioned above. The earlier treatment begins, the better is the chance of preventing delivery. Unfortunately, women having a first child and not expecting problems may not recognize these ominous signs.

The treatment of premature labour

Unfortunately, in many cases of premature labour, either the woman reaches the hospital too late or treatment is ineffective. If the cervix is dilated and thinned, the contractions are rhythmic and regular, and the membranes have ruptured, there is little, if anything, that can be done to prevent delivery.

In other cases, the woman is placed on an intra-venous drip containing substances known as beta-agonists. The most commonly used are Salbutamol or Ventolin, and Ritodrine. The effect of these agents is to inhibit the contractions of the uterus. They are administered until contractions are quietened, at which time the drip may be removed and replaced by oral medication, which may be continued over a period of days or weeks.

The beta-agonists often produce side-effects in the woman. These can be inconvenient and disconcerting, although they cause no harm to the mother or baby. Such side-effects include an increased heart-rate felt as a 'pounding of the heart', a tremor or 'the shakes' in the extremities, and headache and nausea. The severity of side-effects is a very individual matter, varying greatly from woman to woman.

After a period of time when contractions appear to be under control, some women are able to return home. They must rest and not participate in exercise, lifting, strenuous work, or intercourse. Where possible, most doctors prescribe complete bed rest for such patients, and it is advice best followed if at all possible.

In cases where the doctor believes that labour cannot be prevented, only postponed for a period, and the pregnancy is of less than 34 weeks' gestation, the woman may be given two injections of a cortico-steroid known as Betamethazone. This substance is believed to assist in the maturing of the baby's lungs, and hence may reduce the risk of Respiratory Distress Syndrome (RDS) after birth. We shall discuss RDS in more detail later. Many doctors believe that these injections have no effect on lung maturity, and hence do not administer Betamethazone. Others, who may doubt the effectiveness of the injections, still administer them, knowing they do no harm and hoping they do some good.

Where a very premature labour cannot be prevented, most doctors agree that the least traumatic delivery will give the tiny infant the best chance of survival. Doctors may therefore advise mothers of babies of less than 32 weeks' gestation to deliver by caesarean section. Such a procedure puts less strain on the underdeveloped lungs of the premature infant. In vaginal deliveries, an episiotomy is commonly performed to protect the premature infant's soft skull from undue pressure. If necessary, an epidural anaesthetic may be administered to allow for a gentle forceps delivery. Generally, pain-relieving drugs that may depress the baby's respiration are avoided.

Each case of premature labour is very individual, and prevention of it is not guaranteed. This is because of the mystery surrounding the reasons for premature labour and the onset of labour itself. Unfortunately, there is often little that can be done to prevent a future premature labour, although it must be remembered that one such event does not necessarily mean all future deliveries will be premature.

Premature but no labour

In some cases of premature delivery of a baby, the natural onset of labour does not occur. A decision is made to take the baby by induction or caesarean section. This may be necessary in cases where the uterus has become a hostile environment, in which the baby's life is threatened. At times the mother's life may also be in jeopardy, such as in cases of delivery due to severe toxaemia, diabetes, or rhesus incompatibility.

If, after examination of a pregnant woman, it is suspected that a baby's development is retarded, a decision may be made to deliver the baby prematurely. The placenta may not be providing the baby with sufficient nutrients, or a haemorrhage may have caused some of the placenta to detach from the uterine wall. A previous history of growth-retarded babies may indicate that, to ensure safety of this child, early delivery may be necessary.

Some women who have experienced a prior stillbirth between 28 and 40 weeks may, in consultation with their doctors, decide that this baby be delivered early to guard against another tragic outcome.

Whatever the reasons that underlie a decision to deliver a baby prematurely, the event can still be traumatic. In cases where death threatens, the couple have only one course of action; if their premature baby experiences difficulties, they know they had no option. Yet, many such couples may still berate themselves, trying to lay the blame somewhere. 'If only I'd kept my weight down!' 'If only I'd seen the doctor more regularly!'

The couple who elect to have an early delivery may fear that such a decision may actually threaten the life of their child, while to leave the pregnancy continue may see a successful outcome. They must weigh their fears of another loss against possible risks to this child caused by prematurity. If their child does have problems, that guilt can be intense.

Later, some women who have had their children delivered without labour being initiated may naturally feel a bit cheated, envious of others who have had a natural birth experience. Others are simply happy that their child survived.

The premature and dysmature baby

At times, premature babies are defined as those being less than 2,500 grams in weight. By this definition two groups of babies will be included:

a) The pre-term or premature baby is born before 37 weeks' gestation, and is of low birth weight due to the curtailment of development time in the uterus.

b) The dysmature or 'small-for-dates' baby has low birthweight due, not necessarily to pre-term delivery, but to malnourishment in the uterus that curtailed development.

A dysmature infant and a premature infant of the same birth weight will differ considerably, with the dysmature infant having a greater chance of survival. Dysmaturity is generally due to under-efficiency of the placenta. It may occur in multiple pregnancies, where one baby has received more nourishment to the detriment of others.

We shall concentrate in this chapter on the premature infant and its special problems. In discussing premature babies, it is important to realize that there will be vast differences between a premature infant born a matter of three or four weeks early and an infant born some 12 weeks or more early. For the former baby, problems are likely to be minimal. For example, feeding may require patience, as the slightly premature infant may tire and sleep during feeds. In contrast, infants more than eight weeks premature may face a series of life-threatening crises in their first weeks of life. In fact, infants born more than 14 weeks early are unlikely to survive.

What chance does the premature baby have?

The smaller and younger a baby is, the smaller are the chances of survival. Birth weight is an important factor, but it must be considered in combination with gestational age and other factors.

Babies of less than 750 grams have about a one-in-four chance of survival, while those of between 750 grams and 1,000 grams have a survival rate of closer to 50 per cent. Survival rates rise to 85 per cent for those between 1,000 grams and 1,500 grams at birth, and to 95 per cent for those above this weight.[5] Australian perinatal figures suggest that 45 to 50 per cent of babies born at 27 weeks' gestation will survive, while the figure for babies born at 31 weeks or beyond is 90 per cent. From this we can see the importance of attempting to 'buy time' in the womb through treatment of premature labour. Within a matter of four weeks, from 27 to 31 weeks, the chance of survival rises 40 per cent.

Survival chances depend on a variety of factors, such as those below:

a) Birth weight.
b) Degree of prematurity or gestational age.
c) Maturity of the lungs. The administration of betamethazone and the time from administration to delivery can have an effect on this factor in very premature babes.
d) The trauma involved in the delivery and the oxygen supply during delivery.
e) The presence or absence of malformations that in themselves may be life-threatening.
f) The baby itself plays an important role in determining the likelihood of survival. Some very young, extremely-low-birthweight babies actually have fewer problems than some of their older, heavier counterparts. Heredity factors, the history of the pregnancy itself, and the baby's ability to fight may also be factors to consider in the overall prognosis of the premature baby.

Each premature baby is an individual, and therefore it is vitally important that the couple seek the advice of their baby's paediatrician concerning his/her progress and chance of survival.

The most dangerous period of time for a premature baby is the first day. The first three days are still of concern, but if the baby survives these first 72 hours, hope will grow considerably. If the child has survived for the first two weeks, parents can be reasonably sure of eventually taking their baby home with them, unless obvious life-threatening conditions have arisen during that time. This is not necessarily the case with a baby who is on a ventilator. Such babies are never out of danger until they have been taken off the ventilator and are breathing satisfactorily for themselves.

The premature baby

The premature baby is born before it is fully ready to cope with the outside world. Such a baby has lost vital time for development in the safety and security of the uterus. Therefore a premature baby will not behave in the same way as a full-term baby. Many of the bodily functions will be underdeveloped. However, it is important to recognize one vital point: The premature baby is fully formed! Such babies have all their senses, organs, and bodily systems. Some of these systems are simply underdeveloped. If the premature baby survives — as most will — he/she will generally develop normally at a rate similar to that at which he/she would develop in the uterus.

Premature babies differ from full-term babies in many ways that make their progress outside the uterus difficult. Below are some of the characteristics or difficulties that may be noted in connection with the premature infant.

1. The baby is frail and small.
2. When compared to the body proportions of a full-term infant, the head and hands are larger in relation to the body.
3. The skin is thin, allowing blood vessels to be visible through the skin. It may appear red and loose.
4. The baby lacks fatty tissue that normally aids in temperature control. Premature babies often look scrawny. The body temperature is often below normal, and outside intervention is required to maintain it at a constant level.
5. Respiration is often less efficient. The more premature the infant, the more inefficient is the respiratory system. The baby's cry may be feeble, and apnoea (temporary cessation of breathing) may occur at times.
6. The feeding system is often inefficient. Premature infants' sucking and swallowing responses may be underdeveloped, and they tire easily. Babies of less than 34 weeks' gestation must usually be fed through a Gavage tube inserted through the baby's mouth or nose and into the stomach. Babes unable to tolerate milk in their stomachs may have a tube inserted into the bloodstream, often through the naval, to provide them with glucose and water. Mucus accumulation in the mouth may add to the feeding problems.

7. During late pregnancy, the mother transfers immunoglobulins to the baby, which assist the term baby in fighting infection. The premature baby lacks this protection, and is therefore more susceptible to infection. This fact makes it imperative that the pre-term baby is not exposed to infection. Parents or staff with even mild illnesses should avoid contact with the baby or wear sterile masks and gowns. Physical contact with the baby should be preceded by thorough washing of hands and arms.

8. The enzyme systems, particularly those involved with the liver, may be underdeveloped, leading to jaundice.

9. The intestines are unable to absorb fat efficiently. There may be other metabolic disturbances.

10. Blood vessels are fragile, and haemorrhages can occur.

11. Stores of iron in the babe's body are depleted.

12. Very premature babies have underdeveloped muscle strength because they have not developed muscle tone by having had to kick against the confined space of the uterus. In some units, physiotherapists are beginning exercise routines for such young babies once they are out of danger.

13. Eyes may be closed and present problems.

14. Ears are soft and flat.

15. The skull is soft and the fontanelle (soft spots) wide.

16. Fingers are short and may not have nails.

17. Lanugo (downy body-hair) may be plentiful.

18. Kidneys may be immature and function inefficiently.

Even with such difficulties, most premature babies progress well, and the majority can look forward to going home and developing normally.

Dangers that may face the premature baby

Unfortunately, some premature babies, particularly those born more than eight weeks premature, may experience complications that can threaten their lives. We discuss some of these below:

1. Respiratory Distress Syndrome (RDS) or Hyaline Membrane Disease (HMD)

In the mature lungs of a term baby, the air sacs (alveoli) are covered by a phospholipid composed mainly of lecithin and known as surfactant. Surfactant begins to be secreted by the foetal lungs between the twentieth and twenty-fifth week of pregnancy, increasing in amount with increasing gestational age. Insufficient levels of this substance mean the alveoli will collapse when the baby breathes out. Therefore the baby must expand the lungs completely with each breath, and breathing becomes extremely difficult and tiring. In mild cases, the lungs will clear themselves in a matter of days. In more severe cases, the baby may be given extra oxygen. The level of oxygen supplied is carefully monitored.

If increased levels of oxygen fail to stabilize the infant, Continuous Positive Airways Pressure (CPAP) may be employed. In this procedure, when the baby breathes out he/she is forced to work against pressure set up in the lungs. This forces the air sacs to remain partially open. If the baby fails to respond to CPAP, he/she may be put on to a ventilator, which takes over the breathing for the baby. The more premature the baby is, the more likely it is that ventilation will be used.

The administration of betamethazone is believed to increase the secretion of surfactant and hence reduce the incidence of RDS.

Because of the energy infants with RDS expend in breathing, they are generally fed a solution of glucose and water intravenously. Blood samples are regularly taken to determine the concentration of gases and other biochemicals in the blood.

The greater the degree of prematurity is, the more likely the baby is to develop RDS. Approximately half of those of birth weight between 1,000 grams and 1,500 grams are affected. A more severe chronic form of respiratory distress that may strike babies born before 30 weeks' gestation is chronic pulmonary insufficiency of prematurity. It may require oxygen treatment for many days or weeks.

2. Jaundice

A large number of premature babies develop jaundice to some degree. This usually shows itself about two to five days after birth. The most obvious sign of jaundice is a yellow colouration of the skin. Blood tests determine its severity. Severe jaundice in premature babies has been greatly reduced by the introduction of early feeding. Treating moderate jaundice generally involves a procedure known as phototherapy. The baby is exposed to bright fluorescent 'white' light or 'blue' light, which breaks down the yellow substance (bilirubin) in the blood to harmless substances. If phototherapy is unable to control the jaundice, an exchange transfusion is used.

3. Inhalation of feeds

It is more common for a low-birth-weight infant to inhale regurgitated contents of the stomach, which can cause breathing difficulties. This is overcome by carefully sucking contents out of the pharynx.

4. Cerebral intraventricular haemorrhage

In very premature babies there is a possibility that a haemorrhage in the cavities (ventricles) deep in the brain may occur. The condition is serious and life-threatening, but in most cases the haemorrhages are small and disappear without any risk of brain damage.

5. Patent ductus arteriosus

The ductus arteriosus is a blood-vessel of the heart used by the foetus while in the uterus. It generally ceases to function ten to 15 hours after birth. In premature infants it may fail to close, and this can lead to congestive heart failure. This occurs in about 25 per cent of infants less than 1,500 grams. The condition generally occurs within the first two weeks of life. In some cases a drug called indomethacin can be used to try to close off the ductus arteriosus.[6] Surgery may be required if the condition is severe. In most cases, severe patent ductus arteriosus is associated with hyaline membrane disease.

The Special-Care Nursery

Ideally, premature babies should be taken directly to a Neonatal Intensive-Care Nursery or Special-Care Nursery (SCN) following birth. Such nurseries are staffed by highly skilled doctors and nurses who specialize in the care of such babies. They also contain the equipment necessary for dealing effectively with such precious infants.

Unfortunately, many women go into premature labour in areas without direct access to a special-care nursery. In such cases, transfer to a large maternity hospital is vital, particularly where the pregnancy is less than 32 weeks in gestation. If delivery occurs, both mother and baby are generally transferred by road or air ambulance. If a caesarean section has been performed, it may be possible to transfer only the baby. State Health Departments generally provide subsidy for such travel, and details of this are kept by social workers of major hospitals.

Seeing their baby for the first time in a SCN can be frightening for parents. The babies, particularly very small ones, are generally attached to many and varied types of equipment. This equipment may appear ominous, but once their functions are explained the parents can be reassured. Each piece is designed to monitor the important bodily functions of the baby and alert staff to any difficulties, even minor ones. Rather than being ominous jailers of the baby, these pieces of equipment should be viewed as electronic protectors of this tiny precious bundle.

Staff are happy to inform parents of what each piece of equipment does and how it protects the baby, what procedures are taking place, and the baby's progress. Parents' questions are welcome. Sometimes staff who work so closely with premature babies and equipment forget that it can be threatening to the uninitiated. A question from a parent is a welcome chance for the staff to discuss this equipment, which they understand and value highly.

Some of the equipment in the special-care nursery is discussed briefly below:[7]

1. The humidicrib

The humidicrib is commonly known among the general population as an incubator and in medical circles as an isolette. It is basically a perspex box, in which the premature baby may be placed and in which the temperature can be controlled. The baby's body temperature is continually monitored by a probe attached by sticking-plaster to the baby's back. Holes in the side of the humidicrib give the scrubbed hands of parents and staff access to the baby.

2. The head box

A baby requiring oxygen may be catered for by pumping oxygen directly into the humidicrib. Another method involves placing a small plastic box, known as a head box, over the head and possibly shoulders of the baby. Oxygen is supplied from a wall outlet near the humidicrib.

3. Ventilator or respirator

If a baby has severe breathing difficulties, he/she may be helped to breathe by the use of a ventilator. The machine is situated beside the humidicrib, and a small tube is passed down through the mouth or nose of the baby and into the lungs. A mixture of oxygen, air, and water-vapour is then used in the artificial breathing of the ventilator. The aim is to have the premature infant removed from the ventilator and breathing on his/her own as soon as possible.

4. Heart monitor and apnoea alarm

Generally, above the humidicrib is a machine with blinking lights on which numbers may be seen. It may be attached to the chest, arms, or legs of the baby. It is the function of this machine to monitor the baby's breathing and heart-rates. The machine is extremely sensitive; if there is even a slight disruption to the breathing or the heart-beat, an alarm will sound. An alarm sounding may be frightening to parents, but in most instances there is no immediate danger to the baby. If there is a problem, such sensitive equipment means early detection and intervention, which may prevent a more serious problem arising. In most cases, apnoea episodes are ended by a pat on the bottom or a rub on the back.

5. Feeding equipment

As we mentioned before, some babies are too small to suck and must be fed through a Gavage tube. This tube is passed down through the baby's mouth or nose and into the stomach. Breast or formula milk is then fed down the tube via a syringe or funnel. Some very small babies will require intravenous feeding in the first few days of life. The amount is controlled by an electronic pump.

6. Phototherapy lights

As we have discussed, babies suffering from jaundice may be placed under fluorescent lights. Goggles are placed over the baby's eyes to prevent any damage to the retina from the bright lights. The baby is turned regularly to gradually expose the whole body to the lights.

The special-care nursery is a highly specialized area of the hospital, involving a large band of skilled, caring individuals. These individuals, with the use of their special equipment, give a chance of life to babies who even ten years ago would have died.

The nursery staff see parents as vital members of the team caring for the pre-term infant. No amount of specialized medical care can replace the love of a parent. Many nursery staff believe that parental love and contact may be a factor in itself in promoting the well-being of the delicate premature infant.

A question of quality of life

As neonatal intensive care techniques have improved, more babies are surviving at earlier gestational ages. Ten years ago a baby born before 32 weeks had little chance of survival. Today babies as young as 22 to 23 weeks have lived, although survival before 26 weeks is limited.

Some of these babies who are born so prematurely can suffer severe problems. In fact, a small number are left handicapped. The babies most at risk are those born weighing less than 750 grams. But the babies who do survive seem to have a very high chance of normal development. If these babes are adversely affected, it is found that motor and sensory abilities are more likely to be involved than intellectual capacities.[8].

As techniques improve, the question of quality of life will continue to spark discussion. Economic considerations will also impinge on the argument, since a long period of intensive neonatal care is expensive and drains staffing resources.

The question arises as to whether criteria should be determined to guide hospital staff as to when treatment should or should not be continued. Secondly, what are these criteria and who sets them?

For parents, these questions are not academic. This is not a set of criteria lying in a humidicrib fighting for life; this is their child! Unfortunately, prematurity is a condition that often affects the children of the same parents continually. Are these parents to be denied the hope of a child to nurture? Further, medical science has been incorrect in the past in predicting the potential of children classified as 'handicapped' according to medical evidence at birth.

Yet the question of when 'treatment' becomes 'medical heroics' to save a baby whose potential life is of a standard below that arbitrarily set by society as acceptable, will remain a hotly debated question. It is a question that parents and medical staff must answer within themselves, taking into account the facts, their values, and their feelings. This involves a soul-searching process that is often required of parents at a time when their coping is already stretched to its limits. It is a question the concerned staff of special-care nurseries treat with due reverence, for which they must be applauded.

Emotional reactions to premature labour and premature babies

As with other complications we have discussed, reactions to premature labour and premature babies will differ with each individual and will be affected by the situation surrounding the labour. Some of the factors that may affect the severity of reactions include:

a) The degree of prematurity

The earlier the baby is born, the more likely it is that complications may arise and that even death may result. The crises that the extremely premature infant may experience place added strain on the parents. Some parents must not only face the ups and downs of such crises, but may actually grieve in preparation for a possible loss.

b) The time prior to delivery for preparation

Some women, because they have delivered prematurely with a prior birth, are aware of the chance of this recurring in another pregnancy. They have time to prepare themselves. Others are able to prepare for a short period of time, as labour is postponed by treatment. For another group, labour is completely unexpected and is relatively quick. For such couples, the loss of control of the pregnancy must be experienced simultaneously with concerns for their baby.

c) Separation of mother, father, and children

At times a woman and/or the baby must be transferred to an intensive-care nursery of a larger hospital. Such separations from partner, children, and other family members can be difficult for all involved. If the baby is transferred without the mother, the father may follow and find himself divided between his child and his partner. If mother and baby must go, father and other children are left isolated and must make arrangements to deal with a large number of practical problems.

d) The importance of this child

For a couple with a history of previous losses, a premature delivery can rekindle fearful memories. It may even prevent them bonding with the baby, for fear that they will also lose this child. On the other hand, some couples after a series of losses and no term deliveries may actually be relieved by the premature delivery of a live child with a hope of survival.

e) The reactions of hospital staff, particularly those of the SCN

To ensure that parents adjust to this difficult situation, it is important that staff encourage parents to become involved with their child and ask questions.

f) Likely long-term effects, if any

The more difficult a baby's fight for survival is, the more chance there is of long-term effects. Parents may be concerned about the future development of their child. In a small number of cases there may be a degree of handicap, with which parents must cope as well.

Threatened premature labour is a frightening experience for both the woman and her partner. Symptoms may appear over time, and she may not connect them with premature labour. In other cases, the symptoms are severe and cause shock.

> It was a terrible fright when my waters broke at 15 weeks. It wasn't something I was expecting. I'd had a normal first pregnancy and then you think the next one will be a breeze too, but it wasn't. Although I didn't finally have Emma until 33 weeks, it was a very anxious week at 15 weeks not knowing if I was still carrying the baby.

There are fears for the baby's and the woman's own safety, combined with the stress of the emergency situation. Events often happen too quickly for the couple to assimilate successfully. It may be difficult to contact emergency services in more isolated areas. If such difficulties occur, panic may lead to increased discomfort and emotional trauma.

If the woman is transported to a hospital while in premature labour, the situation is assessed. If the pregnancy is less than 34 weeks' gestation and life-threatening situations to the baby have been ruled out as the cause of the premature labour, the woman will be placed on an intravenous drip. Sometimes the drip is inserted after the area has been dulled by a local anaesthetic injection. The woman may experience side-effects of the drugs, but these are monitored carefully by staff. She may also be administered sedatives or pain-killers and, where appropriate, injections of betamethazone. Often the woman, particularly if she has been careful with drugs throughout pregnancy, will be concerned about the effects of these drugs on her baby. Such drugs have been carefully investigated, and the woman can be reassured that there will be no harm done to the baby. Staff must realize these genuine concerns, and reassure the couple.

The woman is generally admitted to the labour ward, where care is efficient and intensive. There is often little time initially to consider the woman's psychological well-being, and many couples feel overwhelmed by the efficiency. Well-explained procedures, a listening ear at a later time, and the company of the father, a relative, friend, or hospital carer can ease pressures generated by the situation. If transferred to the hospital, the woman may be separated from her partner, her main support. She may feel very alone in such a tense situation. The relaying of phone messages — or even better, being able to speak to her partner on the phone — may prove a wonderful morale boost. Where a woman is in her home town, unlimited access to her by her partner, day and night, is important for both. If there is no partner or he is unable to be with her constantly, another person close to her should be able to be with the woman on some extended basis, if she so desires.

Emotional reactions of the woman can be heightened by the lack of sleep, the inability to eat, the pain, and the effects of drugs often involved in episodes of premature labour. Time can lose its meaning as she drifts in and out of sleep and episodes of pain.

> I know I was in the labour ward for two days, yet it only seems
> like a few hours. I know I was in a lot of pain, but it's all a bit of a
> blur now. It's as if your mind protects you from the pain by
> blocking off the thoughts and memories.

If treatment is successful and contractions are eased, the woman
will be transferred to the obstetric unit for complete bed rest. The
drip will remain in place until regular contractions have ceased. It
may then be replaced by oral medication. It is often difficult for
the woman who has experienced threatened premature labour to
be close to new-term babies and newly delivered mothers. This is
particularly true if the gestational age of the baby would make
his/her survival dubious, if born at this time. Sharing
accommodation with another woman facing a pregnancy
complication is preferable if single-room accommodation is not
available.

For many women, threatened premature labour does not consist
of one isolated event. A woman may be faced with a period of
weeks of hospitalization, during which time contractions can
become rhythmic and threatening at intervals. Further episodes on
the intravenous drip may continue to ward off final labour. In the
meantime, each contraction is viewed with suspicion and fear.
The woman may be tense and emotionally charged. She may be
unsure of what constitutes the danger signs. Such fears can be
relieved by patient staff and well-informed explanations.

She may become depressed and bored, particularly if she is
separated from her family and has been unable to prepare herself
with activities for a long hospital stay. At times, many women
wish the baby would be delivered even before its survival chances
are good, 'just to get it over and done with'. If the baby is then
born and suffers complications, the woman may feel guilty for
having had such thoughts.

> When I was in prem labour, I really felt at times as if I wanted
> to give in. But then there were others worse off, like people who'd
> lost babies, and then I felt guilty and tried to pull myself together,
> although I didn't succeed very well. You know you should be
> thankful for every day the baby is in the uterus, but you don't feel
> thankful. You feel selfish for being concerned about your feelings
> rather than the baby's well-being. I really cracked then, after the
> baby was born.

Throughout pregnancy, the couple build up in their minds an idealized picture surrounding labour and their baby. If natural childbirth techniques are to be employed, the couple may have begun attending education classes and practising techniques. They look forward to a fulfilling experience in which both parents are participants in birthing a healthy, mature, cuddly baby, who will soon be home to complete their family.

Premature labour, the medical intervention, a possible caesarean section or hurried delivery, separation of parents and baby at birth, and a long hospital stay destroy this idealized picture. Their cuddly healthy baby may be replaced by a tiny, frail substitute, who hangs on tenuously to life.

> It was the first night. I was very groggy. They took me up to see her, and I can remember being very emotional then. Just the shock of seeing you have such a small baby that looks like a rat. You think: 'She couldn't be my baby. She doesn't look like any of my family.' They don't look like anything, just skin and bone.

The loss of their dreams is a legitimate loss to be grieved. The couple may mourn the loss of their ideal labour experience and the loss of control over the circumstances of birth. They may mourn the loss of their 'perfect' baby and their loss of contact with their baby at birth. They may mourn the loss of a normal post-birth period, during which time other parents may be able to do things for their baby. The woman may also mourn the loss of her final weeks of pregnancy and this time for preparation. She may also feel that the baby is not ready to leave the uterus, and that she has lost part of herself. This may not be relieved until the baby's actual due date passes.

> I lost that third trimester. Now I have an almost magical idea of what happens in the later stages of pregnancy. You miss a big tummy because you never had it, and people used to tease you about it. I didn't put my maternity clothes away for a long time, because in my mind I hadn't really finished my pregnancy. I found I also rushed to lend my maternity clothes to someone else who was pregnant, almost as if I was trying to continue the pregnancy I didn't have.

As with all couples who grieve, feelings can be intense and confused. Once the shock subsides, the woman may experience anger — anger at the baby who came too soon, anger at herself for somehow causing the premature delivery, anger at the staff or doctor or her partner.

Depression is common.

> The second day I was a mess. They told me Jordan would have to go on a ventilator, but not to worry. I was worried. I was so depressed. I couldn't seem to pull myself out of it.

The depression because of loss may be complicated by hormonal changes that follow birth. The crises that may surround the first weeks of life of a premature baby may further depress this mother separated from her child.

The father, too, may feel powerless to help either his partner or his child. If the baby is transferred, he may be the one who is with the baby, torn between time with his partner and time with the child. He is a messenger and support to a distressed partner, while wanting to be close to encourage, to love his child. What time is not spent at the hospital may be spent alone, trying to cope with household and work duties.

> When I was in prem labour, a couple of mornings Rob would get up and set breakfast for me and then remember I wasn't there, and he'd get all choked up when the seriousness of it all came through. He had to be strong. I was so out of it for the first couple of days, so when she went from no oxygen to 70 per cent he had to take all that worry himself, as well as help cope with a wife who'd had a caesarian, as well as all he'd been through before that. It wasn't till a long time after that he told me all about this and how powerless he felt.

Some couples whose baby may be very premature and in a dangerous situation may even mourn in preparation for a possible loss. In fact, some couples become afraid to love their baby in case he/she dies. Unconsciously, they believe that it will hurt less if they didn't love him/her too much. Unfortunately this is not the case, and there is a risk of rejection of this child. This is detrimental to the well-being of both parent and child. A reluctance to see or be involved with the child may be an indication that this is occurring, and requires gentle handling, encouragement, and listening by partner or staff.

Unfortunately, the couple who have had a premature child who lives are often denied the right to grieve these losses we have mentioned. Comments such as 'But at least your baby is alive' or 'You should be thankful he/she is doing so well' deny the parents the right to grieve their losses. Their grief may be suppressed, only to reappear in later depression. Couples should be encouraged to express their real feelings about their situation, both positive and negative.

> Rob couldn't understand why I felt guilty about the premature labour. Also, because you've got a live baby, people don't understand the negative feelings you have. Nobody wants to discuss the horrible feelings. I was angry, too, but everybody thought because I had a live baby I wouldn't feel these things. One of the nursery supervisors realized I'd been through a lot, and she knew it was upsetting. But she said 'O well, we'll leave you alone' the day I was upset. But I'm not sure that's what I needed, and that was the day I needed to talk. It would have helped if someone had said 'Look, I know you're upset; do you have any idea of whether you would like us to leave you alone, or would you like someone to be with you?'

Many women feel that they are a failure, unable to perform adequately the task of pregnancy that appears to be so easy for others. They feel that they have failed their baby and their partner, that they are somehow responsible for the situation in which their baby is now. They may feel guilty that somehow they have caused the pain for everyone involved.

The first visit for the parents to see their baby in the SCN is often a daunting experience. They may be shocked, and even feel some distaste at the sight of this scrawny red bundle, which seems to be covered by electronic devices and needles. This is not the expected contented chubby baby, sucking peacefully at the breast! Instead, this little frail creature seems to be labouring for every breath, without the support of loving arms around him/her. The machines, as we have seen, are not to be feared. But unless this is explained, the sight may further distance the child from his/her parents.

> For the first three or four days I found it very very difficult to go up and see him in Special Care, because it's so foreign. All the tubing worried me. I didn't know what to do or what to think.

If the baby is not critically ill, the parents are encouraged to touch and stroke their baby. This contact can be wonderfully reassuring to parents, and is believed to be of benefit to the baby. When there is so little else a parent can do for their child, such contact can take on heightened importance.

As time passes and the parents become more familiar with the nursery, the daily visits may become less stressful. Parents are encouraged to visit their baby as often as they wish. When the baby is strong enough, they are urged to cuddle him/her. This is vital for the parents, who are often unable to do little else. Many mothers feel that the nurses staffing the SCN are more the mothers of the baby than they are. It is the nursing staff who bathe them, change their nappies, adjust their feeding, and have continued access to them. Mothers must be encouraged by staff to realize that they play a vital role in their baby's well-being through their contact and, just as importantly, through their expressed breast milk.

Breast milk is the best food for the premature infant, for it contains maternal antibodies and is more easily digested by the baby. The expressing of breast milk is often difficult at the beginning, and is also time consuming. For many women it can be frustrating. When a mechanical breast pump is used, some women feel like 'an old cow' rather than a contented human mother.

> Knowing I had to play a very positive role with breast feeding really kept me going. But it was hard, because the milk didn't come in very quickly. I was sitting with other women expressing who were getting bottles full, and I was getting this mere little 10 ml. That was depressing.

Yet it can be a wonderful reassurance for the mother to know she is providing a vital component in the well-being of her baby. If her baby is strong enough, she may be able to hold and feed him/her, or even participate in the tube feeding of a weaker infant.

Unfortunately, the expressing of breast milk can be affected by psychological factors. The stress involved with a premature baby, and the mechanical nature of expressing by hand instead of having a suckling infant, can interrupt the 'letting down' of milk. The mother may then feel a further sense of failure, which heightens tension and further inhibits milk supply. Encouragement by staff and her partner, and a degree of privacy while expressing, combined with a mother's personal attempts at relaxation, may help alleviate the problem. It is also found that seeing and having contact with her baby can assist in milk production.

While in hospital, the mother often feels a strong need to be with her baby as often as possible, and can become obsessed with keeping up her milk supply. The presence of other babies rooming in with their mothers or in nurseries can increase these feelings. She may wish to compensate for all the other things she cannot do for her child. The sooner she is able to do more for her baby, the better.

These needs and concerns are further exaggerated when the baby has been transferred to another hospital. Such a mother may not have even had a good look at her baby before he/she was moved. A photograph may provide some reassurance, as will phone calls to the SCN, day or night. Expressing and transportation of her breast milk to her baby may then play a vital part in her feelings of being involved with her child.

The father may feel even more helpless. Besides touching his child and supporting his partner, he can do little to alleviate the situation. If the baby is transferred, it may be he who develops a strong bond with his child. If that child then dies, he may feel even more intense grief than the mother.

> I spent a lot of time in that nursery with the baby. Anne, after the caesarean, couldn't. She had established a relationship with the baby while she was pregnant. I couldn't really do that. Mine started in a very intense way during those days he lived. When he died, I was devastated because I felt I'd got to know him so well.

It is often common practice for the couple to be approached about the performance of religious ceremonies involving their child. When confronted, many couples panic, fearing that such a request must indicate that their child is in danger of dying. Generally this is not the case, but parents may need reassurance of their child's well-being. Some couples find such ceremonies reassuring. They may be carried out in the SCN by hospital chaplains or clergy of the couple's choice. Other couples may reject the idea, fearing that baptism or other ceremonies may indicate that they are 'giving up' on their child, or may even somehow 'jinx' their child's chances of survival. Others may reject the idea because they see it as yet another 'abnormal' practice taken from their control; they may prefer to wait until the baby is home to celebrate religiously the birth in the usual manner. Yet, they then worry that if the child should die they have denied him/her this benefit, for which they would then feel guilty.

Generally, the premature infant will be unable to leave the hospital until he/she has reached a weight of 2,500 grams or more, and is, in the opinion of the paediatrician, coping well with life outside the humidicrib. There must be evidence of adequate feeding, efficient breathing, and consistent weight-gain. The baby's discharge therefore generally follows some weeks after the mother has been discharged from hospital.

Leaving hospital without their baby may be the most difficult time the couple must face following the premature delivery. Seeing other couples leaving as a family, while they leave alone, can be very distressing.

> I really felt it, not being a normal mother. That feeling coming home was devastating. It was as if you'd cut off a leg or an arm. I felt very down the day I left hospital.

The woman may be torn between wanting to stay in hospital with her child and going home to be with her partner. In fact, often it becomes important to a woman to be able to fulfil her role of wife or partner again, with the reassurance from her husband that she is a success in this role.

> After so many weeks of being in hospital I just wanted to be with Bob that day I left hospital. Unfortunately, my mother came to help out, and by the end of the day I was depressed and took it out on her. I know I shouldn't have, but I couldn't help it. I just wanted Bob and me alone, for him to hold me and tell me he still loved me. I felt as if we had to court all over again. I was like a little girl needing comfort only he could give.

Unfortunately, if her partner returns to work, the woman may feel isolated and experience a deep sense of emptiness without her baby. This may be more pronounced if she has returned to her home some distance from where her baby is being cared for, or is unable to visit her baby when she wishes due to transportation difficulties. If she wants to be with her child, the couple may have to face accommodation and financial difficulties to accomplish this, a situation many couples cannot afford. Government assistance is available in some cases. The separation of the family may then have to continue for weeks, adding further strain.

The daily routine of expressing milk, visiting the hospital, and running a home can be exhausting, particularly if travelling time is quite lengthy and there are other children in the family. The pain of separation each day can also be heart-wrenching. As time goes on, the urge to have their baby at home can become very strong. The woman may even begin to resent being told what she can or cannot do for her baby.

The support given by one partner to the other is vital. Visiting their baby together, particularly early in the baby's life or during crises, can be an important source of support for the couple and a means of their feeling like a family.

Many parents of premature infants find sleeping difficult. The ringing of the phone can become a frightening experience if the baby is very premature and in danger. The parents fear that their child may die while they are not with him/her. They fear that the hospital may not be honest with them or delay calling them until it is too late. Just when they are beginning to relax, their baby may face another crisis. Convincing themselves that most babies of birth weight 1,000 grams or over eventually go home may be difficult. In their depression caused by a setback, they may often feel their baby will never come home.

As time goes on and the baby progresses, the parents are able to do more for him/her. They begin to feel more like parents. The woman, particularly, may then be more willing to share her baby's time out of the humidicrib with others, such as grandparents, than when a cuddle alone distinguished her as the mother.

> If they'd given anybody else beside Rob and me a cuddle when that was the only privilege we had as a parent that distinguished us from the nursery staff and others, I think I would have freaked. It took a lot for me to even let the grandparents have a cuddle.

The day the couple are able to take their baby home is a wonderful day. At last they are a complete family. Strong relationships have often developed with the staff who cared for their child. Saying goodbye and thank you can be emotional for both parents and staff, particularly if the baby was very premature or had to overcome many hurdles to survive.

Although a happy event, home-coming can be extremely daunting for the couple, particularly the mother. In the hospital, the baby was carefully monitored and medical help was always at hand. The couple fear that the responsibility is now all theirs. What if the baby temporarily stops breathing? What if he/she fails to gain weight? All normal concerns can be exaggerated and take on immense proportions. The couple may be tense and highly alert to every change. The characteristics of a premature baby serve only to heighten their insecurities. For example, premature babies, particularly the younger ones, are known to be 'noisy' babies, making persistent noise in their sleep. They are often bad sleepers and feeders, and may cry quite a deal when awake. Therefore, the already tense parents become even more concerned by this baby who does not seem content. Combine this tension in the mother because she feels that she must be 'doing something wrong', her fears that somehow her baby will not be normal due to its prematurity, and the incredible tiredness that accompanies the motherhood of a premature baby, and you have a recipe for depression.

Some mothers, particularly those of very premature babies, find getting their baby to breast feed is difficult, and they may have to express to keep up their milk supply. When a baby is being fed every three hours or so, there seems to be little time to do anything else but feed, change, and bath the baby. At times, the mother can feel herself being devoured by this tiny demanding creature. If there is no relief, she may even come to resent these 24-hour demands placed on her, only to feel guilty about such feelings. These feelings may be more pronounced in the mother who has left a career but has not had time to adjust to being at home before the baby was born. The strains are further complicated if the couple have been unable or not permitted to grieve their loss. Other people may cause more problems, too.

> Even after you get home you can get angry, especially when you're tired. Like: 'Why have I got a refluxy baby?' You give it a feed and it chucks up the whole lot and you've got to refeed it. Yet people don't like you to feel this way about your baby. 'After all, aren't you glad your baby's alive?' So back into guilt you go.

Now that the baby is home, visitors may wish to see the new arrival and call at inconvenient times, such as when the mother is preparing to feed. Invitations to visit others are also difficult to accept when feeding is difficult. A disrupted routine often means a sleepless night for parents.

It is detrimental to both the parents and the premature infant for the parents to become anxious or feel inferior after talking with parents of term babies about their respective babies' progress. It must always be remembered that development is measured from conception, not birth. Therefore, a premature baby's rate of development must be considered in terms of his/her corrected age, obtained by subtracting from the chronological age (from time of birth) the number of weeks he/she was premature.

> You always have the worries, even till perhaps they get to school, that something may be wrong. A friend of mine has a little boy who was born three weeks before my baby was due and those three weeks after he does something it's just a mild panic waiting to see if she will do it, even if you know kids differ in their milestones.

Others may find it hard to accept just how time-consuming a premature baby is, particularly in the early months. Even the male partner may find it difficult to understand how the needs of one tiny baby can fill a whole day, unless he spends a day with the baby. When this is combined with the broken sleep, the depression, the huge adjustments required in the family and household, and the demands of other children, it is not surprising that misunderstandings between partners can grow out of proportion and tempers become frayed. For some women, intercourse may be just another demand on their time and energy. Partners need patience with each other. We discuss difficulties in detail in Chapter 9.

By the end of the premature baby's first year, he/she will be rapidly catching up to match the development of a full-term baby of a similar age. As he/she becomes more independent, and established routines are in play, the family will begin to function as does a family of a full-term infant. We must re-emphasize that every premature baby is an individual, and the degree of difficulties surrounding the baby's first year depend on his/her particular characteristics and the degree of prematurity.

It is not uncommon for parents to be concerned about the future development of their child for quite a few years. If he/she fails to pass a milestone when parents have decided in their own minds that it should be accomplished, they worry. They may see slowness in one area of development as indicative of retardation or physical handicap, instead of as a normal individual variation found in all children. Support for parents is found through Growth and Development clinics that are associated with the SCN of some hospitals; these monitor extremely premature infants up to the age of two years. Parents of other premature babies may provide other indications and information.

Coping with premature labour and premature babies

A. Premature labour

Threatened premature labour that covers a period of weeks can be a tense time, particularly if it involves a period during which the baby, if delivered, would have a limited chance of survival. Unfortunately, the tension involved in this situation is difficult to relieve. Some of the suggestions below may contribute to its alleviation by preventing events making the situation worse.

1. Ask for what you need

Some of the fear of the situation can be dispelled by seeking and getting the information you need. If the couple are unsure of the drugs being given or the side-effects on the woman or the baby, they should ask. If staff overlook a couple's question, it is probably due to their intense concentration. Ask again, of someone else if necessary.

If there is anything that makes the couple uncomfortable or something they wish, they should ask for what they need. If being in a room close to the nursery is distressing, ask to be moved if possible. If the woman wishes the close support or contact with her partner, she should ask for it. Some hospital rules are made flexible for such patients. The staff, rather than being upset, will be pleased that they can do something to help relieve the situation. Where possible, they will agree to a couple's request.

2. Clarify what signs are ominous

After a session of threatened premature labour that has been controlled, every slight ripple in her body may frighten the pregnant woman. Many symptoms, even contractions, do not herald labour. It may be helpful to clarify with your doctor which symptoms should be watched carefully and which are unlikely to indicate any problems. Such a discussion may ease the tension slightly.

3. Express your feelings

The woman experiencing threatened premature labour is entitled to feel afraid, depressed, angry, and hassled. Bottling up these feelings can make them worse. Being able to talk out or cry away some of her feelings can release tension. The woman needn't be ashamed of an emotional display. Staff understand. If she needs someone to talk to and has no relative or friend close at hand, hospitals have staff such as chaplains, social workers, nursing supervisors, and pastoral-care workers whose roles include being an available listening ear.

4. Where possible, maintain constant contact with your partner

Of all the people around the woman, her partner is likely to share her fears most intimately. He may fear not only for his baby, but also for his partner. He feels powerless to relieve her tension and pain. Threatened premature labour may happen quickly, so that neither partner has had a chance of expressing himself/herself to the other. This is worse if the woman is transferred to another hospital. Her main source of support is taken from her. Where possible, the couple should have as much contact with each other as they desire. Hospitals generally are understanding of a couple's need to be together when the situation is serious. Some will provide means for a husband to stay overnight while his wife is on a drip. This may help to relieve her tension. Where a woman is transferred, phone contact or even messages can provide vital support. The couple need to be honest with each other and with their feelings. A partner will usually understand a person better than anyone else.

5. Try to participate in relaxing activities or distractions

While on a drip and contracting, a woman will generally feel like little else but sleeping between the pains. As the crisis is averted and she is sent for observation to a ward, concentrating on her contractions or tightenings becomes a natural reaction. With little else to distract her, she can become obsessed about her condition, which may even make matters worse. Even normal events of pregnancy, such as a baby's movements, can be viewed suspiciously. Sometimes distractions can help alleviate the situation. A television, novels, and handicrafts may help, as may a close friend reading aloud to her. Music may not only help pass the time, but also be relaxing for her. We discuss prolonged hospitalization in more detail in Chapter 8.

B. Premature babies
1. Have as much physical contact with your baby as possible.

As soon as is medically advisable, the couple should be encouraged to touch and stroke their baby. Part of feeling that a child really belongs to them is having contact with the baby. Being able to cuddle their baby can provide a vital bond between the couple and child. It is also beneficial to the baby. The calming effect on a baby is noted by steady pulse and breathing rates during stroking.

2. As often as possible, visit your baby or phone for progress reports; where possible, visit together

Where possible, couples should find time to visit their baby together. This will help them to feel like a family. At times, when the man is trying to act in a strong and supportive manner, the woman may misinterpret this and feel that he is being indifferent and uninvolved. Visits as a family can show each parent just how important this baby is to the other. Frequent visits or phone calls at any time of the day or night help to reassure parents of their baby's progress and help them maintain an involvement with their child.

3. Ask questions so that you know exactly what is happening to your baby

It is important for a couple to know as much as possible about the condition of their child. In this way, they may feel more involved in the decision-making process concerning their baby. If parents don't understand a procedure, the reasoning behind it, or the use of a piece of equipment, they should ask staff. The SCN staff will be happy to answer questions, although during an emergency is not the time. If parents have particular feelings about what is being done for their child or the care given, they should express them diplomatically to staff or their baby's paediatrician.

4. Do as much as you can for your baby as soon as possible

As soon as the baby is strong enough, the couple, particularly the mother, will be offered the chance to do more for her baby, such as feeding, bathing, and changing. Before this time, the expressing of milk allows the mother to be involved in a truly meaningful way.

5. Take the opportunity of living in with your baby for a time before discharge

Before the discharge of a premature baby, a mother may be encouraged to return to the hospital for at least one night to make the transition from hospital to home smoother. If possible, the mother would be well advised to accept this offer to help build her confidence in dealing for a long period with her precious bundle.

6. Once home, don't be ashamed to admit you could use some help if the situation arises

As we have already noted, the premature baby can be even more time-consuming than a term baby. Any new mother will admit that the first few months can be exhausting. Unfortunately, many don't ask for help for fear that somehow this would show that they are an inadequate mother. For the mother of a premature baby, who may already feel less than adequate as a mother, increased pressure to perform as an efficient mother may come from within herself. She may feel overstressed but not ask for help. If help is offered, don't be ashamed to accept it. A truly competent mother is one who has the strength to cope, but also the strength to realize that coping involves knowing that there are limits to human abilities.

7. Don't be ashamed if at times you have negative feelings about your situation or your baby

Unfortunately, as we have noted, the parents of a premature baby are often denied the right to have feelings of anger, depression, or resentment. They are told: 'You should be grateful! Your baby is alive!' 'O, you don't mean that!' Yet, as we have seen, these couples have losses to grieve during and after delivery, which they must be allowed to express.

Once home and facing the demands of a premature baby, the couple may become short-tempered and depressed due to their child's demands. The negative reactions are normal and warranted. The couple should not feel ashamed of having such feelings. They need to find someone who is able to accept their feelings and listen to them. The couple may express these feelings and so loosen the hold such feelings have over them.

8. Seek out the support of other parents of premature babies

The premature baby is a special child, and in the first year of life should not be compared to term babies of a comparable chronological age. Other premature babies can provide a more suitable yardstick as well as reassurance for parents. Parents of other premature babies also understand the special problems of coping with such babies, both before and after discharge from hospital. They can provide not only practical advice but also emotional support and practical help, such as patterns for small baby clothes.

9. Take advantage of regular checks on your baby's development during the first years of life

Where Growth and Development clinics are attached to the SCN, parents should take advantage of the reassurance such clinics offer. In other areas, the baby's paediatrician can provide the expert advice to reassure parents and to recognize any problems before they become serious and while the child is young enough for treatment to be effective.

10. Be assured of your child's future

Unless there has been some permanent damage caused by such crises as an intraventricular haemorrhage, parents can be reassured that a premature baby who survives has a 90 per cent or better chance of normal development.[9] They may suffer more than usual from respiratory illnesses, but generally outgrow any such problems.

Nearly all premature babies grow into strong adults. In fact, many famous people have been premature babies, including Winston Churchill.

Conclusion

Premature labour and a premature delivery can be frightening experiences for parents. They lose control of the situation of their baby's birth. They lose their final months of pregnancy and lose their loving close contact with their baby after birth. Considerable distress can accompany the birth. The baby, particularly if very premature, may face a series of crises in his/her first weeks of life. Parents are tossed between despair and hope. Their situation requires caring and gentle treatment.

Once the family return home together, the time-consuming efforts of looking after a premature baby place strains on the family, and this situation requires adjustments and even outside help.

The first year of a premature baby's life may be difficult, but nearly all of these children will go on to lead normal healthy lives.

References

1. Derek Llewellyn-Jones, *Fundamentals of Obstetrics and Gynaecology*, Vol. 1, Obstetrics, 3rd ed. (London: Faber and Faber, 1982), 103,104.
2. R.C. Goodlin, *Care of the Foetus* (New York: Masson Publishing, 1979).
3. *ibid.*
4. 'Will Your Baby Wait Nine Months?', *New Idea*, July 30, 1983, 51.
5. David I. Tudehope and M. John Thearle, *A Primer of Neonatal Medicine* (Queensland: William Brooks, 1984), 68.
6. *ibid*, 136.
7. *Specialized Care for Newborn Babies* (booklet for parents produced by the Special Care Nursery, Mater Misericordiae Mothers' Hospital, South Brisbane), 8–11.
8. M. Adamson, 'The 24–26 Week Infant: Proceedings of the Inaugural Congress of Australian Perinatal Society, March 12–14, 1983', *Excerpta Medica*, Asia Pacific Congress Series 18, *Journal of Australian Perinatal Society*.
9. *Specialized Care for Newborn Babies, op. cit.*, 5.

6 When Your Baby Dies

In the general flow of events we expect that we will precede our children to the grave. But when our children — and in this case our babies — are lost to us, our whole world — its order, its security — is thrown into utter confusion. Our memories are few. We will never see that child grow and mature. We will always wonder just what he/she would have looked like and what type of person he/she would have become. Our memories may be confined to the realization of a presence as he/she kicked Dad's hand as he placed it on Mum's abdomen, and that small casket at the funeral. It seems so senseless, so wasted, so unfair!

Although couples who miscarry also lose their babies, we shall confine ourselves in this chapter to looking at losses after 20 weeks' gestation, for from this time society, through its legal requirement of cremation or burial, recognizes your baby's existence.

To experience the death of a baby is to be confronted with one of the most difficult times in your life. There is every likelihood that you will never be the same person again. The changes may be both good and bad. Our minor everyday problems and conflicts pale into insignificance after this tragic event. We may meet death close at hand for the first time. Our own mortality and that of those around us is thrown up before our faces. Death is irreversible. Hope is no more for this child. We cannot alter the outcome, but we can give support to those who are left, those who mourn. It was once said: 'For those who mourn, time is anchored in eternity'. When you lose a child you loved, those words seem so very apt. Yet rest assured that you will come through this! The memories will remain very special, and their ability to hurt you will decrease. There will come a time when the love you felt for that child remains the strongest connection to your beloved baby.

Causes of a baby's death

There are many causes of death in babies before, during, and after delivery. In discussing causes, the medical profession uses specific terms, which we shall outline here.[1]

1. **Live birth**. If, after the child has been delivered completely from inside the mother's body, any evidence of life is exhibited such as breathing, the beating of the heart, pulsation of the umbilical cord, or muscular movements, the child is considered born alive.

2. **Foetal death**. If, before the child of any gestational age is fully delivered from its mother, signs of life are not in evidence, foetal death is considered to have occurred. Early miscarriages (early foetal death), late miscarriages before 27 weeks (intermediate foetal death), and stillbirths are therefore considered in this category.

3. **Neonatal death**. If a live-born child dies witin 28 days of birth, it is termed a neonatal death. If this occurs in the first seven days, it is called early neonatal or postnatal death. Between seven and 28 days, the term 'late neonatal death' is applied.

4. **Perinatal death**. There are two different definitions of perinatal death.

a) Perinatal death comprises the deaths of all foetuses after 20 weeks' gestation (or who weighed more than 400 grams) and all neonatal deaths. Australian figures are based on this definition.

b) Perinatal death includes late foetal deaths (after 28 weeks) and early neonatal deaths. That is, all stillbirths and first-week deaths are considered. This is the definition used by the World Health Organization (WHO).

The second definition is more specific. Hence, figures of the incidence of perinatal death according to this definition will be lower than for the first.

5. **Stillbirth**. This term is generally used for the death of a foetus over 1,000 grams in weight at delivery.

These definitions and figures may seem cold and inhuman, as statistics do when you are part of the statistic! What the couple have lost is not a statistic! It was their child! However, these terms are useful in allowing us to interpret the incidence of such losses. In developed nations of the world, the rate of perinatal death is less than two per 100 births. These figures indicate a considerable reduction on those of years ago, due to better antenatal care, medical diagnosis, foetal monitoring during labour, and efficient management of labour.

It may be comforting to many to realize that the figure of less than two deaths in every one hundred births indicates that the chance of bearing a live child after 20 weeks is very high. Even for couples who lose a child, this news is heartening if they wish to try again. Yet there is little comfort in knowing that by losing your child you are part of a small minority!

We shall now look at some of the causes of perinatal death, listed according to when death occurs. We wish to emphasize here that, although perinatal death causes are many and varied, the incidence of such death is *very low*. This cannot be stressed too strongly! Little ever goes wrong, and if it does happen to once, the chances of it occurring a second time are very slim.

Death before delivery or Intra-Uterine Foetal Death (IUFD)

a) Congenital abnormalities

Most commonly, a foetus severely affected by genetic or developmental abnormalities is lost through spontaneous abortion before 20 weeks. At times, the foetus survives beyond 20 weeks and even after birth.

b) Maternal disease

Mothers whose diabetes is not carefully monitored and controlled, those with kidney or heart disease, and those suffering from chronic or pregnancy-induced hypertension (high blood pressure), are more at risk of a foetus dying than the general population. Most commonly, careful observation and treatment during antenatal care can significantly or almost entirely reduce these risks.

Pregnancy-induced hypertension can develop and lead to toxaemia. If the blood pressure of a woman is raised significantly and continually, and drugs and bed rest are not alleviating the problem, the doctor may deliver the baby. This decision is based on the realization that a premature delivery may pose fewer dangers to the baby than if it remained in the hostile environment of the uterus.

c) Placental problems

(i) If the placenta or umbilical cord fails to function effectively (placental dysfunction) even for a short period of time, the supply of oxygen to the baby is disrupted and death can result. This deprivation of oxygen is known as anoxia.

(ii) The fertilized ovum generally implants in the upper portions of the uterus, where the placenta develops. In rare cases, the placenta is found low in the uterus, and this condition is known as placenta praevia. During the final trimester, such a situation may cause vaginal bleeding. Special care is taken during labour; a caesarean section is performed in severe cases. If the condition is undiagnosed — which is rare when antenatal care is sought — the baby can die when the placenta is delivered first and the oxygen supply disrupted.

(iii) In rare instances, the placenta can prematurely separate from the wall of the uterus (abruptio placentae). The baby then dies of oxygen deprivation.

(iv) The placenta reaches maturity at about 32 to 34 weeks' gestation. After this time it gradually becomes less efficient.[2] This is a normal process, but in some cases the pregnancy proceeds past 43 weeks and the placenta declines quickly, or the placenta may degenerate more quickly than is normal. At this time the baby can be deprived of nutrients and oxygen, and death may result.

(v) The placenta may degenerate too quickly or may not have developed sufficiently to supply the baby's needs throughout the pregnancy. This placental insufficiency may produce slow growth in the baby, and he/she becomes known as a 'small for dates' or a 'small for gestational age' (SGA) baby. Generally, the baby fails to grow as expected. Suspicion of placental insufficiency can be confirmed through ultra-sound examination, urine tests, and the checking of the baby's heart rate responses after a Braxton Hicks contraction or baby's movement. This may lead to early delivery of the child before the situation becomes so serious that death can result.

(vi) Areas of the placenta may, through blockage or infection, be deprived of an adequate blood supply. If large areas are affected, then nutrient and oxygen supply is diminished. Generally, post-natal examination of the placenta will show a discolouration in such areas, which are known as placental infarcts.

(vii) A clot or thrombosis can develop in a major blood vessel of the placenta, and once again oxygen deprivation can kill a baby.

d) Infection

(i) Severe acute maternal infection or disease can lead to problems for the unborn child. Few infections can actually cross the placenta, and those that can, such as syphilis and rubella, are now uncommon.

(ii) In some cases, the amniotic fluid or the baby can become infected. Generally, this occurs after the membranes have ruptured prematurely at a time when the baby would have little chance of survival. During attempts to delay labour by the use of drugs and rest, antibiotics are also commonly administered to try to ward off infection. This is generally, but not always, successful.

e) Severe injury to the mother

The uterus is a very safe environment for the baby, resisting all but the most serious injury to the mother. Injury that may cause a loss is of the type involved in a severe car accident. If a mother's life is in peril, the child is also at risk.

f) Rh incompatibility

When a mother with Rh negative blood bears a child with Rh positive blood, the mother's blood does not contain a substance (antigen) that is found in the baby's blood. Therefore, the mother's immune system may produce antibodies that attempt to destroy this foreign substance, resulting in severe anaemia in the baby. Death can occur. Any risk of such problems is detected early. A first pregnancy is not usually affected. But some of this first baby's blood may escape into the mother's system during delivery, stimulating antibody production. Subsequent babies are then threatened with death from anaemia and heart failure (*erythoblastosis foetalis*). An injection of Anti-D immunoglobulin given to the mother soon after delivery 'destroys' all Rh positive cells, so that the woman's immune system does not become 'alert' or sensitized to them, and hence begins to produce antibodies. Death due to Rh incompatibility is quite rare, particularly where antenatal care is sought during pregnancy. There are other types of blood incompatibility routinely screened for in antenatal care, but these are usually not as serious as Rhesus incompatibility problems.

g) Umbilical cord knots

In *very rare* cases, the baby's movements can cause a knot to develop in the umbilical cord, which can lead to oxygen deprivation.

h) Complications of identical-twin pregnancies

Fraternal twins are formed from two separate ova and fertilized by two separate sperm, and they develop separate placentae from which to obtain nourishment. However, identical twins are derived from the same ovum and share the same placenta. A problem arises if one twin becomes dominant and takes an unequal share of the oxygen and nutrients. Generally, this will simply be noted in a heavier birth weight of one twin. In very rare instances, one twin can become so deprived that death can result. In some cases, unless the other twin can be delivered and is at a viable stage, toxins from the dead twin can affect the placenta and the second twin may also be lost.

i) Other causes

There are other very rare causes of death, such as uterine rupture.

j) Unknown causes

Unfortunately, in a large number of cases of death before delivery the exact cause of death cannot be diagnosed, leaving parents and doctors tormented by the unanswered questions.

Death during delivery

Death during delivery of a baby can be related to some of the causes of death before delivery, or may be related to the delivery itself. It is important to remember that these events are rare. The progress of labour is carefully monitored in the hospital by medical staff, and any foetal distress is likely to be picked up early and intervention made before the situation becomes serious.

a) Congenital abnormalities

If a baby is suffering from a severe congenital problem, the baby may already be in a weakened state. He/she may simply be unable to withstand the strain of the birth process and may die during delivery.

b) Complications with the umbilical cord

(i) As we have already noted, in *very rare* instances the cord can become knotted but cause no problems until delivery, when the knot may be pulled tight, cutting off the oxygen supply.

(ii) In *very rare* instances also, the cord may become momentarily compressed between the baby and the birth passage, causing anoxia.

(iii) In some cases the cord may be found to have fallen down below the baby into the birth canal (prolapsed cord). Unless the cervix is fully dilated and delivery easy, compression of the cord or disruption to the placenta can be caused as the baby pushes on the cord, and death can occur.

(iv) The cord may be looped around the baby's neck and may tighten during labour, leading to strangulation of the baby.

c) Placental separation

During delivery the placenta can become prematurely separated before it is no longer required by the baby for oxygen.

d) Birth injuries or 'trauma'

In some cases, the labour itself can become complicated during the second stage. The baby's head may be delayed in the birth passage, or the baby or mother may be showing signs of distress. A forceps delivery may be attempted and is generally successful. In very rare instances, the forceps delivery can fail or the baby can be sufficiently injured to cause death. An excessively long labour can be highly stressful for mother and child. Death of a baby in a long labour was a common cause of stillbirth in the past. Today such prolonged labours are avoided, and a caesarean section may be performed.

e) Unknown causes

In other cases when no indication of any problem has been noted, it is a shock to both parents and doctor when suddenly a baby shows signs of distress or is born dead.

Death shortly after delivery

a) Prematurity

Complications due to prematurity are the most common cause of death of a baby in the first month of life. Chapter 5 deals with the dangers to such babies. In some cases, a very premature baby will be delivered and die before it reaches the facilities of a Neonatal Intensive-Care Nursery. Careful monitoring and recognition of premature labour are vital in preventing such an event.

b) Congenital abnormalities

Some congenital abnormalities make it impossible for a child to survive, and he/she dies shortly after birth or within a few days. Anencephaly and Trisome 18 are two such fatal abnormalities. Malformations or failure of development of the major organs of the heart, liver, or kidneys can lead to death of an infant. Two such conditions of the heart are hypoplastic left heart syndrome and transposition of the major heart vessels.

c) Respiratory Distress Syndrome (RDS)

As we have discussed in Chapter 5, this respiratory problem occurs most often in premature infants but can be found in term babies. In rare severe cases, it can lead to death of a term baby.

d) Haemorrhage

Any severe haemorrhage of the body puts the infant affected in danger of death. Once again, the pre-term infant is the most common victim.

e) Infection

At times, the infant can be affected by an infection before, during, or after delivery. This most commonly occurs where there has been a prolonged period between rupture of the membranes and delivery. Infections such as pneumonia and septicaemia may occur, threatening the life of the newborn. Other infections may be ascending, that is, the bacteria may be present in the vagina of some women and able to reach the baby after rupture of the membrane or during a vaginal delivery. Such is the case of the Group Bβ Streptococcus. In severe cases, death may result after delivery. The immune system of the newborn, particularly the one born prematurely, may be unable to fight off such infections. Mothers in some centres are checked by having a swab from their vagina sent to the laboratory at a late stage in the pregnancy. If this shows Group Bβ haemolytic Strep, then the mother is given penicillin to prevent an infection in the baby.

Death weeks after delivery

a) Sudden Infant Death Syndrome (SIDS) or cot death
Cot death is the most common cause of death of infants between the ages of one and 12 months. This unexplainable death of an apparently healthy thriving baby is made more painful to the parents by the inability of medical science to specify an actual cause of death. There are many theories, but none has been proved conclusively. Medical science can offer no definitive answer, and generally no evidence of any problem is found in the baby. The only factor that is conclusive is that the deaths are definitely not due to neglect.

b) Congenital abnormalities
Death may be due to congenital deformities of the central nervous system or other major organs. For example, during the early 1980s Australians heard a great deal of the disease biliary atresia. This blockage of the bile ducts of the liver leads, in severe cases, to death or a need for liver-transplant surgery. Other organs can also have major development problems which threaten a child's life.

We have discussed a number of possible causes of perinatal death, but it is important to put the incidence of such causes into some perspective. If we remember that perinatal deaths occur in less than two births in 100 or 20 births in 1,000, then this indicates that even the most common cause of perinatal death — that of prematurity at 25 per cent — will claim only about five babies in every 1,000 born.

We have not outlined these causes so that parents are left to fear that something else will go wrong next time. This is simply information parents often seek. Each stage of loss — before, during, and after birth — will involve the common aspects of grief. But each also carries with it unique feelings, experiences, and fears that must also be considered. Many couples who reach the stage of reading a book such as this are searching for information of a comprehensive and straightforward nature. They can't be made more fearful than they probably already are!

The autopsy or post-mortem examination

From what we have just outlined, we note that the possible causes of perinatal death are many and varied. In some instances, what *appears* as the cause of death may simply be a contributing factor. For example, a child born with the cord around his/her throat may be assumed to have strangled, yet may actually have died from a congenital heart defect. In an attempt to ascertain the actual cause of death, the obstetrician or paediatrician may suggest that an autopsy be performed.

An autopsy is an examination of the internal organs of the body. Many parents are initially horrified at the thought of someone 'cutting up' their baby. To be confronted with such a request immediately after the child's death is inappropriate. The couple need time to regain some stability. It is realized that hospitals are busy places, but an autopsy request made too quickly can make the couple feel that the hospital staff want their baby, already forgotten, removed quickly for convenience and discarded as a failure. Autopsy requests should be left, where possible, until at least some hours after the death. The couple should be approached together and privately by someone of seniority who is aware of the feelings the couple may be experiencing. They must then be given time alone to discuss their fears and feelings before an answer is given.

The thought of someone performing an autopsy on your baby is a sickening one. Even now, months after Kate's death, it is a painful thought for us, but we don't regret the decision.

Firstly, the autopsy is performed with all the dignity and respect of any operation. The baby's body is not mutilated. The autopsy is carried out in such a way that the process is not readily detectable later. The baby's beautiful face, a couple's strongest memory, is generally untouched.

Secondly, the pathologists who perform such examinations are people dedicated to the preservation of life, not some faceless ghouls as we sometimes imagine. For them, the autopsy of a baby is usually a painful experience. No one so dedicated to life can remain unaffected by the loss of such a precious little one. We were extremely fortunate that Kate's autopsy was carried out by the pathologist married to our very special general practitioner. It was comforting for us to realize that it was performed lovingly. Perhaps if couples were able to meet these pathologists, their fears would be more easily dispelled.

Thirdly, the autopsy can provide some important information, including:

a) the actual cause of the baby's death
b) reassurance of the health and normality of the child
c) the full identification of any genetic or developmental abnormalities.

Such information can help dispel the fears of the parents as to whether or not their baby was 'really healthy', and perhaps provide them with a cause of death. They may then be less likely to blame themselves for the loss.

> When she was born they said 'No, no hope'. She'd strangled on the cord. We refused an autopsy, more so from shock than anything, and more from the fear of our baby being cut up. It may have been better if we had had the autopsy, because we look back now and wonder if perhaps there was something else wrong.

Emotional reactions to the death of a baby

For the couple whose baby dies, the pain is intense. Grieving is a long process that can linger for two years or more. Years later, anniversaries of the birth and death will still be able to strike at those scars they bear, although their memories will also evoke feelings of love for that lost child.

The days surrounding such losses involve different difficulties, depending on how the loss occurred. Yet each loss still bears many painful aspects in common with other similar sad events.

Death before delivery

When the couple's child dies before delivery, the couple may find their feelings ranging from the depths of depression to hope that the doctors may be wrong. The first indication of a problem may be that the baby fails to move for a period of days.

At 38 weeks Margaret woke to find no movements:

On the Saturday there wasn't much movement at all. I woke up in the early hours of the Sunday morning, and I tried to get some movement, but there was just nothing. I didn't worry Jimmy at that stage. I just lay there. They were the worst few hours, at that stage of my life. About 5 am Jimmy woke and, seeing me, realized something was wrong.

It is not unusual for a baby to stop moving for quite long periods of time, particularly close to term. The baby will begin moving again, but the tension of those times of stillness can be marked. The couple who fear for their child may try to coax it to move or listen for a heartbeat. The mother's pulse may be mistaken for the baby's heartbeat. At times, the baby can be in such a position that the heartbeat cannot be detected even by a doctor. It is to this hope that many couples cling.

When a couple fear that there is something wrong with their baby, it is very difficult for them, particularly the woman, to sit in an obstetrician's waiting room with other obviously happy pregnant women. Many women instinctively know that their child has died, and don't appreciate an overly cheerful and encouraging approach from their doctor before an examination. They need their fears taken seriously, and want to be examined immediately, for only the sound of that foetal heart will resolve the agony.

The tension that has mounted can leave the woman feeling literally sick to her stomach or shaking with fear. These are the reactions of the body to the stress the woman is experiencing, and are not caused by the baby. The longer the examination with the stethoscope, cone, or pendoppler is, the greater the fears become. The final devastation comes when the doctor must admit that he/she cannot detect a heartbeat and must fear the worst, while indicating that this is not a conclusive test. Most doctors will order an ultrasound examination to confirm their diagnosis. That statement sounds simple. Yet for the couple the simple act of having that examination is a shocking ordeal.

They put me on a portable scan, and after having had a scan a week before and seeing the life, Dr D just shook his head. There was no life whatsoever. From there it was just devastating. Jimmy and I knew there was no hope. That was when I didn't want to accept it, even though before that I had. I was probably clinging to

some hope. Then it was there in black and white. I just wouldn't
accept it. I couldn't cope.

Unless the obstetrician has his/her own ultrasound scan, the
couple may have to spend some hours hanging from a precipice,
trying to accept that their baby has died while hanging on to hope
that all is well.

The shock the couple experience may be nature's way of
preventing them from moving over the thin line to insanity. After
the examination, the first obstacle may be leaving the doctor's
office through the waiting-room of pregnant women. Sometimes
the woman must face this without the support of her partner.
Numb and often crying, she must try to negotiate the usually
simple action of walking along a footpath or to a car park. People
take on a new unbelievable dimension. To many couples,
particularly the mother, it is almost as if they are not part of the
world, as if they are under a sentence of invisibility. The world
seems to be revolving without them! They may desperately search
for some understanding in the faces of those they pass. Their
bodies move mechanically, and the familiar route to their home
becomes a blur. The father, if present, may try to suppress his own
pain as he tries to guide his partner through this strange world.

> After the doctor told me, time and the world seemed to stop. I
> don't know how I got to my car. I just remember looking at all the
> faces of the people. They seemed so unconcerned. I felt so alone, so
> very much alone. I hated having such a secret from the world,
> which didn't care.

To enter their own home, which only a short time ago was so
full of happiness and expectation, is a trial. If a nursery has already
been set up, it is even more difficult. Some couples face the pain of
going into the nursery immediately, while others avoid that whole
area of the house.

If the woman has received the news alone, she must face the
difficulties of trying to locate and inform her partner, made worse
at times by switchboards and the finding of her partner at his
place of work. Then, how do you tell your loved one that your
baby has died?

Once the death of the baby has been confirmed, grieving may
begin, if it hasn't already. Some couples, though, are unable to

accept their loss until after the child is born dead. They always hope the doctors may be wrong.

As if the death of a baby is not enough, there is another more harrowing time to face, the delivery. Due to the possible risks involved in a caesarean section or induction of labour, many doctors will send the woman home and hope that labour will begin naturally within a couple of weeks. If labour fails to begin within a reasonable period, then induction occurs.

This waiting time can be unbearable for the grieving couple. Many couples, knowing their child is dead, want the baby 'taken' so the whole agonizing episode will be over. The thought of carrying a dead baby around is terrifying and, for some, repugnant. They may have visions of the baby decomposing quickly within the uterus and becoming some kind of monster, although this is not the case. Others may feel differently.

> The doctor said: 'What can I say? We'll start working on you on Monday, but what I'd like you to do is let me bring this baby on naturally. Will you give me that choice?' I said: 'It's up to you. I just want to have it, finish with it! I don't care.'

The time alone with their thoughts can be demoralizing, but incidents outside the home may be even more difficult to bear. Well-meaning friends and strangers, attracted by the common feelings of protectiveness aroused by the sight of a pregnant woman, ask when the baby is due. 'Do you want a girl or a boy?' they ask. At times, the woman feels like screaming: 'Just don't ask! My baby is dead! Don't you understand? Dead!'

Even if they do tell family or friends that their child has died, they may be greeted by reactions indicating that those whose support they need now are unable to cope with such a situation.

> My parents tried to be understanding, but you could feel they were uncomfortable around me. The atmosphere was stilted. We went home feeling more alone than ever.

Both partners may find it difficult to relate to each other and any other children when there is 'death' in their home. In our society, where we associate death with mortuaries, cemeteries, and hospitals, death in our homes or, even more, in our bodies, seems unnatural and frightening. The woman may even feel a sense of contamination and fear she will die also.

During this difficult time, grieving may begin to work its healing power as the couple begin to distance themselves from this child. They begin to put their feelings for the child into a different perspective. They may begin by packing up the nursery, a difficult task. They may suspend any discussion about the subject, even with each other. Some even begin at this early stage to think about how long it will be before they can try again for another baby. This is a normal reaction, but one often complicated by guilt. The couple may feel that they are deserting their baby and feel themselves to be terrible parents.

Sheryl's baby died at 32 weeks, but she was unable to be delivered until almost full term due to complications:

> The hardest thing to cope with was carrying a baby around inside you that you knew had died, when all I wanted was to get it out. It was starting to get to me mentally, and then I would feel awful and say to myself: 'You awful mother. You shouldn't be thinking like that. It is your child.'

Often they are not reassured that this process is nature's way of helping them cope with their loss and that they *are* loving parents. This is part of what is known as anticipatory grief.

For most couples, it is a relief when labour finally begins. For some, though, it is painful. They feel that soon they will finally lose their beloved child. While the baby is still inside the womb, although dead, it remains close to them. With the beginning of labour, they feel that soon their defenceless child will be taken from those who love him/her to where they cannot follow.

> Personally I wasn't in a hurry to get rid of it. I still wanted to keep holding on to that baby. So the next three weeks weren't difficult having the baby with me.

Labour can often be more difficult under these circumstances.

> By 5 pm things really started going, with sudden onset of contractions. Looking back now, I realize they were probably made worse by the way I was feeling. The slightest pain I just couldn't cope with, but I held out till just after 5 pm. After that it really got beyond me. I just couldn't cope.

Sometimes a couple, who seem outwardly to have accepted the loss of their child, show their confusion by refusing initially to have pain-killers in case they harm the baby. The baby is unable to 'help' in the delivery, and hence progress of labour may be slower. Many women feel unable to push at the appropriate time for the fear of giving birth, not to life, but to death. This prospect can be so frightening that contractions may even cease altogether. It seems so unnatural to associate birth and death. Other women who don't want finally to lose their child may also find difficulties in this final expulsion.

Some women try to cover their feelings during delivery with a false cheerfulness. In doing so, they hope to relieve the discomfort of their partner and staff.

> During labour I was trying to be very, very good. I was making jokes with the nurses, trying to give them a lift. This was for them. I sent my husband away because it was a bad time and he seemed distressed. If it was a very distressing time he may not want to repeat the experience. He may not want to ever try to have another baby. Looking back, I wish I'd had him with me.

When it is known beforehand that a baby is dead, the couple have often decided for themselves whether or not they wish to see their baby. It is a personal decision, although it is believed that for most couples contact with their child will help them in grieving his/her loss. Some couples fear that their baby, who has been dead for a time or is known to have died through some abnormality, will look grotesque. The imagined appearance is generally much worse than the actual reality. In their pain, and because they wish to have the whole ordeal over, they may refuse to see the child. Later they may wish to change their minds, but think that they have lost their chance:

> Jimmy made me sort of promise that I would not want to see the baby. I gave in to his wish. I never saw that little fellow, but now I won't say I've got regrets but I often wonder. Now I've got this beautiful picture of that child because Jimmy's wish was that he would see the baby regardless of what we would discover at the moment of birth. He would then tell me what our child was like. He would rather have me see his picture of the bub, rather than me see something I may not be too happy about.

If parents refuse to see their child initially, they may be offered this opportunity again later in the day or on the following day. The child's body is kept in the hospital mortuary until burial, and parents can see their baby as many times as they wish, even days after the delivery. In hospitals that are attuned to the needs of such couples, photographs are taken of the child that can be given to the couple immediately. If rejected by the parents, the photographs are filed in case the couple wish to have them at a later date. The choice as to whether or not to see their child must remain that of the parents. They should be encouraged, but never forced.

> The death counsellor said to me 'Did I hold the baby?' When I said no, she asked why not. I said I'd never had anything to do with death before, and I was frightened. I very much regret that now. I still have a fear of touching anything dead. She said she would arrange for me to go to the mortuary to see the baby with my husband and two children. That terrified me . . .

If the parents decide to see their child, they should be prepared by staff for the sight of any unusual colouring or deformity. The couple should be given as much time as they wish to hold their baby and cry for it. This time will provide them with concrete memories of their child. If the couple feels it important, siblings and close family members should be allowed to see the child, although this must be discussed carefully. Children, particularly, must be prepared well before the event. For many couples, grieving has been suspended until the delivery. Now the process can begin in earnest, and the distancing that allowed them to survive those difficult days before delivery protects them no longer.

Death during delivery

When a baby dies during delivery, the couple do not have the opportunity to anticipate the loss and so distance themselves from the child. The time leading to the delivery is filled with expectation. The actual birth may become simply a formality that has to be endured before all their plans come into being. The couple talk in terms of 'When the baby is home, we'll . . '

It may not be until the process of labour begins that unanticipated problems arise. At times, staff do not tell the woman of the problems, or de-emphasize them, for fear her anxiety may only serve to aggravate the situation. Most often, the couple sense the concern and become fearful.

Once the foetal heartbeat cannot be found or there is no sign of life at delivery, the suddenness of the event means that shock and numbness may play an important part in helping the parents remain in control. They may show little or no emotion on hearing the news that their child is dead. This is simply shock. Other bereaved parents may initially react more strongly. Some may sob. Others may scream and strike out at staff or loved ones. Others will refuse to believe what they are told. This denial may be stated openly or may appear later, when they may ask to see or feed their baby. This period of shock is not the time to confront the couple with a reality they are as yet unable to face.

Even the male should not be expected to be fully functioning at this time. Often it is accepted that the mother may be unable to cope, and she is dealt with gently. This courtesy may not be similarly offered to the father.

The death is difficult enough for the father, but it unfairly strikes the woman when she is very vulnerable. She may still have to deliver the baby, knowing he/she is dead, a harrowing experience. She may be exhausted after labour, reeling under the effects of pain-killers, and requiring stitches after an episiotomy. If death has occurred just prior to, or during, a caesarean section, she must be confronted with the terrible news as she emerges from the anaesthesia. In this case, she has not been able to see her child and may deny it is dead.

Leith's baby died when she had a massive concealed haemorrhage just before a caesarean section. The death of the baby was not known before the operation:

> It's a really funny thing. I remember nothing of the pain of the caesar, which shows that the sadness was the biggest thing, the most overpowering feeling at the time, all-embracing. It was a shock to everyone. I'd been there in hospital a month with high blood-pressure, and everyone sort of knew me. They were all excited, saying: 'Today's the day'. It certainly was — one I'll never forget.

Death after delivery

As we have seen, the most common cause of death after delivery is extreme prematurity. In such cases, the couple are aware that the possibility of death exists. Similarly, when an obvious congenital abnormality is found, death may be anticipated. For other parents, the joy at the birth of their apparently healthy baby may be suddenly interrupted by the discovery of a problem. The following days are a painful period, during which the couple vacillate with uncertainty between hope and despair. If the child is alive and at risk, the couple may not have the luxury of holding their child.

At delivery, concentration on the baby is so intense that the couple may be overlooked.

> When our daughter was born, she was so tiny. She didn't cry and was quickly taken to the waiting paediatrician. Paul and I had no idea if our baby was alive or dead, or even if it was a boy or a girl. On asking these questions, we received no immediate answers. I was terrified. They finally said it was a girl. I asked three times if she was alive. No answer. I felt desperate when they didn't answer. I knew everyone was preoccupied with her, but I just about went off my head in those few minutes.

If seriously ill, the child may be taken to an Intensive-Care Nursery. If none exists in the area of the couple's residence, the baby may have to be transferred to a distant major hospital. The mother may be unable to follow, and the father is torn between his partner and his child. If the child dies, the couple not only feel this loss but have it complicated by not having been able to hold and look at their baby while he/she was alive. They feel the pain of not even having been able to let their child feel the loving arms of the two people who loved him/her most. They feel the pain that their child died *alone*.

How involved do you become with a baby who is going to die? This is a difficult problem faced by couples who know that their baby has little hope of survival. Some become strongly attached to their child, while others gradually distance themselves from the child and the pain. Each individual will react differently, and this must be respected. There is a strong risk of the parents rejecting the child and then later feeling guilt because of this. Their later grief may then be complicated by these feelings.

Jim and Jannie's daughter Anneliese was born with a congenital abnormality known as Trisome 18:

> Jim went to see if he could find out any more about the baby's condition, and when he returned he was obviously distressed. So many things were affected, both physical disabilities and internal problems. He also told me that the special-care sister was more than willing to bring the baby back to me before I went

downstairs, and encouraged me to accept the offer. It slowly
dawned on me that I was in danger of rejecting her . . . The sister
brought our baby to us, and I touched her. She seemed quite bright
and alert, and gradually I began to relate to her.

The problem is worsened if the parents are confronted by the
decision of whether to allow treatments for certain abnormalities
to proceed or to remove life-support equipment. If the parents
decide that treatment may only prolong their child's agony for a
little time, they may deny its use. They may then later feel guilty
that they didn't do all that was possible to keep their child alive.
Parents are guided by the advice of the baby's paediatrician, and
in some cases, a team of people including medical staff, social
workers, and other persons involved with the care and support of
both parents and child. When a decision does not have to be made
immediately, the couple should be given time to discuss the
options with such a group individually or in a group setting. More
importantly, they need time to talk with each other. The decision
must not be rushed, for it is one with which the couple will need
to feel comfortable for the rest of their lives. To watch their child
die will be devastating enough. Having this complicated by a
nagging fear that their decision was perhaps made without
adequate consideration will only make matters worse.

This is their child. They love this child. This child will die
soon. These facts cause a dilemma we have already mentioned.
Will loving their child without reservation make the time of
parting more difficult? Does the mother risk the pain of
developing that close relationship if she breast-feeds the child as
long as he/she lives? The couple are torn between loving and
wanting to be with their child, and the fear of the pain such
attachment will bring them later. Most couples will generally opt
to risk such attachment in the hope that their love will give their
child strength to face what lies ahead. In most cases they will find
their coping with grief assisted, not hindered, by the attachment.
They will have memories to cling to for many years.

As times goes on and death is inevitable, nature helps parents
by allowing them to distance themselves from their child. This
occurs when they have been able to accept the loss. The same
process occurs for some couples faced with the death of their child
before delivery. Once again, they may feel guilty for such 'loss of

feeling' for their child. They needn't! This same distancing occurs between terminally ill patents and their loved ones.[3] It is nature's way, through the resolution of grief, of helping people cope with the final farewell. Unfortunately, different individuals may reach this stage at different times. One partner may begin to distance himself/herself from their beloved child before the other. This may be seen by his/her partner as not caring about the baby. Resentment may build up as the still deeply involved partner tries to compensate for the other's withdrawal. Couples are at times not assisted in preparing for their loss and are unaware of these natural processes, and hence their reactions are misinterpreted.

It can be very comforting for a couple to be given the opportunity to be with and to hold their child as the end draws near. There has been so little they could do for him/her. They feel so powerless. They are unable to help their child medically, and nursing staff often have more direct contact. But the parents alone can love their child as deeply as they do. At least as parents they can be there for their child at the time he/she needs the greatest love possible. To be able to be the ones who comfort their child in those last hours or minutes sets them apart from the medical staff.

At times, hospitals refrain from contacting parents if their child weakens late at night or early in the morning. Perhaps the child may improve. Yet if the child fails to improve and dies, the parents are deprived of the most important moment in their child's life. On the other hand, some couples will not wish to face this moment of parting. It must be the parents' decision.

> When we were there I could see the gauges dropping back, and it seemed that life was going out of the little chap. I feel the staff were basically keeping him alive for us. We held him after he died. If we'd had the option we'd like to have held him as he died. Yet I didn't, because I felt that was giving up hope. We held him then. We cried.

When a multiple birth is involved and none of the children survives, there is increased grief. If only one child dies, there is a tendency for others to try to console the couple with the knowledge that they have at least one healthy baby. But grief cannot be cheated! Each baby is an individual and as such is entitled to be grieved. The couple may be torn between grief for their lost child and celebration for their live child. Their grief may cause them to resent temporarily the child who has lived and demands their attention. If the baby has feeding problems, the mother may resent the effort required when her other child is dying or has died. Other couples are afraid to become attached to their surviving child for fear he/she will also die. Hence, there is a risk of rejection of the surviving child.

Couples who lose a baby but have other children are expected by many to rally in this thought. But no child can be a substitute for another, and grieving cannot be alleviated by surviving siblings.

> After the stillbirth, people would say to me: 'You're so lucky. You have two others that are so healthy, and some don't have any.' Even though I knew all that, I still felt: 'Yes, I have two others, but she was still my child. I lost her. I still loved her.' This made me angry then.

Parents whose babies are the victims of cot death have experiences similar to those whose child dies during delivery. The loss is completely unexpected, and they have been unable to prepare for it. It is further complicated by the fact that no reason can be given for such a loss of a perfectly healthy baby.

It is final!

We have looked so far at some of the different problems and feelings that may be encountered by couples whose children die at different stages. Once the finality of death has come, couples share many similarities in the days, weeks, months, and even years that follow.

The numbness of shock is often the saving grace in those hours immediately after the baby dies. If the woman is still in hospital, it is difficult for her to return to the ward where the nursery houses the newborns. Women's reactions to other babies can differ. Some find it difficult to face babies and pregnant women, while others simply want to hold a live baby, even if it is not their own. Some fear they are a jinx, and that other babies around them will die.

> At no stage (and I've never had it since, thank goodness) did I find that babies repulsed me. I know a lot of people do feel that. I never had that feeling. I wanted to look at a baby. In fact, some days when I was able to, I found I used to enjoy going past the

nursery and just seeing the other babies. I'd often wonder what Jonathan would have been like. It helped me a lot to be able to accept looking at other children. I would love to have held a little one. I think I can be thankful for that.

Generally, hospitals provide women whose babies have died with the option of a private single room or movement to another part of the hospital. It is assumed that this is what the mother may wish, and in many cases she will. But it must be her decision.

Couples need time to be alone together, to cry, to talk, to comfort each other. It is now they need each other more than ever. The couple feel torn even further when the father is asked to leave. Night is a desolate, lonely time. The wards are dark and quiet, except for crying babies. Even with sedatives, sleep doesn't come easily, and without the support of her partner, the woman can find her grief unbearable. It is often at this time that a woman wants and needs to talk to someone, but cannot. Hospital social workers, chaplains, friends, and relatives are home in bed. The father, probably also unable to sleep, is home. Nursing staff don't 'disturb' the woman, and on finding her awake encourage her to 'try to get some sleep' as it 'will do her good'.

No night seems longer. The woman doesn't have the security of reaching out and finding her beloved partner close. During less serious crises of her life, she has had this security. Even a simple thunderstorm seemed better when she lay beside her partner. Yet at this time of crisis both partners find themselves alone, while the world marches on. Some hospitals today provide a foldaway bed and allow husbands to stay overnight with their wives, or provide staff who are able and willing to talk, if that's what the woman feels she needs.

Her partner may not get this support, and goes home to an empty house. No partner, no child — just he and his grief. He may not yet wish to face family, but may be pleased for the company of a close male friend. It is not only women who need a member of the same sex in difficult times.

> My boss, who is also a friend, had had the same thing happen, and when I phoned him to say what had happened I felt the support link just come through the phone.

> My best mate heard about the death. I had just got home from the hospital and rung my mum. That was upsetting. I was sitting

there all alone when my mate turned up with a pizza and a bottle of beer. He said 'I don't know what to say but I thought we could share these.' It was great. We didn't talk about the death much. In fact we didn't talk much at all, but I needed his company, although before he came I didn't realize it was what I needed.

Perhaps women who have lost babies are the only patients in a hospital happy to have the movements of the hospital begin at 6 am. At least it means the night is over! Some women will wish to be left alone. Staff often find it difficult to cope with such a situation, and are happy to give her privacy. Others, if left, do not feel relieved but abandoned. It is best to ask the woman how she feels about company. She should be given reassurance that it is acceptable for her to summon a nurse if she simply wants to talk or have some human contact.

Most doctors will try to discharge a woman as soon as possible and medically advisable. Most women are relieved to be able to go home. Those who have had a caesarean section or developed postnatal complications must spend more time in hospital. As the days pass, such women may need to talk to someone but may not have the courage to phone a friend. They may feel that they can't use the time of the overworked nursing staff. Here the social worker, hospital chaplain, or members of local support groups may provide important sources of support.

One way that hospitals may help is to assign to such patients a nurse on each shift who has an affinity with, and understanding of, such patients. There is some security for the woman in knowing that during the day there will be someone who knows her situation and is willing to listen.

Unfortunately, communication is at times inadequate in hospitals. It is very difficult for a woman if she is asked by an unknowing staff member why she isn't feeding her baby or if there are any nappies to be collected. Such painful episodes are avoidable and should not occur. Communication may need to be streamlined to achieve this.

Leaving hospital sounds an easy step, but it too can bring pain. For a couple to confront another obviously happy couple leaving with their baby, while their own arms are empty, is devastating. The world around the couple takes on a strange hue. It seems to be going on as usual, but now the couple feel like outsiders, onlookers. They wonder if they'll ever be part of that world again.

> On the way home, everything was so strange. I closed one of my eyes in the lift and half closed the other. I did that till a long way down the road. It sounds silly, but I didn't want to risk seeing other parents with babies. Everything was different. The traffic lights were brighter. The cars were faster and noisier. I felt so alone and strange. The world seemed oblivious to me.

The couple's home, instead of receiving a baby, must be readied for their grieving. Often each step they take in the home is difficult. In the bedroom there are the maternity clothes to be packed away. The kitchen may house the equipment prepared for a baby's feeding. Perhaps the new washer or dryer they bought to cope with a deluge of nappies sits in the laundry. There may still be the washed dishes they used for that happy snack before they left for the hospital. Hardest of all, there is a nursery waiting in readiness for an occupant who will not arrive — at least not this particular occupant. Everything, everywhere, seems to remind them of their baby!

> I was only in hospital for four or five days. The saddest time was the day I came home empty-handed. Not that I'd gone to a lot of trouble with the nursery, but I did have the basics ready. In the meantime, Jimmy and his sister had gone into that room. He threw a blanket over the change table. The baby bath and whatever else was put away into a cupboard. Jimmy did walk me into that back room because I had put up new curtains and such. That was hard to cope with, but it was one of the first things Jimmy did with me. He said: 'Darling, there's something you must do. I want to do it with you, whether it's now or in a couple of hours or what. But I think if you do it as soon as possible it's going to be better.' And he just walked me, arm around me, into that back room. And that was the end of me again!

Even those couples who, perhaps through a previous loss or conscious planning, have not set up a nursery, find reminders in each room — memories of sitting on the couch letting Dad feel the kicks of the baby, or memories of having to negotiate the sliding shower door gingerly because of 'the bump'.

Each couple will have their own special individual memories of their child. The couple may try to put them out of their minds because they cause pain, only to find they can't do this. As we saw in Chapter 2, memories play an important part in grief work. Memories hurt, but they allow one to accept the event's significance. A broken leg may require more pain during its setting and a great deal of concern and concentration initially before healing can begin. Without this early concentration, the leg may not heal correctly or even heal at all. Similarly, with this severe wound of the heart when a baby dies, the body and mind must give the wound full concentration before healing can begin. The mind becomes preoccupied with thoughts and details of the loss. It is difficult to find the motivation to concentrate on anything but the baby. Even the simplest household chores, such as making a meal, getting out of bed, dressing or washing require great effort if they are to be accomplished. The mind and body put all their available energy into protecting the wound of the heart.

Many partners, particularly the women, lose all energy or enthusiasm for any activity, even those they once enjoyed. Insomnia is common, and many lose their appetite. The body may show its distress in many other ways. These symptoms are the body's reactions to stress and may vary considerably. Heart palpitations, dryness of the throat and mouth, constipation, diarrhoea, aching arms, heaviness in the chest, shortness of breath, tiredness, headache, noise intolerance, and muscle tremors are not uncommon. Often the couple may find one or both of them contracting a virus due to their being in a weakened state physically and emotionally.

Even thoughts of suicide may be entertained. For the majority, these are only fleeting thoughts, whose effects serve more to frighten the grieving parents than to cause actual harm.

> Some days I'd be really down. There was one day when I was driving to work. I was driving over this rickety bridge near our home, and I thought about driving off the road and into the river. It was a strange and frightening feeling. I came so close. I've never been able to drive over that bridge since without feeling strange.

A very small number will even attempt suicide. This generally occurs only in situations where the woman has little support or a history of depressive illness.

Bonding with a baby occurs well before the actual birth. And after birth, the woman is in a weakened physical state. Further,

her self-image is affected by her ability to produce children. Therefore, it is not unusual for the reactions of the woman to be more intense and prolonged than those of her partner.

However, this is not to say that the male will not experience intense grief. His grief is combined with a deep concern for the well-being of his partner and his having to keep the routine of the home functioning, while providing an income. Therefore, he may repress his feelings and seem to be coping in the situation. This is also what others expect of him. But grief can't be denied. One day it will have its day. It is not surprising that there often comes a time, just as his partner is beginning to move from her initial deep depression, when the male will become severely depressed or angry. He can no longer resist the grief he has so carefully boxed away while his partner needed him. Unfortunately, many men do not realize that to express his grief will usually help, not harm, his partner.

> I cracked just as Lorraine was starting to pick up. I'd been so busy arranging funerals, looking after Lorraine, and going to work. About three months later, I just went to pieces. I was so tired and depressed. I remember thinking how stupid it was. Lorraine was just beginning to gain some confidence again, and now I was going down the drain. I just couldn't seem to pull myself out of it.

Anger is a common emotion experienced by the bereaved, and can be directed toward many and varied people and situations. One partner may find something wrong in trivial incidents. Relationships between partners can become very strained.

> I put my husband through some very bad times, which I wasn't aware of. I just hit an all-time low. I just couldn't pick up. We went on holidays, and we were really going through a very rough spot. I would say to him: 'Just go! Leave! I don't care. I don't want you anywhere round here. Get lost. Go do your drinking. Go do whatever you want!' I didn't want anything to do with him. I'm lucky I've got a man that stands by me. On holidays it all fell into place. I realized what I was doing to my marriage. From then on, things changed for the better.

There may be feelings of anger toward the doctor, the hospital, and even the baby who has died. Why didn't the doctor realize earlier there was a problem? Why didn't the nursing staff call the doctor earlier? Why didn't the baby put up a better fight? In rare instances, anger toward the doctor or hospital staff is justified. If so, a couple may help dissipate this anger by discussing it with the party concerned in person or in writing. When the couple are in such pain, it is hard to remember that staff are not infallible. But it is best for the couple to discuss their anger, rather than leave it unresolved, which may then prevent them from coming to terms with their baby's death.

In the hope of cheering up the grieving parents, well-intentioned persons may make uninformed statements such as 'There will be other babies'. Being preoccupied with their grief, the parents may lash out in anger, forgetting the intention behind the inappropriate words. Friends and relatives who did call, as well as those who didn't, may all be under attack. Even society is exposed to this anger. Women who voluntarily abort their babies, single mothers, people with little education and large families, spokespersons against IVF programs, and the peoples of Third World overpopulated countries are a few of those who can come under attack. It must be noted that there needs to be some caution about these reactions of such couples. Their reactions must not be assumed by others to be 'sour grapes' on their part. Initially, the anger of grief is involved. But as grief is resolved, their reactions to such social issues may remain the same. At times, a crisis brings new understandings and changes in values, which may be reflected in attitudes to social issues.

Perhaps the most difficult situations in the days, weeks, or months following a baby's death are the encounters with pregnant women and newborn babies. As a woman ventures out into the world to do the shopping or perform other normal duties, it seems as if the whole world is conspiring against her! It seems that every pregnant woman knew she was going to be out at that particular hour on that particular day, and so deliberately decided to go out also! Every second person seems to be pregnant or have a baby or small children. Every magazine seems to be preoccupied with baby-care articles or stories of celebrities and their 'perfect' pregnancies and babies. It is difficult enough for the woman to make herself leave her home. It can become unbearable among pregnant women and babies. She may still have the protruding abdomen of a pregnant woman, which heightens her discomfort. She may still feel so preoccupied with her loss that it may be difficult for her to maintain her composure and concentration, and hence fulfil her task. She can be further exasperated if she meets up with someone offering condolences or another questioning her about her baby, unaware of what has happened. It is often then that her composure is destroyed. If she cries, her discomfort is made worse by the stares of people who offer no assistance, only curiosity.

It was just terrible! Everywhere I turned there were babies, mothers, and pregnant women. I quickly moved down one aisle of the supermarket and escaped into the safety of the next. Sure enough, there was the one woman again. I felt as if she was chasing me! My brain was screaming out! I just wanted to get out of there. Everybody seemed to be looking at me. As hard as I tried, I couldn't keep back the tears. To make matters worse, I got caught at the checkout in a line, and the same pregnant woman came behind me with her trolley. The checkout girl looked at my tear-stained face that I was trying to hide and cheerily gave me the usual line: 'And how are you today?' I felt like screaming: 'How the hell do you think I am? My baby's dead! What do you care?', but instead said nothing. People looked at me while pretending they weren't. I felt so alone. I got out and made for the car, crying all the way. I stood by the boot and sobbed. I didn't notice that there was an elderly couple sitting in the car beside me. When I realized, I tried to choke back the tears and smile at them. Instead of the usual reaction of looking away, the old gentleman got out of the car. He said to me: 'O my dear, you are hurting a lot. Let me help you with your bags.' She took me by the arm, while he opened the boot to put in my groceries. In the meantime, I was sobbing, and she asked me if she could help. I said: 'No thank you'. He opened the door for me, and as I got in he said: 'All the best, my dear. Tomorrow's a new day.' Little did he know how much their kindness meant. I never thanked them. I wish I could thank them now.

Some couples try to overcome such problems by shopping at times such as evenings or Saturday mornings, when working couples and singles, rather than mothers with small babies, are likely to be in the supermarket.

It is also difficult for the couple when there are births among their friends. As much as they may try to be happy for the new parents, and to some extent succeed, part of them is hurt and angry. Part of them may resent or feel envious of the good fortune of their friends, when they themselves have just buried their beloved child.

> It was easy to cope with for a long time because I was the first in a row having their third child. In the back of my mind there was the thought that one of the others would lose their baby and would understand me. But as each baby came along and it didn't happen, it was more difficult. Then one very good friend of mine had her little girl, who was born alive with the cord around her throat like Jemma. I fell to pieces then. I used to watch them stand there and talk, and they had babies in their arms. I became very, very bitter, although I tried not to show it.

In the days following a baby's death, the emotional pain may be complicated by physical discomfort. The pain of episiotomy stitches or a caesarean section are offputting enough when a healthy baby has resulted. The pain seems so senseless and useless when a baby has died! The woman's body seems to play cruel jokes on her by constantly reminding her of the child she has lost. Some doctors will suppress lactation with drugs, while others feel it best not to interfere with nature. The breasts fill with milk and ache, reminding the woman of a beloved baby that will never suckle at them. They leak. The lochia (after-birth discharge from the uterus) is still quite heavy. After-birth pains are other cruel reminders. It is often forgotten that the hormonal changes and post-partum depression that are experienced by many new mothers, also affect women whose babies have died. The whole sad event seems never-ending! Some mothers even experience phantom kicks, as if their child has not been born yet. Her mind and body don't seem to want to forget, even if the woman does!

When a couple's baby dies, they must also cope with physical discomfort, a funeral, daily routine, and difficult incidents. After the funeral, the couple may think the worst is over. Yet, as they try to regain some sort of order in their lives, small incidents can continually send them reeling backwards into the pain of those early days.

> About two weeks after she died, we got a letter from the Office of the Registrar General. Attached to it was a form for the Registration of a Birth. The letter was quite curt, indicating that

we must register our daughter's birth within 60 days. It was difficult contacting this little clerk in the Public Service and trying to explain to him that we also required a Registration of Death form. We both cried as we filled those forms out.

A package of baby goods or a receipt for a payment on baby furniture may arrive. The arrival of photographs, taken during those happy days of pregnancy and sent away to be developed, may be the cause of another painful setback. The list of incidents that cause a couple to experience that intense pain of the first days seems endless!

Difficult as these incidents are, many couples feel a certain confidence in knowing that they have faced them and survived. They believe that things will have to get better as time goes on.

> A friend said something to me that really helped me on Rebecca's birthday. She said: 'This is the last of the worst days. After today there will never be any day or anything that you haven't already experienced. You've experienced your first Mother's Day, your first Father's Day, your first Christmas, Easter, and first birthday. After that, nothing can hurt you quite so much.' That was quite a relief to think: 'Well, I've got this far and nothing's going to hurt quite so much again'.

After a time, many couples realize that they have not just lost a baby, but a son or a daughter. Many people have different special feelings concerning having a son or daughter. They may search their memories or a photograph for any indication of what their son or daughter may have looked like. They may sit and gaze at the photograph for a long period of time. This is generally a comforting activity they may repeat many times, although it is an activity that others may see as morbid and almost repulsive.

As we discussed in Chapter 2, individuals may differ in their ways of grieving. Reactions may range through moderate depression to severe psychological distress. Anger, denial, and physical reactions are all common. As time passes, the individual may enter into a depression that may last for differing amounts of time. In defining depression we will steer away from medical terms for the present. We will simply say that depression is a time when you forget how to laugh. You smile mechanically, but your heart can't laugh. Just as with a broken leg, a wounded grieving heart needs a long period of convalescence during which activity is minimized. Convalescence for a grieving heart is often this period of depression. The days following the death of a baby are often punctuated by sympathetic expressions from many of those around. But soon people stop phoning and stop calling in. Life, for others at least, returns to normal. This can be a time of incredible loneliness for a bereaved couple. Unless they themselves have been bereaved, most people cannot fathom the length of time and the depth of emotion involved in the loss of a loved one. Many assume the incident is forgotten and resolved within a couple of months. If outward signs of grieving continue beyond that time, people can display an embarrassment or uneasiness around the bereaved parent. Some may even curtail their contact with the couple, further increasing their isolation. The bereaved couple may begin to try to hide their emotions in public, to be 'brave', so as not to make others uneasy. Fortunate couples will find family or friends who convey the message that it's acceptable to feel lousy and to cry, for however long it takes. But even their tolerance can become strained if a bereaved person doesn't seem to be 'getting over it' after a certain period of time.

> Another girl, only about six weeks after the baby's death, asked me if I was going to go to the school sports. I said I didn't know, and she said to me: 'You want to remember that you have got other children'. I personally think now that that doesn't let me feel sad. Six weeks later, I think really you're entitled still to be a bit funny.

Many people don't seem to realize that depressed people normally *want* to 'get over it'. They don't enjoy being depressed! They try to talk themselves out of being depressed, force themselves to be happy. But usually this is to no avail. It is possible for a person to want not to come through his/her depression, because it may serve a need for attention or protection. If this is the case, professional help may be required. But generally the bereaved want to feel alive again. If their depression is not understood and accepted by others, it may be suppressed and reappear in other ways, such as in a psychosomatic illness. If the bereaved are accepted and supported, the periods of depression may gradually become shorter in duration and be interspersed with longer periods of well-being. The depressed person may not seem to have the emotional energy to cope with relationships with his/her partner, children, or relatives.

Some couples who have other children pour a lot of time and attention into them. Yet there is still a void that cannot be filled. Siblings cannot replace the lost child. Others feel alienated from their surviving children. Often this is due to fears that they may now lose their spouse or other children. They may be overprotective toward their children, and become tense and nervous when loved ones don't arrive home when expected. These are not easy feelings to overcome, and may persist long after the thick veil of depression has lifted. Often such feelings are never completely dispelled. They simply lose some of their intensity. This is often a person's first encounter with death, and once encountered, death is a reality that can never again be forgotten or denied.

Women may also have an intense fear of their own death. Fear of uterine or bowel cancer or heart disease are made more real by the physical symptoms of grief that may exist. If such fears are reported to a doctor, a person may be dismissed as a hypochondriac, which only adds to feelings of worthlessness. General practitioners often do not have the time to discover that there is intense grief at the root of these symptoms. Many women also fear infertility. They fear that this was their last chance, that they will never fall pregnant again. This may be particularly pronounced in women who have no other children. Fortunately, for the majority, this fear is soon dispelled by a new pregnancy.

Hopelessness and worthlessness are two common feelings of depression. Women, particularly, feel a failure! They feel that they have let down their baby, their husband, their children . . . *everyone*! They see themselves as a failure as a wife, a mother, a woman, a human being! The loss of a child due to any cause can highlight just how much a woman's self-image is tied up with her ability to bear a healthy child. The sexual revolution may have changed the role of women in society to a degree, but the feminine identity of even the most liberated woman is often shattered when a baby dies. Sometimes she may withdraw from her partner for fear of rejection. How could he love such a feeble excuse for a woman? Her partner may interpret this withdrawal as a rejection of himself, and the stage is thus set for misunderstanding and pain.

A bereaved person may try to ignore his/her grief and depression by becoming 'hyperactive'. Following such advice as 'Keep busy so that you don't think about it' or 'Go and do for someone who's worse off than you' may help temporarily. Being extremely busy can help one to *pretend* that he/she has forgotten. In fact, once a couple have worked through their grief, their enthusiasm and energy will return. But to be busy so that one doesn't experience his/her grief is doomed to failure. Other people may applaud the bereaved person, convinced that he/she is coping well. But grief will simply express itself in other ways, such as illness or sleep disturbances. It may simply wait until one can resist it no longer. Some couples who conceive another child almost immediately after the death repress their grief, only to find it reappearing with its full force after the birth of their next child.

Grief is not a logical or predictable process. It doesn't follow a set pattern. Depression can be interspersed with periods of anger, denial, and fantasizing. In time, the couple may be beginning to have some small periods of their day when they can think about things other than their baby. Then an incident may send them reeling into a deep anger or depression. They begin to feel that they'll never be happy again. Generally they need not fear this! As time and healing progress, they will still at times be sent reeling back, but usually not as far back as the last time.

> I had been doing so well. I had been planning to return to work and exercise classes. I really began to see a tiny speck of light at the end of the tunnel. I had become involved in a church caring group. My husband and I had had a particularly pleasant breakfast that Sunday morning, and we planned a picnic lunch after church. I walked into the church, only to be confronted by a baptism. The young mother, obviously proud, was not looking at the minister, but smiling for photos and at the people during the ceremony. It was too much for me. My baby had been baptized by a nurse as she was born. Baptized and buried in a week! The woman didn't seem to understand the importance of this ceremony. I had never seen my daughter's baptism. There was no picnic that day, but many tears instead. Over and over I kept asking: 'When will this nightmare ever end?'

Grief makes us vulnerable, and it may allow other losses, conflicts, and insecurities of a person's life, which have never been fully resolved, to resurface. This is particularly a problem for couples whose relationship was faltering before this pregnancy, or for single women who have been forced to face the pregnancy and loss largely alone. The grief is likely to be more intense where there has been another crisis during the pregnancy, such as marital conflict or separation, death of a close friend or relative, loss of employment, financial concerns, or natural disaster. If a broken heart, like a broken leg, has not had a chance to mend completely, a new break will be more intensely painful. If prior crises are combined with a lack of support, the new crisis and the chronic effects of stress may lead to prolonged depression or ill health. Unfortunately, there are rarely coordinated attempts to identify women or couples whose grief is liable to be complicated by other conflicts. Hence, preventive counselling is usually not suggested. It is often assumed that couples will be able to support one another or find support from family or friends. But this is a dangerous assumption to make.

As time passes, the periods of well-being increase in number and duration, and the set-backs are less devastating. The couple begin to see that although there will be times when they shall feel the pangs of pain again, there is life after grief. It may be a different life, for a changed person, but a life richer for the months of their child's presence. Sometimes the realization is gradual and sometimes sudden.

> One day I found myself watching our new kitten playing on the grass with the ball. He kept trying to bite it as it moved about on the grass. I suddenly realized I was laughing at him, really laughing. It was the greatest feeling in the world!

People will often try to tell a bereaved person that time heals. The statement may be true for most people, but it is inappropriate when there is intense emotional pain. The realization that the day has come when the bereaved parent is able to laugh, really laugh again, is a feeling that cannot be compared to any other.

The funeral

It is difficult enough just to keep on living and functioning in the days following a baby's death, without having to make decisions. The autopsy is one difficult decision, and another soon follows, that of the funeral arrangements.

In most States of Australia, it is expected that a burial or cremation will be conducted for babies of 20 weeks' gestation or beyond or of weight 400 grams or more.[4] It is often difficult in the days immediately following the loss for the couple to accept this loss. A funeral is such a final event, an outward confirmation that their beloved child really is dead. The outcome is irreversible. Many couples are not ready in those first hours or days to accept this. Others are in a hurry to get it 'over and done with', hoping that when the baby's body goes the pain will go with it. Still others feel, rightly or wrongly, 'pressured' by hospitals and relatives to have the funeral, to tidy up the whole sorry, sad event.

There is absolutely no need for the funeral to be arranged hurriedly. The baby's body will remain in the hospital mortuary until the day the family are ready to carry out their final goodbyes. By convention, it is often assumed that the funeral will be carried out within two or three days of the baby's death.

In cases where the mother has undergone a caesarean section, she will be unable to leave hospital in such a time, and hence will not be able to attend. In other cases, she may be encouraged by relatives and friends not to attend because it would be 'too hard' for her. She may decide herself that she does not wish to attend. Yes, a baby's funeral is a very difficult time for a couple, but yet it can be one of the most important and healing experiences in the couple's grief. How can this be?

Firstly, the funeral helps the couple accept that their baby has indeed died. This sounds strange, but it must be remembered that couples suffering acute and intense grief may deny their loss to protect themselves from the pain. Their baby's death and the days following can be so confused and blurred that they take on a sense of unreality. Sometimes there is the feeling that it is just a bad dream, from which they will wake. Shock sends their world spinning, and the realization of what has really happened may not descend on the couple immediately.

Secondly, the funeral provides the couple comfort in knowing what has happened to their child's body. They are able to make at least some decisions in love for their baby.

Thirdly, a funeral allows relatives and friends openly to show their pain, concern, and love for the couple. Often a couple who have lost their child do not feel justified in grieving for a child they knew for so little time. They sometimes simply want a funeral involving only themselves. If this is their wish, it must be respected. Such an act, though, is difficult for their loved ones.

> When Jemma died, we put up this thing: 'Nobody's going to care about her because it's nothing to anybody else. It's only to us.' So we wouldn't allow people that wanted to come to her cremation to come. They would have come, but it was we who put them off. When my neighbour lost her baby, I saw her carry on with her family as if they were all grieving that he was a real baby. I regret not having that now. It was selfish of us. Perhaps that's why they don't recognize her now.

When a couple lose a child, their family and friends often feel helpless and inadequate. They don't know what to say or do to show their concern. Attendance at the funeral allows them to say by their presence: 'We love you. We hurt for you. Your baby through you is part of us. We share your loss.'

Fourthly, a funeral gives public acknowledgment that their baby did exist, that he/she was a real person. Society then gives the couple the right to grieve that is often denied those suffering through infertility or miscarriage.

Fifthly, a funeral allows the couple and their other children to grieve as a family. Often children are not permitted to attend a funeral. They may be sent away to stay with relatives, and denied their grief. But they too need to accept that their little brother or sister is dead. Where it is believed that a child will benefit, he/she should be allowed to attend. We will discuss children and death in more detail later in Chapter 10.

Sixthly, for couples who have religious convictions, the funeral holds deep significance. For them it is a recognition that now their child is with God. This is affirmed in the service. Finally, and most importantly, the funeral allows the couple to say goodbye to their child in a way that is meaningful to them and provides a bond with their loved ones. Generally then, the benefits of a funeral are wide-ranging, even though at the time the pain of the event can be intense.

As we mentioned, the couple should not feel rushed to arrange an immediate funeral. Some couples may wish to see their child again in the days following the death, and this should be arranged if requested.

> After the delivery we were so shocked that we didn't want to see her. But the next day I regretted that. I thought I'd lost my chance, but I asked anyway. The sister told me that they would arrange for us to go to the mortuary to see her. We went down, and it was very hard, but I was glad we did it.

If the couple do not have connections with a Funeral Director, the hospital will generally be able to suggest one who is experienced in the funerals of small babies. Such a director will arrange all details, thereby relieving the bereaved parents. The funeral should be arranged for a time chosen by the couple that allows them time to prepare themselves physically and emotionally.

The couple generally wish to have a small service held. If they have connections with a church, this can be arranged privately. Otherwise, the hospital chaplain, who is experienced in such losses, is able to assist. Often the couple do not realize that they can, if they wish, participate fully in the determination of the funeral. One couple, before the funeral, dressed their baby, who had been a victim of Sudden Infant Death Syndrome. Others have constructed the coffin and participated fully in the service. Perhaps we can highlight this point further by outlining our own experiences with Kate's funeral.

We wanted Kate's funeral to be an expression of our love for her. Our son, lost at 18 weeks, had not received a farewell as we would have wished. We wanted Kate to be farewelled lovingly and meaningfully. Pastor Renner had shared our thoughts. He had been with us throughout those painful days of labour. It was he who had given her the sign of the cross as she grew weaker and finally died. He encouraged us by allowing us to plan our final farewell for her as we felt appropriate.

It was difficult going to see the Funeral Director to discuss casks and costs. We realized that these practical things were necessary, but they seemed so brutal at the time. The support of our loving sister and sister-in-law, who accompanied us to the Funeral Directors, was vital to us.

It was a difficult moment, walking into the church, to see the tiny white casket. We had taken some yellow carnations, from the bouquets we had been sent, to lay upon it. The gathering was small, but we felt the atmosphere of love and protection as we entered.

The service was simple. The reading of John 14:1–4, 1 Thessalonians 4:13–14, and John 10:27–30 were used. When read, the words of Mark 10:14 took on a new meaning at that moment, and will always retain it:

> Suffer the little children to come unto me, and forbid them not, for of such is the kingdom of heaven.

Throughout the times of our previous losses, two songs had provided us comfort. It seemed appropriate that they be played to work their healing power again. After a short address by Pastor Renner, the time of our farewell came, and we were able to say to our daughter those things that were in our hearts. All people who have lost loved ones have words they want to say. If they wish, they can say them publicly in the final farewell, the valedictory of the funeral. Our valedictory written for our Kate is given here.

For Katie — Goodbye from Your Parents

For a few very precious hours we had you to hold;
yet it was more, so much more.
From the day you were conceived, you were loved.
You were wanted and you were ours.
Your arrival was awaited with true love,
but yet we know you weren't really ours;
you belonged to God.
He simply let us have you for a while,
in those few months, and particularly those
    last few hours.
You became a part of our lives that will
    always remain sacred.
God has taken you back with him now.
You have gone from our arms to the stronger arms
    of One who loves you even more than we have.
You are safe. You are secure.
This is our goodbye to you, for we know
    somehow, some way,
you will understand.
You will always be a part of us while we live.
Thank you for what you gave us in so little time,

for what you have given us shows your life in
  no way was in vain.
Please know you were wanted and know you were loved.
You have a portion of our hearts.
There is little else to say, except:
'Rest easy, our little angel.
We will see you again some day in Paradise.'
Heavenly Father, in your strong arms we rest her!
Katie, goodbye!

Michael carried the tiny casket from the church to a waiting sedan. There was no hearse or floral tribute or funeral procession. We wanted simplicity. The burial was a more private affair, short and simple. Our final gift, as the casket was lowered, was a small bunch of pink rose-buds. How appropriate they seemed for one so small and beautiful as she had been!

To this present day, the funeral remains a sad yet joyous memory for us. There was so little we could do for our daughter in life. Her funeral allowed us to show the world just how special she was to us, and how much we loved her. Somehow, there remains a special feeling of closeness to her on that hill-top lawn cemetery, where the gum trees wave in the breeze!

We have outlined our experience here simply to show that through a funeral the couple who have lost a child can be helped in their grieving. For many other couples, the funeral will not hold the same significance. For some, the burial or cremation spot will mean much less than other memories — the photographs, the cards, the hospital bracelet. Every couple is different. Their reactions differ. Their attitudes and beliefs differ. Their family situations and practices differ. What is the same, though, is the love and pain they feel for their lost child. The final farewell is important to the final relief of their pain. Where this farewell occurs — whether at the delivery, the funeral, or the burial — is not important. As long as the couple feel content that it has been right for them and their child, their farewell is appropriate.

In making this final statement, we wish to emphasize that a comforting farewell may be denied some couples. In cases where parents cannot afford the costs of a burial, the State takes over the burial of the child. At times, in such circumstances, the body is removed before parents have been able to say their farewells, either in their own way or in the form of a funeral service. Such parents, who are generally unable to attend their child's burial or to initially mark his/her grave, are often devastated. It is vital that such parents be provided with a chance to say farewell in a dignified, caring manner. Poverty does not mean that parents feel any less for their child. Overworked government officers are not to blame. Society needs to demand compassion for such parents.

Most commonly, the funeral is the time recognized in our society when not only the couple but also family and friends outwardly say goodbye. Hence, a funeral that expresses the love and beauty of their child, can provide a farewell that the couple and their family can look back upon as unspoilt. It was their unique expression and decision for *their* child made by *them alone*.

Stillbirth registration

In some States, the birth of a stillborn child is not registered. No birth certificate or death certificate is issued. This child is not mentioned on the birth certificates of his/her siblings. Officially at least, this child never existed. Yet the same child is buried. A grave for a child who never was! This is a situation parents of stillborn infants find very difficult to accept, and it is a situation that must be rectified. If governments reject the idea of issuing birth and/or death certificates, then perhaps they may consider a certificate of stillbirth. This could then be recorded on the certificates of birth of other siblings, with the notation 'stillborn' or 'deceased' following the infant's name. A stillborn child *did* exist for the months of pregnancy. He/she was real. Parents' love for that child is real. To deny registration of that life is to deny parents another opportunity to express their love for their child.

In 1987, the Queensland government has drafted legislation to see stillbirths being issued birth and death certificates. Some retrospectivity is provided for.

Coping with the death of your baby

No matter how little time a couple spent with a child, the feelings that accompany the death of a child can be as intense as those that follow the loss of another loved one.[5] Grief is a lonely experience, but one's journey through it can be hindered by obstacles. Part of coping and finally resolving grief comes from the removal of these obstacles that hinder progress. Another part involves the healing of the grief process itself. Each individual must travel alone, but below are some suggestions from others who have travelled this rocky road. They may help to provide some cushioning for the journey.

1. Do what is right for you at the time

No matter how many people experience the loss of a child or how many similarities there are between different people, there is no set of symptoms, feelings, or emotions that every individual must experience. One person's needs may differ greatly from others in the same situation. Each person must be true to his/her own particular needs.

Medical staff, family, and friends who must deal with the grieving individual may try to offer comfort and support in ways which have proved helpful to others in the past. In many cases, such support is effective, but there is no general rule. Whether or not to see their child or attend the funeral or leave hospital promptly, are decisions the couple, or even each individual parent, must make. Although such practices have proved helpful to many couples in the past, it is ultimately the decision of each individual to accept or reject these offers. Many hospital personnel realize that couples can later regret decisions they have made, and hence provide a caring service of keeping on file photographs and other mementos of the deceased child.

If a woman wishes to go home rather than to her family to recuperate, or if the couple wish to visit their baby's grave site often, they should. Any other decisions they have to make should be their own. They should be guided by their feelings and needs. Individuals must also remember that their partner's needs may be different from their own, and must be respected also. If others cannot understand the individual's needs, the grieving parent should feel no guilt or embarrassment or be concerned about being 'strange'.

2. Express your emotions without fear or guilt

In the days and weeks that follow the death of a child, a person's whole being may seem dictated by his/her emotions. The bereaved may wonder if they will always feel so wretched. They may feel unable to carry out even the simplest tasks.

> All I did was cry all the time. I cried in the morning, over breakfast, and nearly every other minute of the day. I just couldn't seem to stop.

Crying is a very common expression of grief. It is also a natural way of relieving built-up tension. It actually causes physical changes in the body that promote a feeling of well-being afterwards.[6] Many find a distinction between crying and sobbing. Sometimes in situations that are painful, the tears begin to flow, but, because of the circumstances, one attempts to stem their tide. One may cry in front of a partner but tries to retain some control so as not to upset the other too much. Often it is when a person is alone and the emotional build-up is strong, that the body-wracking, heart-wrenching sobs replace the controlled tears. Not only do the tear ducts work, but the vocal chords may also cry out and the chest heave. Yet the release and calm that follow a 'good sob' can be overwhelming.

Others experience delusions such as ghosts in the nursery, or fantasize about holding and caring for their baby. These reactions are fleeting and normal, and subside with time.[7] Yet the individual may be afraid of being insane, fearing he/she is having hallucinations and is 'hearing things'.

It is often the case that people in the bereaved's family, their social circle, or the general public are uncomfortable with the expression of negative emotions. They prefer to see someone 'getting better', as indicated by fewer emotional displays. Support may be offered in phrases like 'You'll just have to put it behind you and get on with your life', or 'You mustn't say things like that', or 'You don't really mean that', or 'You'll have other children. Cheer up.' The bereaved individuals may begin to feel that maybe they are overreacting and are not coping as they should. Their feelings don't disappear, but they feel guilty and hide such feelings from public display. Their act of 'coping' is rewarded by a return of perhaps strained friendships and social contacts. This reinforces suppression of these negative feelings. But the emotions cannot be denied. They may show themselves in another crisis, relationship difficulties, or physical illness.

Sometimes you acted strong because you wanted people to think you were coping, even when you weren't coping. It was sort of a pride thing I suppose. I wanted people with me not because they pitied me but because they really cared about me.

Many people have yet to experience the loss of a loved one and are therefore unable to understand fully the emotions involved. Therefore, a parent who loses a child must recognize his/her right to express feelings without guilt, irrespective of others' reactions. Of course, the right to express feelings does not include the right to hurt others physically or emotionally.

3. Ask for the help you want

Many people who do want to support the grieving parents are unsure of just what to do or say that will be of assistance. Even if offers of help are not made publicly, most people close to the parents would be only too pleased to do anything requested of them by the parents. If the bereaved parents feel something would help them, they shouldn't be concerned about inconveniencing people. Most will be delighted to feel that there is some way in which they really are supporting the couple effectively. Perhaps it may be that the woman can't cope with household chores. She may dread facing the day alone, or she may wish time to be alone. The couple should ask for what they need, whether it is assistance until the woman recovers from a caesarean section, having someone to talk to, or professional counselling. Rarely will they be denied help by family and friends, or by strangers within support groups or counselling agencies.

4. Create as many memories of your baby as you can

As we have seen in Chapter 2, one of the tasks of grieving involves recalling memories of the lost loved one as a means of accepting the importance of the loss. Unfortunately, to lose a child, just prior to, during, or after birth means that the couple generally have very few memories to assist their grieving in the early stages and to provide a feeling of warmth and closeness later. Many bereaved parents find it beneficial to create memories of their loss, although it seems painful at the time.

It is for this reason that caring hospitals encourage parents to hold and cuddle their child, even if only in death. They are given time to commit those precious features to memory. A photograph provides a beautiful tangible reminder of their child. Some parents are given the child's hospital bracelet, foot or hand prints, a lock of hair, or other small mementos. Today, some hospitals are experimenting with the use of videotape memories of a child, particularly in the case of neonatal death.

Hospitals will often encourage other close relatives, such as children or grandparents, to see the child also. This makes the child a reality in their minds. Shared memories then serve to bind parents to some of their main sources of support. The funeral will also provide other memories to rekindle later.

Where severe abnormalities are the cause of death, the hospital staff will generally prepare parents for what they will expect to see when given their child to cuddle. What parents visualize when told of an abnormality is often much worse than the reality. When they see their child, their fears and frightening imaginings are laid to rest.

Giving the baby a name is an important part of making this child a real person in the minds of all. Often a couple have already chosen a name prior to the death, and may have called the baby by this name while it was still in the uterus. A name is probably the most important thing a couple can give this child, besides their love. It is also something they alone can give him/her. Using the name in conversation can be difficult for some. Yet for others it is vital in the months and years following the death. Friends and family who are also able to use the baby's name freely, are a great source of support to the grieving couple. Use of a name by others shows acceptance and recognition of their beloved child.

Generally, parents are unaware of the value of such memories, or are in such states of shock that they fail to ask for such experiences to be offered them. Therefore, hospital staff must provide opportunities for such experiences for the parents. They should be offered without pressure, yet done so in the knowledge that a decision made now in shock or anger may later be regretted.

5. Talk selectively about the death

Parents who have lost a child often feel a strong need to talk about their loss. They may find themselves relating the details of the event over and over to anyone who will listen. The reactions they receive from others to this may vary. Yet, recalling their memories is vital to their emotional well-being. Therefore, the couple need to find others who are understanding of their need and willing to listen. Friends and family may provide such a support.

There are groups of people who are willing and eager to listen to the couple's story, and are able to recognize the emotions the couple may have difficulty expressing in words. They are support groups made up of couples who have also lost a child. They never tire of each other's stories. For these groups can provide strong support after the death and also in a later new pregnancy. They know the benefit of being able to talk, knowing that one's words will not be misinterpreted and that jumbled emotions are acceptable.

6. Understand something of the process of grieving

Couples, particularly those who have never experienced the loss of a child, do not enter a pregnancy with thoughts of losing that child. Often the loss of a child is the first close encounter with death a couple has. Therefore, they are usually completely unprepared for the intense feelings of their grief. Some of the intensity of grieving can be frightening for the novice, and often they wonder if they are going insane, a terrifying thought. As one woman put it after losing four babies to late miscarriage and prematurity:

> The first time was the most frightening, for I didn't understand what was happening to me. By the third time and fourth time, grief seemed like an old adversary whose movements I could predict. I felt more in control, as I understood my adversary better.

It can help to understand that grief is a process that can involve physical and emotional aspects, that it can be completely irrational, and that it is a frustrating process of ups and downs. Such knowledge removes some of the fear of the unknown. Some preparation and knowledge of grief should be provided to the couple or to persons who will be closely involved with their support.

Support group members can provide such knowledge, since they have made their own personal journeys through grief. Unfortunately, many couples will attest to the fact that they often joined a group only after a time of stumbling around in the unknown world of grief. To understand a little about what they may experience before that time at least removes the fear, if not the pain. Couples don't require detailed information; but a short, meaningful, honest discussion of what may lie ahead, reinforced by the knowledge that it will end, can be reassuring. Information on where support can be found may be offered to the couple when they leave hospital.

7. Remember that others may not understand. Prepare yourself for difficult situations

Some situations, particularly those involving pregnant women and babies, will be difficult to face. It will be difficult to feel happiness when a friend or relative produces a live, healthy baby. A christening or contact with other families can also be difficult. Yet it is often the situations a couple are not expecting that hit the hardest: a chance meeting with a pregnant friend whom they haven't seen for ages, or an introduction to a new workmate with a baby of the age your child would have been. These 'accidents' can hurt deeply.

Often the build-up to an event is worse than the event itself. This is commonly true of friends who have healthy babies after the couple's own loss.

> About six friends had babies in the year after James's death. The weeks before the births were terrible. I felt hurt, bitter, and jealous, and couldn't face them. If I did, there seemed no feelings of friendship in it for me. Yet miraculously, when those babies were actually born, I had to think of them as families, and the pain eased.

Sometimes, as the bereaved parents face continuing situations of this type, such situations become less traumatic. Generally, this occurs as grief is being resolved. Yet for many, such situations will remain as difficult as the first, and will not be ultimately resolved until they have another child. Many parents will dread social contacts where new babies or pregnant women are present. Even months later, invitations that would previously have been accepted immediately may require a great deal of soul-searching and consideration. The bereaved parent realizes that it is not the invitation but the possible appearance of a pregnant woman or baby that frightens them. Guilt at being so 'childish' may then result.

At times, relief can be found by consciously trying to visualize in the mind's eye the situation that is feared. The grieving parent then imagines himself/herself coping well with it and remaining relaxed. Professionals use such processes to help relieve phobias. It may be a case of 'forewarned is forearmed'. We discuss this process in greater detail in Chapter 11.

Expressing fears about these difficult situations to one's partner or a friend who may be accompanying the grieving parent on this outing, can be of assistance. The parent knows that at least someone else is actually aware of his/her pain. The saying 'A problem shared is a problem halved' is true in these situations.

Finally, the couple should not force themselves to face situations before they are ready. Others seem to believe that the sooner one resumes a 'normal life', the better one will feel! The bereaved parents may try to face too much too soon in the hope of cheating grief out of its entitlement. It doesn't work! If a couple refuse invitations, others may accuse them behind their backs of 'feeling sorry for themselves'. Let them! A broken leg cannot have weight put on it until it has regained some strength. If grieving parents know that they are not ready to take on a group of people involving parents, pregnant women, and babies, or a group who want to 'help them forget', then they shouldn't. They should simply refuse the invitation without guilt. One day they will feel they have more strength and will want to face these difficult situations to prove to *themselves* that they can. Avoidance of these painful situations is not a 'cop out' initially. It is a protective measure. Just as an animal protects a wounded paw, at times the bereaved parent needs to protect a wounded heart.

Unfortunately, for some bereaved parents, avoidance and withdrawal go well beyond a protective point. Grief is not being resolved. If, after a considerable passage of time, a bereaved parent still remains isolated and withdrawn, help is needed. It must be offered generously, subtly and carefully, never in a bullying way!

8. Find out as much as you can medically

Some knowledge of why their baby died can provide all involved with a cause of death and an indication of the possibility of such a situation recurring, as well as suggestions, where possible, for preventive measures. Generally, this information is provided by the autopsy and the doctor. Caring hospitals now arrange a conference with bereaved parents six to eight weeks after the death of their child, during which the autopsy report can be discussed fully and suggestions on any future treatments made.

Some parents refuse an autopsy, but most feel that it means a great deal to them to be relieved of the burden of wondering what actually caused the death. The importance of this knowledge is highlighted by the plight of parents of SIDS babies and those intra-uterine foetal deaths where a cause cannot be found.

Knowledge can often remove fears for a future pregnancy. To know that a stillbirth was caused by a complication that is very unlikely to recur can be somewhat — although not fully — comforting. Investigations that diagnose a chromosomal abnormality can suggest what chance a couple may have of a recurrence. Tests such as an amniocentisis can then be suggested to alleviate concerns in a later pregnancy.

Structural abnormalities of the reproductive system can be investigated and corrected. Maternal disease or conditions unrelated to, or associated with, the pregnancy can be monitored and managed.

Unfortunately, there will remain a group of parents for whom a definite diagnosis cannot be made. Possibilities may be suspected, but medically the case remains a mystery. Careful observation of a later pregnancy is all that can be offered in these cases.

Hence, knowledge of the cause of death may help in the resolution of grief and also assist in providing the couple with a prognosis for a later pregnancy.

9. Sort out other difficulties that may hinder grieving

The death of a baby is difficult enough in itself, but grief may be further complicated by other crises and fears.

If there is anger toward a doctor, hospital, relative, or partner over some aspect of the death, it is important to voice this so that it can be dealt with appropriately. Problems of financial burdens of hospitalization, employment, or children need to have solutions found. There are many and varied minor crises that can make grieving more difficult. As we suggested earlier, if others can assist, ask them to!

There may be other fears, not specifically related to the actual death, that need to be tackled to relieve tension. A woman may blame herself for the death of her baby, or may fear infertility and the future, particularly if the death is of a first child or preceded by other losses. An understanding doctor can help alleviate some of these fears. The six-week postnatal check-up may be helpful in this regard.

Crises of communication within a relationship, or unresolved past losses, will complicate grieving. Help, including professional counselling, may need to be sought in such cases.

10. Be nice to yourself

A bereaved parent needs tender loving care, not only from those around, but also from himself/herself. The past has occurred and cannot be changed. To punish oneself with guilt and recriminations of 'If only I'd done . . .' is destructive. It is best to avoid tormenting oneself by looking at the unfairness of the situation. Life isn't fair and never made any guarantees to be so! One needs to accept himself/herself as human, a person who is justifiably upset over a great pain. Those who are bereaved shouldn't force themselves to be brave if they don't feel so. They should pamper themselves a little and pamper their partners too. In general, bereaved persons needs to be gentle with themselves and not expect too much too soon.

11. Initially at least, take one day at a time

In the days following a baby's death, the bereaved parents will probably wonder if they will survive the pain of the next hour, let alone the whole day. The future seems to stretch out terrifyingly before them. At this stage at least, the future is often something they feel unable to face without their baby. Perhaps it is best not to think about the future. Aim to plan no further than one day, or even one hour, ahead. The future that they fear will only happen one hour at a time.

12. When it feels right, find activities that provide an energy outlet and meaning

As we mentioned, some people become hyperactive to overcome grief. This is not successful. Yet, as time and grieving progress, the bereaved parent may find that meaningful activity is helpful in providing diversion, a new perspective of the world and the future, or a release of tension. Some people find relaxation in sport, music, craft, or literature. Many are able to return to work, and if they are involved in a satisfying occupation with companionable workmates, find this a meaningful outlet. Some have remarked that becoming involved with others in similar situations, or in community or social groups, provided some sense of re-entering humanity and giving life some meaning and normality again.

Emotions are raw after the death of a loved one, and can interfere with the logical thought required in making major decisions. Decisions made in such a time can be regretted.

> After my two miscarriages and now a stillbirth I just couldn't face it again. I demanded the doctor tie my tubes a few months later. He didn't want to, but I demanded it. Now I'm desperately trying to have it reversed. I should have listened to him.

13. Think carefully before making major decisions

Even the decision to have another baby must be made with caution and forethought. Returning to, or leaving work, moving house, or adoption are also decisions that should not be made while the couple are experiencing the early intense grief. As time progresses and grieving is being resolved, the emotional burdens of such decisions may be lessened and informed decisions can be made. The couple will be better able to see their situation in the broader perspective of their lives as a whole, rather than simply their lives as parents.

Pregnant again

A new pregnancy following the death of a child is met with some relief and happiness, but is often overshadowed by the fear of a painful recurrence of the loss.

Many couples, particularly the women, feel an intense desire to become pregnant immediately after the death.

> I was very, very hard on my husband, because from the minute I lost the baby I went into 'I'm having a baby immediately. I am not waiting. I am going to get pregnant this month.' Five months went by before I did fall pregnant, and I felt terrible. Everytime I ovulated instinct told me I hadn't conceived, and during intercourse at that ovulation time I would burst into tears, which didn't help my husband to have me crying through this act.

On consulting their doctor about when they should begin trying to conceive again, the couple may receive ambiguous advice. Medical evidence is unclear, but some doctors intuitively feel that the uterus should be 'rested' for six to 12 months before another pregnancy. Others believe that once menstruation has resumed and any wounds from a caesarean or episiotomy have healed, there is no physical reason for delaying.

Generally, doctors feel that a time delay is required to allow the couple to grieve the lost child before embarking on a new pregnancy. This is sound advice. Each pregnancy, particularly where there has been a prior loss, requires immense courage and fortitude. Emotional drain is further complicated by the physical changes of pregnancy. Intense grieving produces incredible strain in itself, without the added burden of pregnancy. In fact, over time, the intense desire to fall pregnant again can ease. On the other hand, some couples find that the resolution of their grief comes more easily during a second pregnancy. Once again, each couple is different, and each case must be viewed individually.

There is one important danger in embarking without careful consideration on a new pregnancy soon after the death of a child. The new child is *not* the dead child, and never can be. This sounds a ridiculous statement to the conscious mind, but subconsciously there can be an attempt to replace the lost child with this new one. This is common enough to be termed 'the replacement child'. Just as an adopted child can be an attempt to take the place of the dreamed-for biological child, so the replacement child can be in danger of being seen not as a unique individual but as a substitute. Unless this is resolved, this unique individual, who cannot ever measure up to an idealized standard, will suffer.

Five months after Jemma was born, I fell pregnant again. I went into that pregnancy to replace her, as I hadn't got the anger or jealousies out of my system. So when this little fellow came along and was a little boy, I rejected him for the first eight months of his life. Hence, today he is emotionally a handful because he didn't get that security from me when he was a baby.

If carefully considered, a new pregnancy can help to heal the loss of a beloved child. Each child has the right to be an individual: the dead child the right to be grieved and remembered lovingly, the new arrival the right to be loved and treasured for himself/herself and his/her safe arrival.

Many couples can't believe that they will be so fortunate as to have to consider such needs of another child. Many fear that they will never have another child to love and hold. They fear infertility or further miscarriages, stillbirths and neonatal deaths. Although evidence and statistics suggest that, unless a specific unremediated problem exists, this sad event is extremely unlikely to recur, any new pregnancy is viewed suspiciously and watched carefully.

With Michael, every movement and every non-movement nearly drove me out of my head.

Couples may not be reassured by figures. Careful vigilance by medical staff, including more regular antenatal visits and careful examination of any worries expressed may be more reassuring. This vigilance, combined with the understanding of family and friends, may make this time just a little easier.

Conclusion

Between one and two babies in every 100 will die before, during, or shortly after birth. The causes of such deaths are many and varied, but most are unlikely to recur in later pregnancies.

The grief that follows the death of a child can be as intense as that experienced by others who lose a loved one. Others are often unaware of, and unable to accept, the intensity of such grief. Parents are entitled to feel their pain and to express it. Not only do they grieve a beloved child; they must also face their own mortality, perhaps before they are ready.

As they work through their pain, many couples discover that the life that was with them for so short a time has blessed them. They find new depths of meaning in their lives and the world around them. No life is in vain, not even so short a life. We sincerely hope that you, as parents who have lost a child, as we have, will finally see the beauty, not only the pain of your dreadful loss.

Our thoughts are with you!

References

1. Derek Llewellyn-Jones, *Fundamentals of Obstetrics and Gynaecology*, Vol. 1, Obstetrics, 3rd ed. (London: Faber and Faber, 1982), 427,428.
2. Gordon Bourne, *Pregnancy* (London: Pan. 1979), 291.
3. Elisabeth Kübler-Ross, *On Death and Dying* (London: Tavistock, 1969).
4. These criteria of 20 weeks' gestation or 400 grams birthweight may vary in different States and countries. In fact, in Queensland at the time of writing this, these criteria are under review.
5. Catherine M. Sanders, 'A Comparison of Adult Bereavement in the death of a Spouse, Child, and Parent', *Omega*, 10(4) (1979–80).
6. Joan Moody, 'Crying: the Experts Say It's Good for You', *Woman's Day* (July 8, 1985), 52.
7. W. Dewi Rees, 'The Bereaved and Their Hallucinations' in Bernard Schoenberg, Irwin Gerber, Alfred Wiener, Austin H. Kutscher, David Peretz, and Arthur C. Carr, eds., *Bereavement: Its Psychosocial Aspects* (New York: Columbia University Press, 1975), 66–71.

7 When There Is Something 'Wrong' with Your Baby:
Congenital Abnormalities

As pregnancy progresses into its later stages, couples begin to think of the time following the birth, with its enjoyment of the baby, the closeness of the family, and the sharing of their joy with others. For some, this will not be the case, for there will be something 'wrong' with their baby. Knowledge of a problem may come before birth, immediately after birth, or even weeks or months after birth. Their child's infancy may be shadowed by periods of worry and depression.

Fortunately, many problems that a newborn may have are able to be corrected by nature and time alone, or by medical science. Other children may have a mild permanent impairment. For a small group the problem is severe, and the child is labelled physically or intellectually disabled. In quite rare cases, the problem means that the child's bodily functions cannot support life. Hence, the child will die after a period of hours to months.

The joy of the birth and the anticipated perfect child are lost. This is a loss that must be grieved. This grief must be recognized and resolved before parents are able to tackle successfully the problems of their disabled or ill child.

A clarification

The range of possible problems and their severity is broad. The less severe ones, or those that are 'curable', may not affect the life of the family to any great degree. Others will cause great upheaval. It would be beyond the scope of this book to look at all possible problems or discuss problems in any depth. It would also require many books to discuss the bringing up of a disabled child, a subject which we do not feel qualified to discuss. We shall therefore confine ourselves to the basic causes of problems in the infant and the period surrounding the birth.

Before discussing the issue further, we wish to make a statement concerning our beliefs and use of terms. Most minor or curable problems with which an infant may be born will be accepted and treated with understanding and sympathy by our society. This is particularly true if the problem does not mar the baby's appearance. Unfortunately, a problem that is more severe and will affect the child all his/her life may not be viewed so compassionately. This is because there still lives in our society a fear or even distrust of things that are different.

Very soon after birth a child with a severe physical or intellectual problem is labelled 'abnormal', 'disabled', or 'handicapped'. A 'child' and a 'disabled child' are seen as almost two different creatures. For the 'child' the future is viewed with anticipation of great things. The future for the 'disabled child' may already be seen by many as mundane at best, and as hopeless at worst. The problem with which the child is born is labelled an 'abnormality'. It brings with it the social stigma attached to anything imperfect. In a society in which we strive for perfection and value achievement and success, the 'abnormal child' must fight a battle from the day of birth onwards. A child labelled as 'abnormal' is often similarly labelled in the minds of people as inferior or not normal. Yet, who decided what constitutes 'normal'?

Is a normal person one who has physical attributes within a particular range? Do normal people have a certain intelligence or skin colour? Are there normal habits one must have, or normal speech patterns? If we look around us at the people we pass on the street, we could probably find something 'abnormal' in each if we compare them to our 'perfect' selves. We all vary in so many different attributes: height, weight, intelligence, talents, speech patterns, energy levels, eating habits, and vices, to name but a few. Who then is 'normal'? Is the person who has no use of his/her legs or is unable to perform certain daily functions less 'normal' or inferior to a person who abuses his/her children in a drunken stupor? Yet the latter may be 'normal', while the former is labelled 'handicapped'!

Normality is an arbitrary concept, with no set of accepted criteria in all cultures. For example, the deformed feet of the Ostrich people of Africa are normal to them. By extending our definition of normal to encompass all peoples, we may help to remove some of the unnecessary stigma. We are all normal, and simply lie on a continuum of what help we require to function as independent beings at a particular time. At one end of the continuum lie those restricted by intellectual functioning, illness, age, or accident to dependence on others for their basic survival needs. At the other end are those blessed with health and efficient intellectual functioning, who are not only able to provide sufficiently for their own needs but also to serve the needs of others. Somewhere on that continuum all of us, the 'normals', lie.

However, within this chapter we shall use the term 'abnormal' or 'abnormality' simply because these terms are used medically and socially, and so will cause less confusion. But we have a very specific definition of 'abnormal'. An abnormal child is one who is born with a condition (the abnormality) that is not commonly found in babies in general. This condition may cause them some physical or functioning problems, and may or may not be able to be affected medically to relieve its effects. Hence, there is no value judgment made of the innate worth of such a child. Children are children, all innately valuable in themselves.

Causes of abnormalities

An abnormality present at birth is known as a **congenital** abnormality. It is on such problems that we shall concentrate. Major abnormalities occur in about three babies in every 100, with up to another four per 100 being affected to minor degrees.[1] The two major types of abnormality which we shall discuss have different origins. These types are Genetic/Chromosomal and Structural Abnormalities.

Genetic/chromosomal abnormalities

Body structures develop according to the patterns set down in the genes. Genes are found on long spindly thread-like structures which are found in the nucleus of each cell and are known as chromosomes. All the characteristics of the body, and perhaps parts of the personality, are determined by these genes. Each cell in the human body, except for the sperm and ova, contains 46 chromosomes. At fertilization, the ovum and sperm, which should each bear 23 chromosomes, combine to form a new life, a cell containing 46 chromosomes. The 46 chromosomes are arranged in

23 pairs. The arrangement of the chromosome pairs and the genes on each pair is specific. Any problem within this first arrangement will be repeated in every cell of the body.

The problems that occur in the genetic structure of the new individual may be inherited from one or both parents, or may be caused by an initial random error in the arrangement of the chromosomes. The former are known as **inherited disorders**, while the latter are termed **chromosomal abnormalities**.

(i) Chromosomal abnormalities

The sperm and ovum are formed during a process called meiosis. During this process, the 23 pairs of chromosomes in a particular cell meet in the centre of the cell. Half the chromosomes will go to one of the new germ daughter cells, and half to the other. These new daughter cells are the ova or sperm. In this way, each new sperm or ovum has only 23 chromosomes.

Sometimes the pairs do not separate in time, and one of the daughter cells ends up with the two chromosomes of this pair and the other with none. This is known as a **non-disjunction**. In other cases, part of one of the chromosomes breaks off and is added to the other of the pair, before each then joins one of the daughter cells. This is known as a **translocation**. Both of these chromosomal mistakes can lead to congenital abnormalities.

Non-disjunction.[2] If a sperm or ovum suffering from a non-disjunction is involved in fertilization, the resulting fertilized cell will not have the usual 46 chromosomes. If the sperm or ovum used had an extra chromosome, the fertilized ovum will have 47 chromosomes, one of the 23 pairs having three instead of two chromosomes. The resulting condition is known as a **trisomy**. The most common trisomies are Trisomy 21 or Down's Syndrome (in which the cell has three chromosomes instead of the twenty-first pair), Trisomy 18, and Trisomy 13. In some cases, the extra chromosomes may be carried in the sex-determination pair, that is, the XX gene pair for a girl and XY gene pair for a boy. Extra genes on these pairs can lead to fertilized ova in which the sex determination pairs are now XXY (Kleinfetter's Syndrome), XYY, or XXX super female.

If the sperm or ovum that is missing a chromosome is involved in fertilization, spontaneous abortion generally occurs. In the case

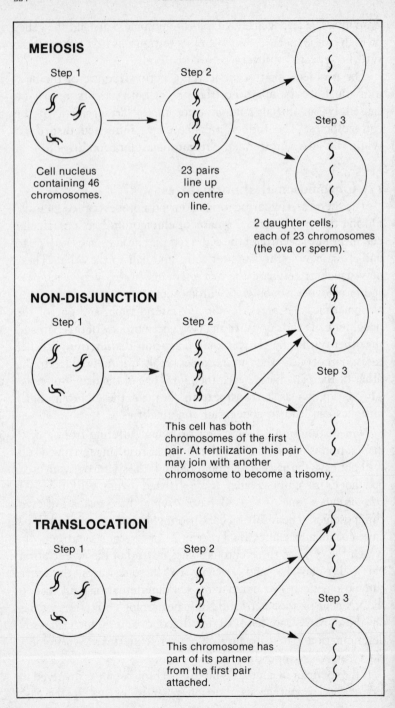

MEIOSIS

Step 1

Cell nucleus containing 46 chromosomes.

Step 2

23 pairs line up on centre line.

Step 3

2 daughter cells, each of 23 chromosomes (the ova or sperm).

NON-DISJUNCTION

Step 1

Step 2

Step 3

This cell has both chromosomes of the first pair. At fertilization this pair may join with another chromosome to become a trisomy.

TRANSLOCATION

Step 1

Step 2

Step 3

This chromosome has part of its partner from the first pair attached.

where only an X chromosome is present, the sex determination pair is then XO, and Turner's Syndrome results.

Translocation.[2] The addition or deletion of parts of chromosomes is rare. It is possible for a parent with a translocation known as a balanced translocation not to show any overt symptoms of this problem, although the condition appears in his/her offspring. The translocation can also happen by accident.

(ii) Inherited disorders

At times, one or both parents may carry a gene on their chromosomes for a particular condition which may be inherited by their offspring. The genes may be of a dominant or recessive nature. If the gene is dominant and carried by the parent, the parent will himself/herself display the condition. If the gene is recessive, the parent will not show the condition and may not even be aware that he/she carries a gene for the abnormality. Yet it may be passed on to offspring.

A word of warning

The determining of whether or not a child will be affected by an abnormality is not an exact science. We will mention percentages of children who may be affected by an abnormality, but it cannot be stressed too strongly that these are only the probability of an event occurring. If we say that there is 25 per cent chance of a child suffering from an inherited abnormality, this doesn't mean that if you have four children one will have the abnormality. A small exercise may help highlight this point. Take four pieces of paper. On three, draw a black dot, and on one a red dot. Roll them into balls. The red dot, the one piece of paper in four, will indicate a child with an abnormality. Put the four paper balls in a dish, hold this above your head, and pull down one ball. Open it and see the coloured dot, and then replace it. Then draw again. Do this a few times. You could end up with a great variety of outcomes for four draws, for example: a red dot, black dot, black dot, red dot; or a black dot, black dot, black dot, black dot. The first case would indicate that the first and fourth child would have an abnormality, while in the second case none of the children would have the condition. The probability of an abnormality is still one chance in four or 25 per cent, but the actual outcome in a specific case cannot be so easily determined.

Where abnormalities are of a genetic/chromosomal nature, the condition is determined at fertilization. Every cell of the body will display the genetic structure of the condition, since after fertilization only genetic copies of the original nucleus of the fertilized cell are made.

Genetic counsellors are persons specializing in the area of genetics, and they can fairly accurately determine the probability of any subsequent children being affected by the same condition. They perform tests to determine the character of the abnormality and the genetic structure of the child and parents. During pregnancy, tests may be performed to determine if the foetus has certain abnormalities.

At this stage, medical science can only identify the condition and advise on treatment and future pregnancies. Geneticists can only speculate on whether or not a child will have a condition; they cannot prevent the condition.

It is believed that most foetuses affected by chromosomal abnormalities are lost early in pregnancy through miscarriage, nature's own form of quality control. Hence, the actual incidence of chromosomal abnormality may never be known without investigation of all spontaneously aborted foetuses.

There are some tendencies surrounding inherited disorders:

a) If the gene for an abnormality is dominant and one parent carries the abnormality, there is a 50 per cent chance that the child will also have the abnormality. Such disorders that are inherited in this way include Huntington's chorea, some forms of finger anomalies, and polycystic kidneys.

b) In other cases, neither parent will show signs of the abnormality, as they carry a recessive gene for the condition. Where both parents carry a recessive gene, there is a 25 per cent chance of it appearing in the offspring. Two out of three of the offspring who don't show the abnormality may carry the recessive gene.

c) If one parent shows the condition, which is carried on a recessive gene, and the other parent, not showing the abnormality, also carries a recessive gene for the condition, 50 per cent of the offspring will have the abnormality. The others will be carriers of it.

d) If only one parent carries the recessive gene, 50 per cent of the children will carry the condition, although none will show it.

The most common recessive-gene disease in Australia is cystic fibrosis. Another is phenylketonuria (PKU).

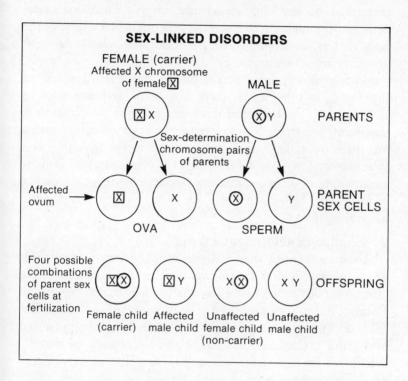

SEX-LINKED DISORDERS

FEMALE (carrier)
Affected X chromosome of female ☒

MALE

PARENTS

Sex-determination chromosome pairs of parents

Affected ovum →

PARENT SEX CELLS

OVA   SPERM

Four possible combinations of parent sex cells at fertilization

OFFSPRING

Female child (carrier) Affected male child Unaffected female child (non-carrier) Unaffected male child

Sometimes disorders are carried by an abnormal gene on the X chromosome. Such disorders are known as sex-linked. The female carries the abnormal gene.

Half of the girls born may carry the abnormal gene, although they will not show the condition themselves due to the influence of the other X chromosome. Half of the boys born may have the abnormal gene, and will show the condition. Therefore, the female carries the gene for the abnormality, which only appears in male offspring. Conditions affected by this type of inheritance include haemophilia and colour-blindness.

There are other rarer genetic/chromosomal conditions that are due to different abnormal processes, but we shall not try to discuss them here.

Structural abnormalities

Other congenital abnormalities that originate after fertilization are not linked to the chromosome or genetic arrangement. They are caused by outside agents such as drugs, maternal disease, or chemicals, or are due to chance errors. These structural abnormalities only affect a certain structure or structures of the body that are developing at the particular time when some agent or agents are acting on the embryo.

Most commonly, this occurs during the first 12 weeks of pregnancy. In other cases, there may occur a chance error in development. The timing of this interruption in development is important. For example, a case of rubella at six weeks' gestation may have more damaging effects on the foetus than the same infection may have on a foetus of 11 weeks' gestation. This is because more of the major structures are developing rapidly earlier in pregnancy. Below we shall look more closely at the possible harmful agents:

1. Chance development errors

The causes of many abnormalities cannot be specified, and these are then put down as chance events. Every body system of the child is formed in the first 13 weeks of pregnancy. This growth from one cell to a complete human body in its earliest stages in just 13 weeks is almost unbelievable. The fact that more doesn't go wrong due to chance errors in these weeks is perhaps the miracle, rather than the fact that things can go wrong. Errors that do occur may affect internal or external features.

2. Drugs

Although the placenta is impermeable to many drugs, some, if taken early in pregnancy, are able to cross the placenta and may cause abnormalities. The most infamous drug able to have such an effect is the drug thalidomide. This sedative was often prescribed for pregnant women, and most commonly caused limb absence or limb deformities, ear deformities, and defects in the cranial nerves in children born to these mothers. It was most damaging when taken by the mother within the first two months of pregnancy.

A second drug, diethylstilbestrol (DES), was taken by many women in early pregnancy in the 1940s and 1950s in an attempt to prevent miscarriage. There is now found to be a link between DES and a rare cancer of the vagina, benign abnormalities of the cervix, vagina, and uterus, and child-bearing difficulties in daughters born to DES mothers. Even links to infertility and abnormalities of the testicles in the sons of DES mothers have been noted.

Progestogens, such as ethisterone and norethesterone, taken by the mother in the first ten weeks of pregnancy can cause masculinization of female children. The taking of antimitotic agents, such as folic acid antagonists, can result in multiple congenital abnormalities. Antithyroid agents taken by the mother may lead to an enlargement of the thyroid gland in a child. Other drugs, such as the anticonvulsants, anticoagulants, and narcotics, are suspected of leading to varying abnormalities, although evidence of this is not conclusive.[3] Most other drugs are believed safe for the mother to take in pregnancy, although doctors generally work from a golden rule that no drugs except those absolutely necessary to maintain the health of the mother should be taken during pregnancy. This is of particular importance during the first trimester. Over many years, doctors have found alternative drugs or ruled harmless those drugs most commonly required by mothers to control maternal disease such as epilepsy, diabetes, and thyroid conditions. Women should be guided by their doctor's advice, and take no prescribed or over-the-counter drugs not sanctioned by him/her.

3. The easy access drugs: alcohol, nicotine, and caffeine

Many people forget that alcohol is itself a drug. It was not uncommon for couples to celebrate the confirmation of a pregnancy with social drinks over a few days in early pregnancy. Today it is believed that even this practice may be dangerous to the foetus. It has been recognized that a collection of abnormalities may appear in the babies of women who drink heavily during pregnancy. Problems included facial abnormalities, giving it a flattened appearance, retardation of growth, abnormalities of the skeleton and body organs, and possible mental retardation. This collection of symptoms has become known as Foetal Alcohol Syndrome (FAS). Doctors now advise women to avoid alcohol completely during pregnancy, or at least during the first trimester.

The nicotine found in tobacco also has its dangers. It can lead to the retardation of growth in the foetus. Nicotine constricts the blood vessels, and so reduces the blood-flow in the uterus and placenta. It also increases the level of the dangerous substance carboxylhaemoglobin in the foetal blood system.

Many medical authorities also believe that large intakes of caffeine in coffee, tea, and cola drinks may also damage the foetus.

4. Infections

Some infections, both viral and bacterial, are able to cross the placenta and may cause abnormalities. But it must be remembered that, even if a woman contracts an infection, her child will not necessarily suffer from some abnormality. Contracting the infection simply means that there is an increased risk of some abnormality occurring.

a) Rubella. The most common virus affecting the foetus has been the rubella virus, commonly known as German measles. Depending on when the virus was contracted, rubella may cause cataracts, deafness, heart problems, growth retardation, and kidney problems, to name but some of the possible effects. The distinctive feature of rubella is a rash. Feelings of definite ill health are not necessarily present. A woman can be tested for her immunity to rubella before pregnancy. This involves a simple blood test, and is advisable for all women contemplating pregnancy. Today, girls between the ages of ten and 14 are routinely vaccinated against rubella, which should significantly reduce the incidence of abnormality caused by this virus in the future. It is still advisable, even after such an injection, to have the blood test before pregnancy to ensure that the woman does indeed have an immunity to the virus.

b) Toxoplasmosis. This infective agent is believed to affect approximately five pregnant women in every 1,000. Approximately one foetus in four of these affected women may develop some congenital abnormality, ranging from eye problems to defects of the central nervous system. Such abnormalities generally only occur if the pregnant woman has suffered a severe acute attack of the infection, in which symptoms such as gland enlargement and fever are obvious. Although contracting the virus is rare, there are simple steps that can be taken to avoid the virus and provide a couple with peace of mind. The virus is most often acquired through contact with cat faeces or from eating raw or grossly undercooked meat. A pregnant woman should therefore wash her hands and utensils thoroughly after handling raw meat, and any meat eaten should be cooked thoroughly. She should have someone else empty cat litter boxes daily, or use disposable gloves if she must do the task herself. She should avoid unknown cats, and keep her own away from raw meat or rodents.

c) Cytomegalovirus. This uncommon virus may, in rare cases, affect a pregnant woman, although she may be unaware of it. The foetus may also become infected. Fortunately, affected foetuses generally show no problems, but a very small proportion of affected babies may suffer from brain damage.[4]

d) Syphilis. This is a dangerous sexually-transmitted disease, which requires urgent treatment in a pregnant woman. If it is untreated, the baby can be affected by the disease, leading to many problems and even death. If the disease is noted and treated before the fifteenth week of pregnancy, the foetus is unlikely to be affected.[5]

e) Other infections. Other infections are suspected of causing abnormalities in the foetus, but once again evidence of such effects is inconclusive. These infections include chicken-pox, Coxsackie B, Hepatitis B, and mumps.[6] There is believed to be little danger from other infections. What danger to the foetus there is is determined by the severity of the illness itself and its effects, such as high fever and dehydration. Congenital abnormalities are not associated with the common viruses. Although it is best for the foetus to develop in the body of a healthy mother, common illnesses such as colds and gastroenteritis need not be feared by the pregnant woman.

5. Other agents

In looking for causes of abnormalities, researchers have considered many other agents. Results surrounding most of these agents are still inconclusive. X-rays have not been conclusively shown as causing abnormalities, but are best avoided in the early weeks of pregnancy. The Vietnam war veterans' seeking of compensation for birth abnormalities and health problems, allegedly associated with the insecticide 245T found in Agent Orange, has brought into focus the possible effects on the unborn child of chemicals used in our society in industry and as pesticides and herbicides. The possible genetic and structural effects of nuclear fallout and waste have also been considered, after noting increased incidences of miscarriage, stillbirth, and congenital abnormalities in communities close to dumping sites and also in the population of Hiroshima.

6. Birth injuries

In extremely rare cases, during birth the baby is deprived of oxygen for an extended period of time. In a small percentage of such cases there may be some neurological damage, and in this small percentage are a proportion of babies who then are found to suffer from cerebral palsy or severe mental retardation. In today's era of modern obstetric care such instances are extremely rare, as the baby's progress during birth is monitored and early signs of distress are considered seriously, and intervention of some description takes place where necessary.

7. Heat

Recent research has suggested that excessive heat, such as that caused by high fever during the early stages of pregnancy, may cause some abnormality. Excessive heat from very hot baths or saunas, or extremely rigorous exercise, may also be suspect.

8. Maternal disease

Uncontrolled diseases in the mother, such as diabetes and hyperthyroidism, can lead to abnormalities in the baby.

Some abnormalities — a more detailed discussion

Chromosomal

a) Trisomy 21 (Down's Syndrome)

This is the most common chromosomal abnormality. The syndrome used to be known as Mongolism, because the affected children have a fold of flesh over the join of the eyes, giving the eyes a slanting appearance similar to that found in Asiatic races. Some of the other characteristics of the syndrome include a short head, short hands with small fingers, deposits of fat in the cheeks and on the back of the neck, a flat broad nose, squarish ears, a larger upper than lower jaw, dry skin, a body lacking in muscle strength, and some degree of mental retardation.

As we mentioned, the 46 chromosomes of the human cell are arranged in 23 pairs. In the common form of Down's Syndrome there is an extra chromosome connected with the twenty-first pair, hence its medical name Trisomy 21. The chromosomes then number 47. In a rarer form there is a translocation of the extra chromosome to join the head of chromosome 15, leaving the total chromosome count at 46. This second form accounts for only about three to six per cent of all Down's Syndrome affected children, but is perhaps more serious. This is because the more common form of Down's Syndrome is unlikely to recur in any subsequent children, while if the condition is caused by the translocation there is a 30 per cent chance of recurrence. Chromosomal studies may be carried out on both parents of a Down's Syndrome child to determine which form it has taken.

Currently, Down's Syndrome can be identified through the use of a test known as an amniocentesis, carried out at about the fifteenth week of pregnancy. The test is generally offered to women over the age of 37 or those who have previously had a Down's Syndrome child. This is because the incidence of the condition is higher in older mothers and fathers. Before 35 years of age, the incidence of Down's Syndrome is about one in every 700 births. By age 35, the incidence has risen to about one in every 300 births; at 40, to about one in 100; and at 45, one in every 40 births.

Due to recent research, a simple blood-screening test for Down's Syndrome may be available in the near future. The test would be carried out during the early weeks of pregnancy.

b) Trisomy 18 (Edward's Syndrome)

This rare severe chromosomal abnormality occurs mainly in female infants, and generally culminates in death, since the child fails to thrive. Trisomy 18 is due to an extra chromosome on the eighteenth pair. Its characteristics include: mental retardation; muscular tension with clenched hands; deformities of the hands, sternum, and pelvis; facial abnormalities, including low-set, malformed ears; prominence of the back of the head; and heart and kidney defects.

As with Down's Syndrome, amniocentesis can be carried out in any subsequent pregnancy to identify this abnormality, which is unlikely to recur.

c) Haemophilia

This disorder is sex-linked. Haemophilia is characterized by a lowered ability, or an inability, of blood plasma to coagulate or clot. Hence, haemophiliacs who begin to bleed externally or internally may bleed to death. They must have regular injections of the clotting agent, Factor 8, which is derived from the blood donations of others.

d) Metabolic disorders

(i) Phenylketonuria. In this condition there is an inability of the body to dispose of the phenylalanine in the body that is produced from foods containing protein. If left untreated, this condition leads to irreversible mental retardation. The condition is very rare, and is preventable if detected at birth. A blood-test, which detects the condition, involves the taking of a drop of blood from the newborn, and is routinely performed on all newborns. Treatment of the condition involves a diet low in protein and an avoidance of breast-feeding.

(ii) Cystic Fibrosis. In this inherited disorder there is a dysfunction of certain glands of the body, including the mucus-producing glands. This usually leads to chronic lung disease. In some States of Australia, newborns are tested for this condition through a blood-test, which may be followed by a sweat-test if the condition is suspected. This condition occurs in about one in every 2,000 live births.[7]

Structural
a) Neural-tube defects

The brain and spinal cord comprising the central nervous system form a tube-like structure of neurones in the embryo, known as the Neural Tube. At times, this development from the neural tube is adversely affected, leading to severe abnormalities of the brain and/or spine.

(i) Anencephaly. This is the most severe neural-tube defect. The child is incompatible with life and will usually die within hours of birth. An anencephalic child is born without the upper part of the brain (cerebrum) and a large portion of the lower brain (cerebellum). Often the flat bones of the skull are also missing. In fact, the gross abnormality of the anencephalic child may prove to be unpleasant viewing for the parents. Caring staff often wrap the child, allowing only the face to show. This may help to make bonding between parent and child easier.

(ii) Spina bifida. At times during the development of the spine, the bony vertebral canal fails to close properly and the membranes covering the spinal cord protrude through the canal. On the back, most commonly in the lumbosacral (lower back) region, there appears a membraneous sac containing cerebrospinal fluid and sometimes nervous tissue. Some severely affected babies will die, while others will remain handicapped. The extent of the handicap will depend upon the position of the protrusion; if it is low on the back, only the legs may be affected. Many spina bifida babies undergo an operation to alleviate the condition, and may in time develop significant use of their limbs and control of body functions. The condition occurs in approximately one birth in every 1,000. [8] Spina bifida is the name under which a number of medical conditions are grouped, including myelomeningocele, meningocele, lipoma, and myelodysplasia.

(iii) Hydrocephaly. This condition is more commonly known by the general population as 'water on the brain'. The brain has inner space, called ventricles, that are filled with cerebrospinal fluid. In hydrocephalic babies there is an excess of such fluid, which is unable to escape from the ventricles or be absorbed into the venous system. This build-up of fluid places pressure on the surrounding brain tissue, and can cause varying degrees of damage to the brain, with a resulting loss of functioning. The abnormality may be detected before birth during an ultrasound examination, suggested at birth by difficulty in delivering the head, or suggested by the appearance of spina bifida, with which the condition is often associated. It may also appear as a complication of extreme prematurity.

Examination of the baby's head will show a greater-than-normal head circumference and bulging fontanella (the membranous space found between the bones of the skull in a newborn). In many such hydrocephalic children, a shunt (an artificial bypass) from one of the ventricles to a neck vein is inserted during surgery, to allow drainage of the excess fluid.

(iv) Microcephaly. This rare condition is characterized by a very small head when compared to the average baby's head circumference. There is generally underdevelopment of the brain, and the baby is mentally retarded.

Severe neural-tube defects, such as spina bifida and anencephaly, can sometimes be detected by a blood-test at approximately 15 weeks' gestation. The test measures the level of alphafetoprotein in the mother's blood. This substance is produced by the foetus. If the level is greater than two-and-a-half times the normal level produced by a foetus of the same gestation, a neural-tube defect is suspected. Such a result would be followed by ultrasound and amniocentesis testing to confirm such a diagnosis, as other causes, such as a multiple pregnancy, can lead to higher levels. The alphafetoprotein test is only one tool in detecting neural-tube defects. It does not accurately diagnose closed-neural-tube defects, and is not completely reliable for open defects either. Other tests must be carried out to confirm a diagnosis.

b) Cleft palate and cleft lip

A cleft palate occurs when there is a failure of the closure of the facial processes of the embryo, leaving a gap in the palate, the roof of the mouth. The gap may be complete, extending through the hard and soft palates into the nose; or partial, affecting only part of the palate. A cleft palate involving the hard palate may create feeding problems. A cleft palate is often associated with a cleft lip, which is a gap in the upper lip. Cleft palate and lip sufferers are adamant in their preference for the use of the term 'cleft lip', rather than the more commonly used term 'harelip'. The use of such a term in the past has only served to increase, rather than decrease, social stigma surrounding the condition. There is some evidence to suggest that there may be a genetic component involved in some way in this condition. Today, very successful operations can be performed on the cleft palate and cleft lip, which leave little indication of the problem that existed.

c) Heart problems

(i) Hypoplastic left-heart syndrome. In this rare condition, there is an underdevelopment or absence of development of the left side of the heart. The baby becomes extremely blue due to a lack of oxygen (cyanosis), and eventually the child dies of heart failure. In July 1984, Holly Roffey, a tiny English baby, was born with this problem and underwent a heart-transplant operation. She lived only 28 days, but future refinements of such techniques may indicate some hope for such babies.

(ii) Hole in the heart. Some babies are found during the paediatric examination to display a heart murmur. In some cases, this murmur is due to a small hole that is to be found between two chambers of the heart. Most murmurs will disappear in the first year of life, as the hole closes itself over. In more severe cases, drugs may be used or surgery may become necessary. The results of such measures are extremely promising.

Tests used in the recognition of abnormalities

A. Antenatal measures

Some abnormalities are suspected prior to birth or are found when tests are carried out for other reasons. The most common tests used prior to birth are discussed below.

a) The ultrasound scan

The basic principle underlying ultrasound scanning is that sound waves are able to travel through a liquid and are reflected at varying intensities from solid materials, depending on the density of such materials. In early pregnancy, the fluid medium through which the sound travels is provided by a full bladder. There is a variety of ultrasound scanning machines. Most commonly, the woman lies on her back, and a clear gel is smoothed over her abdomen. A probe with a flat surface is then passed over the gel. The sound waves are reflected, and appear on a screen as varying shades of black, white, and grey. The trained eye can identify the various features of the foetus. The procedure, which is painless, is performed while the woman is fully conscious, allowing her also to 'see' her baby. Ultrasound scanning is useful in detecting conditions such as hydrocephaly, spina bifida, and deformities of the heart and kidneys and their associated features. Ultrasound scanning also provides measurements of the chest, crown, rump, or abdomen. These may indicate growth retardation or some internal abnormalities at early stages. Ultrasound scanning is used for many other purposes besides detecting abnormalities, such as determining foetal age, multiple pregnancies, and the presence of an ectopic pregnancy, and in conjunction with the test amniocentesis.

b) Amniocentesis

Amniocentesis involves the insertion of a hollow needle through the abdominal wall and uterus into the pregnancy sac, thereby allowing for the removal of a sample of the fluid surrounding the baby (the amniotic fluid). This test is usually carried out at approximately 15 to 16 weeks' gestation. It is generally offered to women over the age of 37, those with a history of a genetic disorder in the family, or those who have previously had a child with particular congenital abnormalities. Ultrasound scanning is used to locate the placenta and guide the positioning of the needle so as to avoid any possible damage to placenta or foetus. The woman is given a local anaesthetic while the procedure is carried out. The risk to mother and child in experienced centres is extremely low. In very rare cases, the procedure has been known to lead to miscarriage. Amniocentesis can also be used to assess the well-being of a rhesus incompatible foetus, and to test for respiratory maturity. The fluid can be examined and cultured to detect chromosomal abnormalities, such as Down's Syndrome and inherited disorders. The presence of high levels of alphafetoprotein in the fluid can also confirm the suspicion of a neural-tube defect.

c) Radiology (X-rays)

X-rays should never be used in early pregnancy, but may be used at a later stage of pregnancy to detect skeletal abnormalities. They are most commonly used when ultrasound scanning is not available, and can detect anencephaly, hydrocephaly, and spina bifida, among other conditions.

d) Chorionic villus sampling/DNA sampling and blood testing[9]

In some cases during early pregnancy, a small sample of the chorionic villi, which is composed of tissue identical to that of the developing foetus, is taken. There is some slight risk of damage. The presence of certain abnormalities can be detected from testing such a sample. It is hoped that in the future concentrated blood samples containing cells from the placenta will fulfil this purpose.

B. The paediatric examination

After birth, many congenital abnormalities are noted during the routine paediatric examinations carried out on every newborn. The examination is an in-depth observation and testing of all parts of the body. Newborns, or neonates as they are medically termed, may be screened for a number of congenital metabolic diseases as part of the thorough examination.

C. Later developments

Unfortunately, some abnormalities may not become apparent until weeks or even months after birth. This period can be extremely trying for parents who may suspect an abnormality but are unable to identify specific symptoms, or those who must wait for further developments to occur before a condition can be positively diagnosed.

One of the most obvious signs of a possible problem is a failure of the baby to put on weight, accompanied by limited periods of activity. This failure to thrive may indicate a physical problem, but not necessarily. Prolonged delay in a child passing milestones of development, such as sitting up, crawling, walking, and talking may suggest some degree of retardation. Parents are best advised to seek medical opinion if they feel there may be something 'wrong' with their child. If necessary, seek out a professional in the area of your concern.

Possible treatments of congenital abnormalities

The types of treatment of congenital abnormalities and the levels of success of such treatments are dependent on the form and severity of the abnormality.

A. Surgery

Neonatal surgery is a very specialized field of medicine. The newborn's body systems are extremely small, and they are highly susceptible to problems such as respiratory problems and bacterial infections. Yet, newborn babies have astonishing abilities to recover from surgery. They heal very quickly, and their bodily systems act more efficiently in some ways than do those of adults.

Many congenital abnormalities can be corrected or relieved through surgery. Most commonly, surgery is used to correct structural defects, such as heart problems and intestinal blockages. Other conditions can also be relieved. The placing of a shunt to relieve pressure in hydrocephaly, and the correcting of a cleft palate and cleft lip or other external abnormalities, such as webbed toes and fingers, are possible. Surgery of a more delicate nature is also being carried out on conditions that were previously untreatable, including liver and heart transplants and 'deep freeze' surgery. Surgery has even been performed on foetuses with congenital abnormalities while they have still been in the uterus.

B. Drug therapy

A number of abnormalities such as some cardiac problems, including Patent Ductus Arteriosis, and metabolic problems, may be relieved through the use of drugs. Some conditions may require lifelong drug treatment.

C. Diet

Some metabolic disorders such as phenylketonuria, the body's inability to digest fats and proteins, or its rejection of carbohydrates, require a specialized diet throughout life to avoid continuing problems and further damage. Some children even must be fed intravenously for a period of time.

D. Continuing physical and educational therapy

With congenital abnormalities that involve neurological impairment or severe physical defects, there is a need for continuing therapy involving physical, social, and educational aspects. Evidence seems to suggest that the earlier intervention occurs the better. Some programs involve stimulation of the brain through a combination of intense physical and educational activities. Doctors, support groups, universities, specialist centres, and neonatal units may be able to provide training programs or contacts with such programs in local areas.

Emotional reactions to abnormalities

The intensity of parents' emotional reactions to an abnormality in a child depends on a number of factors. These include whether or not there has been prior knowledge of a possible problem, the severity of the abnormality, the prognosis, the experience of the couple with abnormalities, and the type of abnormality.

The news of an abnormality may come as a terrible shock to parents who are expecting a normal, healthy child. This idealized child, who has lived in their minds throughout pregnancy, has suddenly become a child 'with a problem', whose future may be affected by this problem. Their dreams of the birth and the nurturing of their perfect child in the days after birth are shattered. The child may be placed in intensive-care facilities and may have to undergo involved medical procedures, including perhaps surgery, during the time that was supposed to be so blissfully happy.

Parents who find out about the abnormality prior to birth through routine tests or tests specially indicated from their past history are also shocked. Even if there has been a child born previously with the same condition, and couples intellectually acknowledge a possible repetition, deep in their hearts many don't want to accept this possibility. Hence, the news of an abnormality still comes as a shock.

Whenever parents find out about an abnormality, whether it is before, at, or after birth, shock and disbelief are common. These parents grieve. They grieve a very significant loss. They grieve the loss of their 'perfect' child, their dreams, and their hopes for that child. They may grieve the loss of a future in which they are in control, since they realize that their own freedom will be affected by the demands of their child. They may also grieve a loss of a sense of themselves as 'pure', feeling that in some way they must also be 'defective'. They also grieve the loss of enjoying birth and infancy as others do.

In cases where the abnormality is fairly minor and able to be corrected, this grief may be soon resolved. For other couples, whose child suffers from a severe abnormality, grief may go on for many years. For example, the parents of a severely retarded child may feel some renewed grief as their child fails to reach each significant milestone at a time comparable to other children.

If the abnormality is severe enough to cause death, the couple must then grieve as do other couples whose child dies. Their grief may be even more intense when this same child has survived prior surgery and other difficult treatment. The parents may then have to experience their grief when they are already emotionally drained by such experiences. They may feel further remorse at having put their child through this pain with no result.

Being confronted with the news of an abnormality is traumatic, and breaking the news must be handled with care. Ideally the news should be delivered to both parents together, who are then able to support each other at this time. It should be delivered by the doctor whom the couple know, or who is in charge of their child's case with the support of the known doctor. Parents need a simple, direct explanation of the problem and what will be done. They may be unable to absorb too much detail initially when they must face the shock of the news. An openness to questions and greater detail will be appreciated by them at a later time.

> We were so excited about James. He was such a beautiful baby. When they came and told us that there was a problem with his heart it was so hard to take. He seemed so alert and well. I know the doctor was talking, but I can't remember much of what he said. It just kept going through my mind 'He might die! He might die!' We had to get the doctor to repeat everything he had said later on. At that time my brain just couldn't take it all in.

Some parents may try to deny that their child suffers from some abnormality, particularly when the baby appears alert and contented. They may fantasize about treatment making their child 'as good as new', when treatment will only improve the abnormality, not completely cure it. When frustrated, unrealistic expectations can lead to intense depression and anger toward the doctors, who are unable to fulfil the parents' fantasies. The parents may become angry at themselves, their partner, or their family if there is a traceable genetic abnormality. They may even feel angry at the child himself/herself. This is normal grieving.

> When I realized that the problem was carried by me, I felt devastated. I was angry with myself for carrying it and at my family for having the problem. I was specially angry at my mother, who never told me about this strange thing that had been in our

family. It was a kind of skeleton in the cupboard. If only she'd told us . . .

Depression is also normal. The circumstances surrounding the birth may help to make depression more intense. Instead of the greetings and enthusiasm following a normal delivery, the birth of a child with an abnormality may be greeted by uneasy silence from others. Most are unsure of what to say, whether to offer congratulations or condolences. Rather than risk upsetting the couple or fearing seeing the child with the abnormality, people stay away, further increasing the isolation of the couple and making them feel even more undesirable.

The couple may already feel extremely self-conscious about being the parents of a deformed child. They, along with others, may fear abnormality and hence even 'fear' this child. At times, this fear may leave the parents feeling unable to relate to the child. Some couples may refuse to see or hold their child.

If the abnormality is life-threatening, such a reaction may also be based on the wish not to get too close to a child who is going to die, for fear that attachment will make the parting more difficult. There is a possibility of the parents rejecting this child. This is more common in situations where the abnormality is severe and obvious, such as in anencephaly. Part of the rejection may also be rooted in the feelings of guilt or failure the parents are experiencing. Seeing their child may only remind them of their involvement in the conception of this child. Staff gently encourage couples to see their child to prevent this rejection, realizing that the reality is often much easier to bear than the imagined appearance. Obvious abnormalities are, where possible, camouflaged by the wrap in which the baby is held. On seeing the baby, parents are often relieved at the sight of their child, whose facial features and body are often near perfect. Many parents remove the wrap to see the abnormality, but this must be their own decision. As they spend time with their child and the abnormality becomes familiar, they are often able to relate to the child as a child in his/her own right.

Their acceptance or rejection of their child is often influenced by their feelings about abnormality. If the prospect is abhorrent to them, acceptance may come only slowly or never at all. Acceptance of a child with an abnormality is not a process that comes immediately to all. Some need to grieve for a period of time before they can concentrate on their child rather than themselves. Parents should never be forced or pressured into contact with their child, for this may lead to further feelings of guilt for being a 'heartless parent'. Such guilt may hinder, rather than enhance, the acceptance of the child. Gentle encouragement and open shows of acceptance of the child by staff and relatives will be of greater help in this regard.

> They told me my baby had a problem that meant he would die. He was grossly deformed. The doctor explained what he would look like, and asked me if I wanted to hold him. I said 'No'. I just couldn't face the thought of this horrible creature I had in my mind. They told me they would welcome me in the nursery any time if I changed my mind. I felt kind of dirty that I could have produced such a monster. Then I felt so awful because everyone else was so concerned about him. Every day, for the two days he lived, the nurse would come and tell me how he was. By the afternoon of the second day, I decided to see him. I was really scared. The nurse knew I was coming. I waited while one of them wrapped him up. She was talking to him and smiling at him. She said he was everyone's favourite. She didn't seem bothered by how he looked. When they gave him to me only his face was showing. He had beautiful eyes. He seemed to look at me. My arms were shaking. I held him for about ten minutes. He certainly wasn't beautiful, but I was glad I'd seen him. I'll always remember those eyes. I gave him a name then — Peter — because of those eyes.

At times, parents are hardly able to recover from the shock of the news before they are required to make difficult decisions. Immediate surgery may be necessary, and parental consent must be gained. Parents must weigh up the advantages and disadvantages of the surgery. Where it is urgent, the parents may feel out of control, as everything seems to be happening so fast. Fathers whose partners have had a caesarean section may be confronted by such major decisions while they also worry about the partner who may not even be fully aware of the drama. Crisis seems to follow crisis, and the emotional energy of parents is drained.

> After Catherine was born they soon realized she had a heart problem that needed surgery. Jill was not fully aware for 24 hours or so, and was in a lot of pain. I wanted to be with her, but

Catherine needed me too. They decided to transport her to another hospital on the other side of town for the surgery. Jill was almost hysterical about not being with Catherine, and I couldn't stay to calm her as the ambulance was waiting. I felt so torn and hassled. Everything was happening too fast. I felt like screaming: 'Stop! Hang on a minute! Let me get myself together first!'

For parents the waiting can seem interminable. Tests are often carried out to confirm a suspected diagnosis and determine treatment and prognosis. They take time, leaving the parents trying to accept the worst while desperately hoping for the best. Then there is the waiting to determine the success or otherwise of surgery or other treatment. For some there is the waiting to die.

In some cases, the abnormality is of such a nature that death is inevitable. Death may come quickly. For others, the child may survive for a period of days or weeks. In some cases the waiting can go on for months. In extremely serious conditions where imminent death is likely, the parents may request the withholding of all treatment that may simply prolong life for a short period, and allow only attention to basic survival needs. At times, they must decide whether or not to remove life-support systems. Parents of a severely affected child may even pray for death, for an end to the suffering of their child, as well as their own suffering. These feelings may frighten them. They may feel guilty and even ghoulish, wondering what kind of parents they are to wish their own child's death. When death does occur after they have refused life-prolonging treatment, they may also feel guilt, wondering if they made the right decision.

At times, parents feel guilty about other normal reactions involved in grieving. When death is inevitable, parents often grieve before the actual event. In this way they share the same reactions as those who face their own death or the loss of a loved one through terminal illness. If grief is allowed to proceed in an atmosphere of support and encouragement, the parents may come to accept the inevitable loss. Doctor Kübler-Ross outlines the stage in which there is a process of 'letting go'. There is a movement away from the intense preoccupation with the child. Some parents may feel this emotionally as a lowering of the intensity of their feelings about the child and his/her impending death. Some may visit less frequently, yet show a great deal of caring with each visit. This is not rejection of the child, but rather a fuller acceptance of the situation and a means of coping with the loss that is to come. Each parent may reach this stage at different times, which can lead to conflict. For example, the parent who arrives at this point may seem uncaring and cold to the other parent still intensely involved with his/her grief. The latter may see the less frequent visits and the reduced need to talk about the baby as not caring or not loving the child. Anger may result, and the other in turn may feel guilty for being a 'bad parent'. Astute family, friends, and hospital staff who are aware of such variations in grief, can often help to ease such conflicts by reassuring parents that their individual feelings are normal.

Where the abnormality is not life-threatening, the parents must face a future in which there may be some difficulties for their child and their whole family. In some instances there may be a need for an operation or a series of operations to correct or relieve the problem. Difficulties of repeated hospitalizations, recuperation, and separations must be dealt with. With the birth of a more seriously affected child, the new parents may have to face significant changes to their lifestyle and their family structure. Contemplating these changes can be extremely difficult.

If the parents have had no previous contact with a handicapped child, they may be unaware of the practical difficulties that may present themselves until the child is released to their personal care. Feeding difficulties may mean that days are simply filled with feeding, washing, and preparing for feeding. In time they may become aware of the limits of their child's abilities, and in the rare moments available for reflection, they may fear for their child's and family's future. In times of depression and extreme fatigue that occur, they may resent this child who puts such demands on them and has changed their life so drastically. Tiredness, constant effort, and a lack of time for even the most ordinary or personal tasks can leave the parents feeling extremely depressed. They may find their own relationship becoming strained by the constant pressure under which they find themselves. In fact, the breakdown rate of marriages among couples who have a child with an abnormality is high.

In some cases of abnormality — particularly mental retardation, blindness, or deafness — the abnormality may not be noticed immediately at birth. It is often a mother, who spends so much time with the child, who first suspects that there may be a problem. Often she keeps her concerns private at first, not wanting to acknowledge the problem, hoping she is wrong. Yet when she can ignore the problem no longer and voices her concerns, she may be treated offhandedly by others, leaving her feeling as if she is being 'neurotic'. When symptoms are vague, this may be a more likely reaction.

In some cases, parents are painted a pessimistic picture of their child's prognosis. There have been many cases of children who were expected to be little more than 'vegetables', who developed skills allowing them to function fairly competently as individuals. At times, handicapped children are limited by the negative expectations and behaviour of others. There is often a concentration on what they can't do, rather than on what they can do. Doctors can only speculate on the future abilities of an abnormal child. These speculations must not be considered absolute dictates. Early intervention programs set up by educationists are proving many of these early speculations incorrect. Yet parents should not disregard the speculations of doctors, for their words are based on experience. Unreal expectations of the child, even positive ones, can be harmful to both child and parents. Doctors need to provide parents with simple, direct statements of what is known about the condition, while emphasizing to parents the highly individual nature of each case and the broad range of possibilities.

Parents who must face the situation of their child requiring extended treatment or immediate surgery must deal with the added feelings of helplessness and powerlessness. How difficult it is to see and hear your child in such pain! Little eyes seem to plead for the pain to stop.

Some parents may find themselves unable to cope with their child and his/her abnormality. They may have found difficulty in coping with their lives before the birth, or may have little or no support. Realizing that they can't cope can be extremely difficult for them to accept. They may resent this child who is so demanding and makes them feel more inadequate. There may come a time when the needs of all involved are best served by the child being institutionalized or put into foster or adoptive care. Such a decision can leave the parents feeling extremely guilt-ridden. Parents need understanding and support when faced with such a decision. If practical home-support is all that is lacking, then provision of this may avert the situation. It is easy for others, who don't have to live under such pressure constantly, to criticize parents for needing a period of relief from a severely affected child. Instead of practical assistance, they offer criticism.

Parents who are informed that their child will be, or has been, born with an abnormality have a loss to grieve. They require understanding of their feelings and support from those around them, from the time the news is delivered on through perhaps a lifetime, as they battle to prevent this problem destroying the hope and contentment of themselves and their child.

Coping with abnormality

It would be impossible here to try to discuss the ways in which people cope with rearing a handicapped child. We shall simply discuss here coping in those first few difficult weeks after birth.

1. Allow yourself to grieve

Parents of an abnormal child do have a loss to grieve and hence a right to grieve. They have a right to feel shocked, numb, angry, and depressed. They should express their feelings as they occur. Cry or scream or talk! Even when the problem is able to be corrected, it is acceptable to feel depressed at being separated from one's child or being in this situation. If the abnormality will affect their child over time, the parents need to accept that grief may return even when others feel that they 'should be over it by now'.

2. Get to know your child

In this case the old saying 'Familiarity breeds contempt' is quite wrong. The more time parents spend with their child, the more the individual child, rather than the abnormality, will become the foremost feature. In fact, in time the abnormality may even 'disappear' in the eyes of the parents, although it remains obvious to others around. If death is inevitable, the parents may then have beautiful memories to cherish, rather than feelings of distaste and fear. Knowing the child may even help the parents come to accept death more peacefully. When the child's life is not threatened, knowing the child can help to put the situation into a more optimistic perspective and help parents to find some hope for the future.

3. Concentrate on what your child can do, not what he or she can't do

The innate potential of *any* child is an unknown quantity at birth. This is particularly true of the child born with an abnormality. A too-pessimistic picture painted of such a child can cloud parental reactions to that child. Children, even those with no abnormality, will perform at a level expected of them by significant people in their lives. An optimistic but realistic view of the child, with a concentration on enhancing the skills he/she can develop while seeking to improve his/her diminished capabilities, may be the best therapy a parent can offer a child battling an abnormality.

4. Seek out as much information as possible on the condition

A sound knowledge of the characteristics, the problems, the limitations, the possibilities, and the treatments of a condition, provides the parents with a firm foundation on which they can make decisions concerning their child. Doctors are often the first source of such information. Others are also available, such as social workers, State health departments, support groups, educational establishments specializing in such handicaps, disabled persons' organizations, education, psychology, or medical faculties of universities, major children's hospitals, and other parents.

5. If necessary, seek out a genetic counsellor

Couples whose child's abnormality was of a genetic nature may feel great anxiety that the condition may recur in subsequent pregnancies. In many cases, specialized people in the field of genetics (genetic counsellors) can give couples an informed opinion on the possibility of such a recurrence. Their opinion is based on their knowledge of the chromosome structure and the rules of inheritance that nature appears to follow. As we have already discussed, they cannot guarantee a particular outcome. Unfortunately, each new pregnancy is a gamble. The parents must take the final gamble, but they can be armed with the knowledge of whether or not their chances of a favourable outcome are high.

6. Meet with other parents of children with abnormalities

The easiest way of finding parents who have faced or are facing a similar situation is through support groups. Most States have support groups for parents whose child has a particular abnormality. Support groups concerned with more common abnormalities are only too happy to welcome parents of children with rarer abnormalities, who are not able to find support groups concerned with their specific problem. The abnormalities may differ, but the support needed and the feelings expressed are the same for parents. People outside major centres are kept in contact with others through regular newsletters. These groups not only aim to provide support and encouragement, but also offer up-to-date information on the condition and its treatment. Other parents of children with the same abnormality are usually better able to understand the feelings, fears, frustrations, and practical needs of the family of such a child.

7. Make time for your partner and other children

A child with an abnormality requiring constant care or treatment can be extremely time-consuming. It is easy when under such pressure to forget one's partner or other children. Other family members may then feel rejected and resentful of the child who requires all a parent's attention. Parents need to make a conscious effort to set aside specific times during the day for each individual child in the family. Parents, too, need time simply to spend together, to build up their relationship, to spoil each other with love and attention. This is more than making the other feel good; this is survival! Finding time to do this can be difficult, hence the importance of the next suggestion.

8. Ask for help and relief

The birth of a child with an abnormality does not automatically endow the parents of such a child with superhuman powers. They remain mortal! An affected child can be extremely demanding of parents. Some people need assistance in their homes even to run a 'normal' family. It should therefore come as no surprise if the family of a child with an abnormality requires some assistance in the practical aspects of care and in the emotional aspects of coping. Ask for help without shame! If parents are fortunate, family and friends may offer help without asking. Don't refuse it out of pride! Those who offered may feel rejected and never ask again, even at times when it is obvious that one could use such help. Neighbours and community groups such as service clubs and church groups may be only too pleased to be able to provide parents with some relief.

Besides practical help, parents under such pressure need understanding and a listening ear. At times, they may even need some help from a counsellor skilled in the area of crisis intervention or relationships. Don't be ashamed of needing help! The difficulties of having an abnormal child are more than enough reason for feeling strained. Counselling is to prevent problems becoming insurmountable at a later time.

9. Know yourself, and your limitations

The parents of a child with an abnormality have suffered a severe blow to their self-esteem. Even when assured that the event could have happened to anyone, they may still feel that they are in some way defective or faulty. They may feel inferior to those around them who have healthy 'normal' children. They may also feel guilt toward their child for 'having done this terrible thing to them'. To try to make up in some way for their perceived mistake, they may try to overcompensate for the loss. To the outside world they may show a front of extreme efficiency and an amazing ability to cope with the problems. No cracks appear in the facade, in public at least. The parents may deny their right to grieve because they were the cause of the problem. In cases of genetic abnormalities this feeling may be stronger in the partner through whom the anomaly was transferred to the child.

Yet parents are not superhuman, devoid of emotion and needing no one. But it is often difficult for them to recognize their own limitations and accept help. The parents of a child with an abnormality, particularly a severe one, often have little time to sit quietly and get in touch with their own feelings about themselves, their child, and the situation, without the interference of others and society in general. Knowing one's self, needs, feelings, values, and emotions can help in dealing successfully in relationships with one's child, partner, and others.

10. Try to ignore society's concept of 'handicap'

It is difficult for the parents of a child with an obvious abnormality to cope with the stares and guarded whispers of a society which finds it difficult to accept any deviation from what is considered 'normal' and 'acceptable'. This is particularly true in the case of parents who are battling with feelings of inferiority, and have not yet fully accepted their child's abnormality themselves. They can become withdrawn, depressed, or angry. Parents may need to develop a new perspective for viewing everyday thoughtless incidents. They need to do this for their own sake and that of their child. A new perspective comes by first accepting that society is often wrong in its attitudes. Many, including the sick and the mentally disturbed, have suffered wrongly at the hands of others throughout history. Their illness was seen as a punishment or demonic possession. Although intellectually we realize today that this is not the case, perhaps many in society still hold unconscious thoughts of some 'evil' involvement in abnormality. Many in society also need to bolster their own feelings of inferiority by comparing themselves favourably with the person with an abnormality, and feeling pity. Perhaps the greatest gift the parents of a child with an abnormality can give their child is an understanding of society's inability to cope with 'special' people, combined with a pride in themselves and their worthiness. This gift can only be given by parents who themselves have come to accept their child's innate value and the problems of society. Understanding and acceptance, rather than anger, will provide their child with the best chance of being accepted into society. Contact with other parents of abnormal children and handicapped people themselves can provide parents with a glimpse of such a new perspective.

A new pregnancy

For a couple who have had one child with an abnormality, the prospect of a new pregnancy is often frightening, particularly where doctors suspect that the abnormality was more than a chance event. These feelings they share with other couples who have suffered a loss in pregnancy. What if it happens again?

Where tests are available to detect the abnormality in the first half of pregnancy, the period of waiting for testing can be very trying. Couples may be afraid to become attached to this new life, for fear that they may have to face the prospect of an induced abortion or a death due to abnormality. Waiting for actual test results can bring days, or even weeks, of sleeplessness and tension. Every change in the pregnant state may be viewed suspiciously.

> I had only met Jenny a few times. I didn't know about her daughter having had Trisomy 18. With this condition the mother is at times very large, due to an excess of fluid. She was 31 weeks' pregnant at the time with her next child. It was winter, and being fairly short she looked quite large. In small talk I asked her when she was due. When she said nine weeks, I said 'You will be a size!' She was very put back by this remark, and explained about the fear of excess fluid and recurring Trisomy 18. She handled it well, but it must have upset her. I just wished I could have fallen through the floor.

If test results indicate no abnormality, the couple may feel extremely relieved. Yet they may still harbour some doubts, unable to truly believe there is no problem until after their child is born.

The couple who fear another abnormality are, like other couples who have lost, offered a clear-cut choice: They either try again or don't try again! There is no option of trying again with the certainty of a favourable outcome.

Very difficult decisions

Because of modern refinements and advancements in the medical treatment of neonates, many babies with abnormalities who would have died in the past are able to be saved. When we consider this development, together with the debates surrounding abortion and the rights of the child to life, the expense of treating severe abnormalities, and the debate about euthanasia and quality of life, we can soon see that parents and doctors are often faced with an extremely difficult task. In 1973, two doctors in America wrote an article in *The New England Journal of Medicine* in which they admitted to the withholding of treatment from abnormal babies until they died, as a management option.[10] In the early 1980s a case known as the case of Baby Jane Doe highlighted the legal and emotional aspects of such cases. Baby Jane Doe was a Long Island child born with spina bifida, whose parents refused operations to close the spine and insert a shunt. The US federal government sought to review the medical records of the baby to decide if she was being discriminated against. After losing a number of court battles, the federal government altered legislation on child abuse to include as abuse denial of medical treatment or nutrition to infants born with life-threatening conditions. Treatment considered necessary did not include the mere prolonging of the process of dying. Although this case occurred in the United States, Australia must also consider the legal, ethical, moral, social, and emotional aspects of the question of whether or not infants born with treatable or manageable handicaps should be 'allowed' to die. The issue will not disappear. It is already with us.

A second development involves the refinement of tests able to detect abnormalities early in pregnancy. If an abnormality is found, do the couple continue with the pregnancy or seek an induced abortion? This brings parents and doctors right into the middle of the abortion controversy. In most States of Australia the presence of certain severe abnormalities is recognized as grounds for a legal induced abortion. There is a striking difference between the couple who face an abortion on the grounds of an abnormality and those who undergo the procedure as a means of terminating an unwanted pregnancy; the first couple often wanted this child and this pregnancy a great deal. Deciding to undergo a test for the abnormality has often been a difficult decision for couples to make. They realize that they may then be faced with deciding what to do from there.

Whereas terminations generally occur before three months, couples who must wait on the use of amniocentesis may have the test done at 15 to 16 weeks. They may have to wait another two to three weeks for results, by which time many have begun to notice foetal movements. Suddenly this 'baby', up till now an intellectual idea, is a distinct reality. The mother may be 'showing', which then makes it so much more difficult for her as she waits for the results of the tests. Others around her may enthuse about this new child. How alone she feels, as she may smile sweetly, realizing that she may have to face either an induced abortion or the birth of an abnormal child. Knowing of the existence of an abnormality and deciding to continue with a pregnancy can be a very difficult and painful decision. Some couples will elect to continue with the pregnancy on religious, moral, or other grounds. For this reason, many doctors advise against having the tests for abnormalities unless the couple plan to take the action of seeking an induced abortion if an abnormality is indicated.

Fortunately, only about five per cent of foetuses tested show an abnormality. Tests may therefore be very comforting for a couple who have had a prior affected child, for the mother who has contracted a severe case of rubella or other virus, or for one who has been exposed to serious environmental hazards or drugs.

The range of abnormalities able to be detected by tests is limited. Some conditions, such as some genetic conditions that are known to be sex-linked, cannot be confirmed, but only suspected, in a male child. Hence, the couple who find out that the child is male must then decide whether or not to risk having a son with the abnormality or risk aborting an unaffected child, which would leave them with severe feelings of guilt and frustration.

A couple who decide on an induced abortion may feel very strongly about the word 'abortion'. They may morally reject the idea of abortion as a means of terminating an unwanted pregnancy, and may fear that others will assume that they didn't want their baby or only looked for 'the easy way out'.

Many couples who face an induced abortion report to friends and family that they have had a miscarriage, and may even invent a feasible set of circumstances to surround such an event. They must therefore hide their real feelings, further extending and complicating their grief. Many fear being 'found out' and shamed, not only for undergoing an abortion but also for conceiving a 'defective' child.

The actual induced abortion itself is a terribly traumatic experience. Labour may be induced for a more advanced pregnancy, while a dilation and evacuation may be used in early pregnancy. The actual labour may be more painful, as it is associated with a great deal of grief, fear, and anxiety. Hospitalization can also complicate matters if staff are not well informed. Attempts to monitor a foetal heart, or the presence of normal delivery equipment or cribs in the room, can be very distressing for the mother.

Dignified treatment of the foetus after delivery is still vital to the couple, for it was still 'their child'. Whether or not the couple see the foetus must be their decision, and such a situation must be handled very carefully. Many are simply relieved that the incident is over, and wish to forget. Others are relieved to see that although there is an abnormality, their child is not the hideous malformed creature they may have imagined.

Unfortunately, the incident is not fully over. The mother's breasts and vaginal discharge remind her of the child. The couple who have had to face an induced abortion encounter many of the same feelings as those who face a miscarriage, but their grief is often compounded with extreme guilt, intense isolation, a destructive blow to their self-esteem, and a fear of a recurrence in future pregnancies.

In both of the above situations, the parents are forced to make a decision of great complexity at a time when, due to shock and grief, they are least able to make such a decision with which they are sure they will always feel comfortable. Community leaders, experts in ethics and morals, theologians, lawyers, vocal organizations, and governments may heatedly debate the issue, often from the comfort of their own life-situation unaffected by handicap. Community discussion is important, but should be accompanied by a willingness on the part of the community to become involved financially, practically, and emotionally with the difficulties of the parents who must make these very difficult decisions and possibly face the financial, emotional, and physical burdens of rearing a child with a severe abnormality. In other words, our society must be concerned not only with its rights but also with its responsibilities.

Conclusion

The birth of a child with an abnormality often comes as a terrible shock to parents who grieve the loss of their 'perfect' child. A small proportion of babies born will be severely affected, although the range of severity of abnormalities is large. Many will be able to be treated successfully. A small group will be affected moderately or severely throughout their lives. Such a situation can place a great deal of strain on all family members. Parents and child require understanding, support, and acceptance from those around them, while living in a society which has itself not successfully come to terms with the concept of 'handicap' or 'abnormality'.

References

1. David I. Tudehope and M. John Thearle, A Primer of Neonatal Medicine (Brisbane: William Brooks, 1984), 109.
2. Hank Pizer and Christine O'Brien Palinski, Coping with a Miscarriage (London: Jill Norman, 1980), 59–64.
3. David Harvey (ed.), A New Life: Pregnancy, Birth and Your Child's First Year (London: Marshall Cavendish, 1982), 38,39.
   Gordon Bourne, Pregnancy (London: Pan Books, 1979), 237–242.
   Derek Llewellyn-Jones, Fundamentals of Obstetrics and Gynaecology, Vol. 1, Obstetrics (London: Faber and Faber, 1982), 444,445.
4. ibid., 254.
5. ibid., 255.
6. Tudehope et al., op.cit., 59,60.
7. Cystic Fibrosis: A Summary of Symptoms, Diagnosis and Treatment (booklet prepared by the Cystic Fibrosis Association of NSW, Burwood NSW).
8. Australian Spina Bifida Association, Spina Bifida: A Handbook for Parents (South Australia: Australian Spina Bifida Association, 1982), 6.
9. Penny Wolf, 'Chorionic Villus Biopsy: The Earlier Test for Genetic Disorders', Parents and Children, Jan./July 1985, 13–15.
10. Raymond Duff and A.G.M. Campbell, 'Moral and Ethical Dilemmas in the Special Care Nursery', The New England Journal of Medicine, 1973, 289,890–894.

8 When You Are Disappointed More Than Once

The loss of a child in pregnancy is a terrible blow to the prospective parents. A new pregnancy is then thwarted with fears and anxiety. Fortunately, for most couples who experience a loss, their new pregnancy will produce a live, healthy child, and their fears and anxiety are soon dispelled.

But there is a small group of couples who will experience a number of losses. A period of infertility may be followed by, or follow, a perinatal death; a series of miscarriages may occur; or a stillbirth may follow a previous premature labour. Fortunately, this will happen only to a small number of couples. It is to these couples that this chapter is dedicated. It is difficult enough to find courage to try once more, but to have to find it over and over, is, in a word, devastating. For some, it becomes too much, and they don't try again.

The medical literature often discusses losses as singular entities that are in themselves ripples on the surface of a reproductive history. It is reasonable to assume for most couples that their sad event will not recur. Hence, there is cause for optimism in a later pregnancy. But when there are a number of losses, the words of encouragement seem to have a hollow ring to them. It is little comfort to a couple who have been part of the small percentage who lose a number of children, to be told that each pregnancy is a new one and that statistics are on their side this time. Many of the statistics quoted concerning certain losses in pregnancy involve the same couples in a number of figures. Pregnancy losses are not necessarily spread evenly among the population; many experience no losses, while others seem to have an unreasonable share of them. When you have become a statistic that brings such unhappiness, figures and general trends mean little.

In this chapter we wish to discuss the intense feelings that are part of such a couple's life when they lose more than once. These couples know personally what the words fear, pain, and tension mean. They require special care and understanding, and some recognition of just how much emotional strength it requires for them to try yet again.

Possible causes of repeated losses

The repeated losses couples must experience are generally due to a combination of factors, or are a mystery to all involved. It is virtually impossible to give a list of definite causes of repeated losses. The histories of such losses can be so varied. For example, some losses all occur at approximately the same stage of pregnancy, while in other cases couples experience infertility followed by miscarriage, stillbirth, or abnormality. Some losses may be related to others, while other losses may be completely independent of each other. In cases where losses are varied, it is best to refer to the specific chapters on those different losses for their possible causes. Often the basic cause is simply bad luck, fate, or whatever you may call a series of disasters. Here we shall look at factors that may contribute to repeated losses.

1. Chronic maternal disease

Some chronic diseases, if not treated and controlled during pregnancy, can lead to an increased possibility of losing a child.

a) Diabetes

Today diabetes can be effectively controlled. It is of vital importance that strict control of the diabetes be maintained during pregnancy if a baby is to be successfully carried through to term. Insulin dosages may require modification, but with constant careful medical supervision repeated disasters need not occur.

b) Chronic hypertension

Raised blood pressure is unusual in a normal healthy woman of child-bearing age, unless it is the result of some chronic condition. Hypertension can reduce the blood supply to the uterus and the placenta. If this occurs, the baby can, at best, be small and dysmature, and, at worst, may be lost. The danger is increased if pre-eclampsia begins to develop. A woman must be extremely careful during her pregnancy to rest and avoid increased blood pressure. If this is achieved, success may be likely. Once again, it must be stressed that she remain under the constant supervision of her doctor.

c) Chronic kidney disease

Chronic kidney conditions, such as chronic nephritis, can predispose a woman and child to danger. Once again, a doctor will monitor such a pregnancy closely.

d) Untreated venereal disease

VD, particularly syphilis, can be serious, as this disease can affect the foetus from the twentieth week of pregnancy and cause damage to the child, and even death. It is a curable disease through the administration of antibiotics, and hence, where suspected, should be tested early in antenatal care.

2. Tendency to develop pre-eclampsia

Pre-eclampsia is characterized by a raised blood pressure, excessive swelling of the feet, ankles, or hands (oedema), the presence of protein in the urine, and commonly an excessive weight-gain in pregnancy. It is seldom seen before the twentieth week of pregnancy, and can usually be diagnosed before any severe problems arise if regular antenatal checks are being carried out. The height of the mother's blood pressure indicates the danger to the babe. Premature labour may occur or premature delivery may be effected to save the lives of mother and baby. This may put the child at risk. Once again, careful monitoring is necessary. Pre-eclampsia usually occurs only in a first pregnancy. If it does recur in a subsequent pregnancy, it is likely to be less severe.

3. Uterine structural defects

Some women are born with congenital abnormalities in the structure of the uterus, and these can contribute to repeated losses. Other abnormalities can occur after prior intervention, or may develop naturally.

a) Uterine tumours

Although they are extremely rare, it is obvious that malignant tumours in the uterus are a danger not only to the child but also to the mother. Life-saving treatments are required. More commonly, benign or non-cancerous tumours, commonly known as fibroids, have been suspected as a cause of repeated losses.[1] Unfortunately, evidence is inconclusive, since many women with fibroids carry a pregnancy successfully. They may be significant in the losses of some women, but not others. It is felt that what may be important is not how large these fibroids are, but their position in the uterus in relation to the pregnancy.

b) Müllerian abnormalities

During the development of the female foetus, the uterus is formed when two tubal structures, Müllerian ducts, join together. Malformations may occur during this development. A unicornate, bicornate, or septate uterus may result. See Chapter 4 for more details on these conditions. In a mildly bicornate (or heart-shaped) uterus, the uterus is stretched with each new pregnancy and is better able to accommodate a pregnancy. Eventually a pregnancy will reach near or full term. Doctors may prefer this natural course of correction rather than surgery. Unfortunately, babies may be lost before the condition is corrected. Once again, these abnormalities seem to be significant in some women and not others.

c) Asherman's Syndrome

Sometimes, after a too-aggressive curetting or uterine surgery, or as a result of pelvic infection, the wall of the uterus can be scarred. Fibrous tissue (known as adhesions) may develop. Such adhesions can obstruct the uterine wall and make implantation of a fertilized egg difficult, leading to early miscarriage.

4. Hormonal imbalance

Insufficient levels of progesterone and other hormones have been suspected as causes for miscarriage, as we have seen in Chapter 4. Their effects, if any, on repeated losses are debatable.

5. Rhesus incompatibility

In Chapter 4 we discussed Rhesus incompatibility as it pertained to possible causes of miscarriage. It is also believed that incompatibility may be a factor in repeated losses.

6. Tendency to premature labour

Some women, because of problems such as an incompetent cervix or excessive uterine irritability, are inclined to go into premature labour, leading to such dangers for the child as are involved in premature delivery. A number of women tend to go into premature labour for no discernible reason. One such episode can suggest that such an event may recur. Therefore these women must be monitored carefully in later pregnancies. A lack of the hormone relaxin in the systems of such women is also believed to be a possible cause.

7. Genetic anomalies

As has been discussed, either the mother or father may carry a gene that may produce in a child a genetic abnormality. Each pregnancy has a chance of being affected. Hence, successive pregnancies may be lost or an abnormal child delivered. Some congenital, non-inherited problems are more likely to recur in a couple who have previously had a child with the complaint. Today, through tests such as amniocentesis, many problems can be diagnosed relatively early in the pregnancy.

8. Possible congenital and environmental problems

Recent research on daughters of women who took DES (diethylstilbestrol) during pregnancy suggests a higher incidence of pregnancy loss in such women than occurs in the general population. This has brought renewed speculation on the possible effects of other drugs prescribed in the past. The effects of pollution, such as bromide, and occupational environments are also under consideration.

9. The body's immune system

A foetus contains some material that is genetically foreign to the mother's system, since it is that of the father. Yet, the immune system generally does not reject the foetus, as it does other foreign substances that enter the body. The mother's body produces a substance that stops rejection of the foetus. This has been called the 'blocking factor'. As yet, research into this area is in its infant stages, but shows promise. Could some women have a lack of blocking factor that causes the body to reject the foetus? Could women who experience long periods of infertility, followed by pregnancy loss, have an immune system that is determined to reject the male's genetic code wherever it is found? This is an area that may lead to exciting new developments.

10. 'Cause unknown'

Unfortunately for many, the causes behind successive pregnancy losses are not clear and can only be speculated on. Medical knowledge is not exhaustive. The human body is a complicated, awe-inspiring working system. In some cases of repeated losses, the causes will remain a mystery. But generally at least one pregnancy will overcome the difficulties and produce a live baby, and so the couple do not need to lose hope completely.

Emotional reactions to repeated losses

Fortunately, most couples embarking on a first pregnancy do not know about most of the complications that can arise. They then enjoy the experience. From the time the news is received that the woman is pregnant, many couples begin to think about babies' names and a nursery. Their days are full of thoughts of a baby, until the day the baby arrives with no problem and their dreams become a reality. Pregnancy is a beautiful, happy time!

However, for a couple who have lost a child once, there is a loss of this innocence, and pregnancy becomes a time of fear and anxiety. Happily, at term this anxiety is alleviated by the birth of a healthy, mature baby. Future pregnancies, though tainted, may recoup some of the happiness.

For the couple who have experienced repeated losses, there is often little joy left in pregnancy. The confirmation of the pregnancy is clouded by a fear of failure.

Marg had experienced two miscarriages and a stillbirth:

> I've become very negative now. I don't feel confident at all in the fact that everything will be all right. I dread pregnancy. We wondered whether we will or not. Let's face it: age is running out, if not run out, on me. We'd like to try again, but I am frightened as to what's going to happen. I think perhaps a man cannot fully understand how you feel.

At times, the couple feel that the question 'Will it work this time?' is even too optimistic. They feel more like asking not 'If . . .?' but 'When will it go wrong this time?' After a few disappointments, hope can be knocked out of them, or, at best, severely shaken.

Many doctors believe in the importance of a positive outlook for a healthy pregnancy, and hence try to encourage optimism in such couples. Words such as 'Cheer up! It'll work this time!' or 'Chin up!' somehow don't help. Optimism is a difficult state of mind for the couple to achieve, as there may be many factors that have contributed to their present feelings of fear and failure. Let's look at some of these factors and their effects on the couple:

1. The couple have had to experience grief over each loss. The months following any loss are very difficult, as we saw by the complexity of the grief process in Chapter 2.

2. These couples have not one loss to contend with, but a number, often within a relatively short period of time.

3. In many cases where an actual foetus is lost, the female feels strongly that she is to blame, not her husband. If the couple are not infertile, she feels that her partner has done his part satisfactorily. After a number of losses, she may develop a distrust of her body. This may sound insignificant, but to lose trust in one's body to perform as expected can be a severe blow. Persons suffering from degenerative diseases in which functions are gradually lost will attest to that fact.

4. Tied closely to distrust of the body is a feeling of failure. The woman may feel that she has failed as a mother, a woman, a wife, and consequently, a person. She can lose complete confidence in herself. Unfortunately, a woman's self-image is often closely tied to her ability to reproduce. Her feelings of failure can generalize into other spheres of her life, such as work and personal relationships. Essentially, she begins to see herself as a womb with a person inside rather than a person with a womb.

5. The whole lifestyle of the couple can be affected. For example, they may delay moving to a new town for a promotion if specialist obstetric care is not available. A woman may take only temporary work in case she falls pregnant again. She may resign from her job so that she can rest for a new attempt. Whole areas of their lives in which they gained self-respect can be lost to them. They can feel that they are living 'in limbo', where whole years of their lives seem to revolve around pregnancy.

6. They may wish to become pregnant, to try again as soon as possible. Hence, they work very hard at attaining this, perhaps too hard. They often fear that they may now be infertile and there will be no more chances. This fear may be linked to past pregnancies. They wonder, for example, what damage may have been done by a D and C, an infection, or a

cervical suture, even when such fears are unfounded. For some, this anxiety may contribute to infertility problems through ineffective sexual intercourse.

7. At times, intercourse may become a mechanical action that must be carried out as planned by the couple according to cycle lengths, temperature, or mucus changes. Intercourse can lose its spontaneity and its meaning as an expression of love, and so affect the participants, their relationship, and its ultimate effectiveness in attaining a pregnancy. The male can resent being called on for what he may see as 'stud' purposes, while the female may be so concerned that he ejaculates that the act is in no way special for her either.

8. Each month in which pregnancy is not achieved, they experience the intense disappointment that follows a month of hope. They also have their fears of infertility renewed.

9. Even when pregnancy is achieved, the couple are more aware of what can go wrong — not just at the particular times when they have lost prior pregnancies, but all the way through a pregnancy to birth and even to the time after birth. Pregnancy then becomes a frightening, stressful experience for them.

10. Many couples who experience repeated losses are yet to have one live child. They can't even be consoled with the thought that they have at least one child to love. They lose children, and they also lose their dreams of the future. If we define infertility as being unable to have a child, then they are actually 'infertile', with its associated strains.

These factors by no means apply to all couples who experience repeated losses. Some couples are able to remain positive. Others are able to divorce pregnancy from the other aspects of their lives. Yet these factors often affect the feelings of such couples. They are listed here to highlight the mixed emotions and stresses that these couples bring to a new pregnancy, usually without the knowledge of the doctor.

By considering these factors, we can perhaps picture the couple who come to see their doctor to embark on yet another pregnancy. They may be two people whose self-confidence has been severely shaken. They are people trying to come to terms with grief during a time when there is intense pressure on their sexual and general relationship. Their whole lives also seem to be in limbo, revolving around the prospect of attaining a pregnancy, which to them is simply another frightening time. When we consider this, is it any wonder that such a couple appear tense and emotional, and find it difficult to accept a doctor's reassurance that all will be well this time? Their past experience may have served to breed in them a cynicism about a medical profession who 'said the same thing last time'.

Once the new pregnancy is confirmed, the couple may find it difficult to feel excited about the prospect. It is a real 'wait and see' game for them. They don't want to be happy, for fear of being hurt once again. Every detail of the pregnancy, no matter how common or innocent, is viewed with suspicion. Any indications of back pain or wind pain are a source of concern. If the baby moves too much or too little, if the mother gains weight too slowly or too quickly, or has a cold, a headache or any discharge, these can all be interpreted as signs for concern.

Unfortunately, others may be inclined simply to label these couples — particularly the female partner — as being 'neurotic' or overstressed when they voice their concerns. Of course, most of their worries are unfounded, but for the welfare of mother and child they should be treated with concern and understanding, for sometimes they do herald problems. To exemplify this possibility, we quote our own case.

After our first miscarriage at 18 weeks, the general practitioner in attendance believed the abortion was complete. We were sent home without a date for a check-up. Fortunately, we had read enough about miscarriage to realize that infection was a possibility, if all the products of conception were not completely removed. Each day Judith recorded her body temperature. Five days later it rose 0.5°C. We immediately headed to the doctor, who was sceptical. He prescribed oral antibiotics 'to be on the safe side'. He felt that there was no problem, but said that we could see the Flying Surgeon, who was coming to town the next day. He doubted if any action would be taken. The surgeon was understanding, but also felt sure there was no problem. He gave us the option of a D and C, which we accepted. After the procedure, the surgeon returned to us shaking his head, and told us that he had taken, in medical terms, copious currettings from the uterus. It is understandable that medically the first doctor did not anticipate trouble. But what affected us more was the impression he gave that he thought that we, particularly Judith, were 'overreacting'. The doctor could see that this was understandable under the circumstances, yet he still instilled the feeling that she was being 'neurotic'. We were continually encouraged by being told: 'Lots of people have one miscarriage'. Later experiences with our second loss engrained the 'neurotic' label in our minds.

Feeling that we must be truly overreacting, in our third pregnancy we were determined not to be so sensitive. We tried hard to ignore these unusual tightenings, sure that our concerns were making them seem more than they really were. When five occurred in the space of an hour at 16 weeks, we rang our obstetrician at home, feeling embarrassed and decidedly 'neurotic'. Instead of openly admitting that we feared something was wrong, we trivialized the whole event, telling the doctor that it was probably nothing but that we just wanted his reassurance. We didn't convey a feeling of anxiety, and hence he didn't realize how strong they had been. He was understanding, and we now know he would not have treated us as 'neurotic'. It is a point to ponder whether or not at this stage the doctor could have been alerted to the fact that all was not well, and the pregnancy managed to a happier ending. We didn't give him the opportunity. We can look back philosophically on quotations of letters from other doctors suggesting that we were 'very apprehensive' and that 'such should never occur again', and wonder.

In referring to these incidents, we are not trying to blame anyone for losses that no one could prevent. What we wish to highlight here is the importance of finding the fine line between overreaction to the situation of repeated losses and real knowledge, perhaps even subconscious knowledge, of the mother that all is not well.

When I started to bleed at 33 weeks, I went straight to the hospital. It had only been a little bit of blood, but somehow I knew all was not well. I couldn't explain my feeling, but it was very real. I begged the doctor to take the baby, but he said he felt it was too early and would wait a few days to see what happened. The bleeding stopped within an hour, and was barely enough to fill a pad. After a week in hospital, during which time nothing more occurred and the baby's heartbeat was strong, I was told I would go home. They had found I had no placenta praevia, and felt there would be no further problem. Still I had this terrible feeling. I begged them to keep me in the hospital and take the baby now. My husband was convinced by staff that this was not the best action, and he took me home. Four days later, I had no movements. It was later found that I had had a massive concealed haemorrhage that day. Somehow I knew all was not well. There wasn't any medical evidence to back up my fears, but I knew, somehow I knew!

Some doctors already respect a woman's intimate relationship with her unborn child. A woman's stress can show on the heartbeat responses of a foetus. Perhaps one day science will be able to show a reverse situation, and a woman's 'intuition' or 'gut feeling' of what is going on with her child will have a scientific basis.

It must be remembered that a woman who has suffered a number of losses has a severely shaken self-confidence. If her concerns are dismissed in an offhand manner, or in a too-optimistic manner not accompanied by medical examination, she may feel that the doctor thinks she is overreacting, and is patronizing her. She may feel this even if it is not the attitude of her doctor. As many doctors will admit, there is often little that can be done medically for couples suffering repeated losses. For these couples, it is the emotional and psychological support that is important. It takes a special doctor who can give honesty, compassion, respect, and hope to such couples all at once. Yet such would be the *second* greatest thing they could offer; a healthy child would always be number one.

By discussing each fear and thoroughly examining the possibilities underlying such fears, the doctor will show these couples that he/she respects their opinions, the woman's knowledge of her own body, and their right to be severely stressed in such a situation. We in no way suggest that every presenting complaint is a sign of trouble. Fortunately, the vast majority arise from an oversensitivity of the woman to her pregnant state. But investigating each complaint cannot harm a doctor and can show respect for a suffering couple. For this effect, the effort is worthwhile. In addition, where there have been repeated losses, signs of trouble must be taken seriously from a medical viewpoint, for these couples have often learnt the real danger signs through bitter experience.

Apart from reacting to physical signs of pregnancy, the couple may try to ward off any possible later feelings of grief by not allowing themselves to expect anything from each pregnancy. They feel that by trying to ignore the pregnancy they can deny their joy and hopes, so that they will not have so far to fall if this one also fails. The couple may, consciously or unconsciously, decide not to discuss the pregnancy or babies' names, or refuse to set up a nursery, until the baby is born. They may not tell anyone of the pregnancy until it is obvious. At times, such an action may be taken to avoid difficult situations. Other people may make well-meaning comments like 'Some people aren't meant to have children' or 'Don't you think you've had enough?' or 'Why don't you let it go for a few years?' or 'Why put yourself through it again?' Such people don't realize just how much courage that couple must find to try again. Instead of being helpful, such comments introduce a feeling of guilt for their being foolhardy or obsessional about having a baby.

The new pregnancy can be beset with fears, lack of sleep, and tension, particularly as each important stage marking prior losses and developmental milestones are reached. The fears can accompany the couple right to the moment of birth. The incredible relief and joy of such couples at producing a live, mature child may not have a parallel anywhere in human happiness. Unfortunately, the previous months and years of anxiety can rob them of some of their ecstasy.

With normal births, many mothers experience post-partum depression or 'baby blues' a few days after the birth. The mother who has had repeated losses prior to this birth may have such depression intensified when her old grief for her 'lost' children is rekindled.

> The second miscarriage I had after the stillbirth was particularly difficult. I had accepted it until I came out of the D and C anaesthetic. I just cracked again. After Michael was born, I cried and cried when I thought of Jonathan. I should have been happy, but I was so upset.

The anticipation of this baby may be followed by a real anticlimax. No event, not even birth, may be able to match the emotional input the couple have put into this baby over months, even years. In extreme instances, the mother can even resent her child because he/she survived while her other children didn't. Such responses are often the result of unresolved grief. This most often occurs when the new pregnancy was embarked on shortly after another loss, as is often the case with couples who suffer repeated losses.

> I think that with all the miscarriages and everything else being in the last six years, I hadn't got over one lot of grief before I started on a new one. It all piled up. I think I only started working on my grief after Damien died. After the death was the first time I'd really been allowed to grieve.

Some couples' grief is never relieved by the joy of the birth of a child. After a series of losses, they are not prepared to be hurt again, and so they don't try again. They feel that emotionally and physically they and their family cannot cope any more.

A man may resist a new pregnancy because he cannot accept his partner, the woman he loves, experiencing the physical and emotional strain she must go through. The male may try to reassure his partner that it doesn't matter to him, when in fact he too may want a family or an addition to it. Some of these couples consciously begin using contraceptive measures, with some even seeking sterilization as a guarantee that the pain will not be repeated. This too is a valid response, but only if the decision is made through careful consideration after grief has been resolved. It is a decision that should not be made when the pain is acute, for it is a decision that either cannot be reversed or takes extreme measures to reverse.

The decision to opt for voluntary childlessness is a very difficult one to make. The couple have a new loss to grieve in addition to their previous losses. They must now also grieve those losses experienced by an infertile couple, the loss of their dreams and their future as they had envisioned it to be. They may also bear a certain resentment for all the time they wasted in pregnancy, only to be still where they started, in a state of childlessness. If a fear of genetic abnormality has prompted the decision, the feelings of self-denigration must also be dealt with. These couples must grieve so many losses before they are able to make plans for the future. A decision for voluntary childlessness is not something one should rush into when grief is new and painful.

> After Damien died, my husband didn't want to try again. So we compromised on trying one more time, and then that was it. When I was in hospital with Shaun, my doctor, after four weeks, said I could go home and rest. We talked about that, and decided because this was our last shot we'd do the best we could, so I stayed. It was a hard decision to make, but I realized I wasn't being fair to Brendan and my husband. Basically we were trying to create a family and destroying the family that we had . . . I made the decision not to have any more children too early for me, as I was really depressed when I did it. I think you need to be unpressured before making such a decision.

Couples, particularly the woman, may harbour a guilt, and because of their shame they may be afraid to discuss it. The woman may feel guilty for the anger, jealousy, and bitterness she may feel toward those who have no problem bearing a child, particularly recent mothers and mothers-to-be. She seems to see pregnant women everywhere, who are excitedly buying nursery equipment and are obviously extremely happy and content in their pregnancies. In her very low moments, she can secretly wish the loss of a baby on a pregnant woman with whom she has contact. It doesn't seem fair that they should have a baby without problems! These types of thoughts are frightening to a woman, and she can feel extremely guilty for wishing harm on another woman and her baby. She begins to wonder what kind of terrible, ghoulish person she is. These feelings are seldom voiced, yet they can cause great distress. There are explanations for these frightening feelings that women, so worn down by stress and grief, may experience. As we recall from Chapter 2, anger is a phase of grief, and it can be directed toward anyone. Such anger may be the cause of these feelings toward other pregnant women. But there may also be another cause.

Women who have suffered repeated losses don't necessarily wish harm on another, but simply wish for the pregnancies of others to disappear, for the world to stop until they achieve their dream of a child. They want some time to catch up on the happiness the rest of the world seems to have. As children, we don't like other children to get a treat first when they were behind us in the line. They should wait their turn until those ahead have got their treat. That way it is fair. Perhaps in adulthood this feeling in us hasn't changed; we feel the unfairness of a situation in which we have been trying so hard, and others, who have only reached the line, seem to be rewarded before us. Like children, we strike out at the ones ahead of us. Yet what we are striking out at is not the people personally, but what seems the incredible injustice of the situation. Of course, if these feelings become extreme or constant, rather than fleeting thoughts, help is needed. In general, they are fleeting, uncontrollable thoughts, followed by guilt and remorse. Such feelings do not indicate that one is satanic in any way. Rather, they indicate that one is deeply hurt by the situation. Perhaps, too, there is the feeling that if others lost their baby they would be more understanding.

No matter how many losses a couple experience, each new loss comes as a shock and brings with it renewed grief. Contrary to what some believe, no one gets used to losing a child! Each loss hurts just as much. Over time, a couple may simply become better equipped and more experienced in handling the associated grief. Yet the loss is still painful. They are still shocked, somehow unable to believe that this has happened again. They feel out of control of their lives and their future, a very disquieting feeling for anyone.

> I felt a strong sense of being out of control of my life and my future. I had already had seven losses. Lying in hospital with Shaun I remember thinking, 'This kind of thing doesn't happen so many times to one person, so this one's going to be all right'. Then when it didn't, it was really a shock.

Isolation can be intense for couples suffering repeated losses. They may never meet another couple who have experienced similar tragedy. Even couples who have lost only one child may be shut out by these couples with feelings of: 'Of course you can tell me it'll be all right next time. It was for you. You only lost one. You don't know what it's like to lose again and again!'

A couple's whole world seems to revolve around pregnancy and all its associated aspects. Constantly going from heights to depths in a seemingly never-ending cycle can create incredible strain on a person. Couples may make conscious decisions to forget about it, but that is almost impossible if they sincerely want a child. They feel that they have always been pregnant, thinking about pregnancy, trying to get pregnant, or recovering from pregnancy. Sometimes they just get sick to death of the whole thing! We can almost see the heads nodding in agreement with this last statement. It is harder when others don't understand. Many couples who contributed to this book *do* understand and want you to know that!

A parent or not?

Within this group of couples who experience repeated losses, there is a subgroup composed of those who are trying to realize the dream of their first child. As we have already noted, they share a common sense of loss with those who face infertility, that of losing their dream of being a family. Yet they differ from the infertile couple. For the couple who suffer repeated losses there has been an actual entity, a real child to consider, no matter how far along in development that child was. This is not to discount the right of the infertile couple to grieve as intensely. What we highlight here is that there was a pregnancy, or a number of pregnancies, recognized by society as a developing child. This recognition is more apparent when a child is lost through late miscarriage, stillbirth, or neonatal death. If lost, the child is allowed to be mourned legitimately for a time.

The couple are parents in the strict sense of the word, as defined by the Oxford Dictionary: 'father or mother: thing from which others are derived'. Unfortunately, when there is no child running around the house, couples do not receive recognition of their status as parents. Common social questions, such as how many children they have, are difficult for such couples to answer. If they say 'None', they feel they are denying these children they loved. Yet if they try to explain or use the answer 'None who are living', they feel uneasy about the reactions of others to such an answer. To society at large they are childless, while as far as they are concerned they are parents.

Other people who have families may avoid discussing the topics of pregnancy and children with these couples. They may even deny the couple's experiences by assuming that they have no knowledge of such matters.

I was sitting with a group of what I thought were friends. They all had babies or young children. They were exchanging stories about their experiences of labour. Not one of them asked me how I had found certain things like pain killers, postural positions, or caesarean deliveries. I felt so isolated. They assumed that because I had no child around me I had no experience of such things. Yet some of them knew my history. After two late miscarriages and a still birth, I probably knew more than all of them put together. You know, since then, I've noticed that there is nothing more conceited or patronizing than a cocky, first-time mother.

Couples who experience repeated losses should never be ashamed of their feelings for their lost children. If they have photographs of them which they wish to have out on display, they should do so, irrespective of what others may think or say. They should use their babies' names freely and discuss them if they feel the need. If others are uncomfortable, that is their problem and not a problem of the couple. Their lost children will always remain very special to a couple, no matter how many others they may have who live. These were their children, and they were their parents!

Coping with repeated losses

The only way of ultimately overcoming the pain of repeated losses is a successful pregnancy. Unfortunately, herein lies the problem. The months or years before this occurs are a time when stress is immense. Therefore, there are no prescriptions that can be given for the cure of the pain. The following suggestions, in conjunction with other chapters on specific losses, may help to alleviate the stress to some extent.

1. Be satisfied medically

As we have noted, it is virtually impossible for couples suffering repeated losses to forget about pregnancy. Instead of trying, it may be best to face it. The couple can make significant moves toward giving a new pregnancy its best chance of success. They may not prevent another loss, but at least they can feel that they did all that was humanly possible to contribute to the success of the new pregnancy. The first step may be the medical one.

The physical condition of the couple must be faced and dealt with. Firstly, they should think carefully about all aspects of their prior losses that confused or concerned them. They should note these and formulate them into questions for the doctor. Perhaps discussions with other women whom they may know through social contact, or support groups, about their particular histories and treatment, may stimulate other questions the couple may wish to ask. Then they should visit their doctor and ask them.

This sounds a straightforward procedure, but often it is not. Many women, especially if their confidence is shaken, will not ask questions of their doctor for fear of being seen as ignorant. Rather, they undertake his/her suggested treatment without question. Some doctors encourage such behaviour by their clinical, aloof manner, which discourages discussion. At times, women accept this situation even when it causes them distress.

> My doctor was very good, but he never explained anything to me. I wasn't happy about that, but never considered going to another doctor. I felt as if I'd be a traitor. I was afraid I'd go into hospital under a new doctor and run into Dr P. and feel very embarrassed.

It can be important for couples such as we are discussing to feel involved in the decision-making, fully aware of the basis on which such decisions were made. Many couples have complete confidence in their doctors, and don't wish further involvement; but others who wish more information or two-way communication should not be ashamed of this. Most doctors will attest to the fact that doctors do not understand all the causes of such losses. Many are relieved to have the couple cooperate in decision-making. They are also happy to refer couples to specialists in the area or to other doctors of similar experience for a second opinion. Ultimately, they acknowledge that final decisions must be made by the couple, and that decisions with which people are most content are those made in the light of all available information.

Couples, then, are best to seek out a doctor who can provide emotional support, expertise, honest responses, an openness to new information, and a respect for the rights of the couple to be fully involved in their management. If a couple are happy simply to follow the suggestions of their doctor and fear that too much information could depress or frighten them, then by all means they should continue as they are, knowing that they are doing what is right for them.

Couples feel more confident knowing that they are receiving all possible treatment, and that what treatment they are receiving is in their doctor's and their own opinions the best possible alternative. This is particularly important when a definite diagnosis of a problem cannot be made.

A doctor may further help a couple during a new pregnancy by giving them time. The usual month between antenatal checks is a very long time for a couple who fear even the innocent signs of pregnancy. Fortnightly or even weekly visits may help the couple express their fears more freely, and so prevent them being bottled up, only to grow out of proportion. Frequent visits help to put the mind at rest. Alternatively, the doctor may specify a special time each week when the couple, the doctor, and his/her receptionist know that the couple are welcome to ring the doctor if they have any worries or simply require reassurance.

2. Take care of your physical well-being

A pregnancy that is the result of the union of two healthy bodies has the best chance of success. Couples can feel that they are contributing to success by devoting the months prior to conception to making their bodies as healthy as possible.

The depression these couples feel can show itself in lethargy and a lack of concern for physical appearance and fitness, which may not lead to the healthiest body in which to begin a new pregnancy. To rebuild their physical strength, the couple must first plan a healthy diet, including all the necessary food groups.

Combined with a healthy eating plan, an exercise routine should be carried out regularly. If they have the opportunity, the couple may wish to join an exercise or sporting club of their choice. Of course, before doing so, they should undertake to have a full physical checkup. At times, the exercise may seem a chore for which they have no motivation. Then they just have to grit their teeth and say: 'I'm going to do everything possible, even exercise, to give my next pregnancy the best chance'.

A word of caution! Be sure that once a woman does become pregnant she checks with her doctor as to whether or not she should continue with her exercise program. Chapter 11 discusses physical well-being in greater detail.

3. Take care of your psychological well-being

Besides a healthy body, doctors believe that a healthy mind also benefits a pregnancy. Unfortunately for a couple facing repeated losses, a calm, relaxed mind is much more difficult to attain than a healthy body.

Activities to enhance the body's health can contribute to one's psychological well-being. The feeling that they are doing something tangible to aid their next pregnancy can reassure a couple that they are regaining some small measure of control over their situation.

The woman, particularly, may feel a failure. It is important for her well-being to find ways of boosting her self-confidence. To do this, she may need to relook at herself as a whole person, who has one part involved in childbearing. There are many other areas in her life in which she is vital to the people around her. She must face the same issues about her childbearing role as women confronted with infertility. See Chapter 3 for more detail.

A woman's importance as a person does not end when she has problems producing a child. Other aspects of her person and her contribution to her family and society make her special and unique. A couple need to investigate their other talents, and put them to use, while they keep working on their dream of a child. A woman who holds a job or is involved in many activities has an advantage over one who must cope with repeated losses without such outside diversions. The woman who gets out is forced by circumstance to face people and situations, and to show her talents and contributions. Too much time on her hands to think about her situation can be as destructive as becoming hyperactive to deny grief.

How can a couple find some of their other talents? Experiment! If they work, they may become involved in new projects. They may work part time or become involved in activities outside work that they enjoy or used to enjoy. Learn a musical instrument. Take a cookery or a home handyman course. Learn to type or learn about computers. Knit or macrame all the Christmas or birthday gifts for one year. Take up voluntary work or become a helper in the local school. Opportunities are only limited by imagination and a couple's confidence.

It is often difficult to find the courage to join a new group composed of people one doesn't know. The couple may go together or interest a friend in going along. The couple could make up a short list of questions they could ask someone to begin a conversation.

An important point to remember is that the days of men marrying for an heir are gone. The vast majority of men find a partner whom they love for herself. Children are an added bonus. There are many aspects of the woman with which her partner fell in love, not just her ability to have children.

Relaxation also aids psychological well-being. In Chapter 11 we discuss relaxation as a contribution toward a person being able to cope with a stressful situation.

Although many couples wish to become pregnant as soon as possible after one loss, there is a case for having a break between pregnancies if a couple are confronted with repeated losses. If the couple are over 30, they may feel that they do not have the luxury of giving themselves this time. Yet even a few months when pregnancy is not contemplated can provide a breathing space. A break can help the couple get off the crazy roundabout they seem to be on. It can give them a chance to spend time concentrating on each other and building strength into their relationship, before it is exposed to pressure again. How sad it would be if wanting a child to complete a family serves to destroy the very foundation on which that family is to be built!

It is vital to remember that one's partner has to remain the most important person in the life of his/her partner. This is because the security of children is based on that bond. Perhaps there comes a time when a person's priorities must put his/her partner above a child. This must be a conscious decision, for it is a very, very difficult decision to make. A couple's inclinations are to keep trying until they succeed in having a child. One partner may decide to take that job promotion to a new city or new firm. If a woman has held off going back to work or study in case she became pregnant, perhaps she should hold off no longer. Even taking a holiday, during which they will not try to fall pregnant, can provide the chance to get off the roundabout.

Ultimately, whatever a couple feels is best for them, after considering the alternatives, is best for them.

4. Talk out your concerns; don't bottle them up

Fear is a terrible thing, for it saps the energy of a person. Small worries, if bottled up, can, under the influence of fear, become terrifying hurdles. The couple who have experienced several losses, and particularly those whose new pregnancies do not proceed smoothly, are plagued by such fears. One way to disarm the fear is to talk it out. Both partners will have fears, although the woman who actually carries the pregnancy may experience them more intensely. It is important that each partner discusses his/her fears, feelings, and frustrations with his/her partner. Trying to be brave for the other doesn't really help if the fear remains bottled up inside.

An important source of support may come from other couples who have experienced a number of losses. Such persons may be connected to support groups that are concerned with death, premature babies, or miscarriage. Contact with support groups about such couples may be made by phone or letter, or by attending a meeting of such a group.

Even a caring friend or family member who is able to accept the negative feelings and is willing to listen can be a vital support link.

Prolonged hospitalization

Where a woman has suffered repeated pregnancy losses, and a definite diagnosis is not available, the doctor may advise a prolonged period of hospitalization. In other cases, it may be prescribed in a new pregnancy when any sign of a difficulty becomes evident.

Prolonged hospitalization can be trying for the whole family. It can be difficult for the woman, particularly if she is separated from her family by distance. For the male, it can be exhausting, if he now must add to his already busy day regular visits to the hospital. If other children are involved, the practical problems of maintaining a house, minding children, and overcoming separation fears of children can be daunting. Where grandparents, other family members, or friends can step in, the burden is eased. At times the children must be uprooted to achieve this, which can add to their fears. Very young children may become distressed at being separated from their mother. Yet in time they may attach themselves to their new care-giver; seeing a child secure and being called 'Nan' or the name of the care-giver can add to the feelings of depression and isolation a mother may feel.

Depression and boredom are two common problems experienced by a woman facing prolonged hospitalization. She may be depressed at being separated from her partner and family, at being denied the chance to carry on with activities she enjoys, at being in a strange situation and environment, at being confined, and at being out of control. If the woman is also experiencing acute difficulties with her pregnancy, her depression will be added to by medical procedures and by her fears of losing also this child. A willingness on the part of medical and hospital staff to accept her feelings and listen to her can help alleviate some of this depression.

Hospitalization, while creating some depression, may actually relieve other feelings of depression. Knowing that she is being carefully and constantly monitored and that she will see her doctor nearly every day, can relieve some of the woman's fears. At least in the hospital any danger signs will be noted and, where possible, intervention be made before the situation becomes more serious.

Boredom can also be a problem. There are only so many books to read or so much television one can watch before the novelty wears off and boredom sets in. One way a woman can overcome this problem is to find a time-consuming project to work on. Such a project should involve not just a week's work but months of work. What the project is, is not important, as long as it is of interest to the woman. Some women interested in handcrafts, such as knitting or patchwork, don't just work on one small garment, but set about a whole bedspread, nursery ensemble, or other piece that may take weeks to complete. Others take up correspondence courses in different areas, ranging from higher education to computers to business to hobbies. The education departments of each State have correspondence sections in secondary and further education that offer such courses to adults. Others write poetry, take up sketching, or teach themselves to type or to acquire some other skills. Some, like us, write books.

The advantages of having a project are numerous. Firstly, a project helps to fill in the long hours of the day. Days seem longer when they have no structure and one drifts aimlessly from one activity to another. A project provides routine to the day, thereby providing it with some structure. Having a set time to shower, work on the project, rest, and do other activities based around the hospital routine can really make days seem shorter. It may be difficult for a woman to discipline herself to carry out a project, but it is worth the effort!

Secondly, being busy can even take a woman's mind off her pregnancy, for some time at least. Thirdly, a project gives one a sense of accomplishing something, which can help a woman feel some confidence in herself. After her baby is born, she can look back on her time as doubly productive. If, sadly, the pregnancy fails, she may not see the time of her prolonged hospitalization as completely wasted. It may even lead her into a new, exciting area of life or occupation.

Prolonged hospitalization in a maternity hospital can be emotionally difficult. The woman constantly encounters newly-delivered mothers and babies. If her own pregnancy is not secure or has not yet reached a viable stage, this can be extremely trying. Sharing a room with new mothers can add to such a difficulty. Some hospitals try to arrange it that such long-term patients are provided with a room of their own for some period of time, or are able to share with other long-term patients. This can be helpful for all such women, as they can work at raising each other's morale. Even introductions by staff of one long-term patient to others can be reassuring. Many build up strong friendships and 'visit' each other regularly, helping further to pass the time. If a woman is uncomfortable in sharing with new mothers, she should ask a senior sister if there is any way this can be changed. If possible, the hospital will organize this.

Facing the outside world again after prolonged hospitalization can be quite daunting for the woman. Firstly, she may feel weak due to inactivity of the muscles. To relieve this, physiotherapists will generally provide exercises for the woman to do. Secondly, she can lose her sense of perspective. Once she is outside the hospital, ordinary things seem different. The cars seem larger and faster. Lights seem brighter. Crowds of people can be frightening, and even familiar places seem strange. Some liken these feelings to a mild form of those experienced by an agoraphobic person.

Generally, they pass in a few hours or days, but can be prolonged.

Prolonged hospitalization can be extremely trying for a couple. Displays of affection are often stifled, and their lack of privacy can be upsetting. They require understanding of their feelings. Feelings of resenting this very-much-wanted baby who is responsible for the hospitalization may occur. Others may feel a strong sense of wanting it 'over and done with', even if delivery of the baby at such a time would be life-threatening to the child. These negative feelings must be understood and accepted by others, to prevent the woman experiencing unnecessary guilt.

Much of the coping with prolonged hospitalization must come from the woman herself. Personalities are different. Some people are better able successfully to adapt to new situations. Hence, reactions to hospitalization may vary widely. The woman can help herself if she tries to take only one day at a time and work hard at being busy and remaining positive. If negative feelings are allowed to take her over, the strain on her, her family, and this baby are increased. It does take a bit of 'guts' to cope with this stressful situation, but it is well worth it!

Conclusion

We have not suggested that a couple who have suffered repeated losses forget about pregnancy. If they *are* able to put it into the back of their mind and get on with life, congratulations and our best wishes! If not, they needn't feel guilty because they can't relax as prescribed. Instead, they should face their fears and prepare in the very best ways they can to give the new pregnancy its best chance:

1. Eat well.
2. Exercise regularly.
3. Be satisfied that your medical treatment is adequate and the best alternative available.
4. Seek out a doctor with whom you are able to communicate.
5. Discover or rediscover your talents in other areas.
6. Seek out others in your situation with whom you can discuss your fears.
7. Concentrate on loving and pleasing your partner.

8. Go out and enjoy the activities that you will find it more difficult to take part in once your baby does arrive.
9. Practise relaxation.
10. Consider a break from pregnancy, so that you or your partner can complete a worthwhile project.
11. Think carefully about why you want a child or more children.
12. Consider what other alternatives exist for you and your future.
13. Consciously train yourself to think no further than one day at a time.

These suggestions may actually help a couple to ignore pregnancy, even for a short period. They may also provide them with the confidence of knowing that they have given something its 'best shot'. Herein lies a vitally important point: A couple *are* doing what is humanly possible, and that is *all* they can do! The final outcome of a new pregnancy is now out of their hands. This is a very difficult situation for human beings to accept. But sometimes, no matter how hard we try, things don't work out as we want them to. To accept that you are ultimately not in control of a situation can be frightening. Yet this knowledge can make the fact that each pregnancy is a new one heartening. There is always hope! Even if it doesn't work this time, maybe their efforts will be rewarded next time. Each pregnancy is a new one, a clean slate! It is important not to put a time-limit on success. Years ago, a couple who had suffered repeated losses were given little hope of producing a live child. Today, evidence suggests that this is not the case and that such couples have a good chance of achieving their ultimate goal of a child, although it may take time and a lot of patience. Patience is probably the most difficult state for these couples to achieve. We know! If we could bottle patience and take a dose as required, how easy it would be!

Each new pregnancy is a worry. An old lady once remarked to us that worry is like a child's swing. There is a lot of activity and energy expended in pushing it, but it never goes very far. Worrying about a pregnancy serves only to upset our whole system, and yet it cannot prevent another loss. It may even contribute slightly to making matters worse. Yet how do couples dissipate worry and remain hopeful?

One couple took toilet rolls. Each day of the pregnancy they tore off a sheet. The days when they were fairly content they put the sheet in one basket. The days when they became concerned and nothing adverse happened, they noted the fearful symptom on the sheet and put it into a separate basket. Soon they saw that there were many more days they spent in fear than were necessary. After a couple of losses, they had learnt the real danger signs as distinct from the innocent symptoms, which they now ignored. If the woman became concerned about a symptom, her husband asked her a set of questions they had devised that helped them differentiate the dangerous from the innocent signs. Fewer sheets went into the troubled basket with each pregnancy. They refined their symptoms list. They learnt to share the pain and the worry. The husband felt that he could really contribute to his wife's well-being in a significant way, rather than by simply paying lip-service to her fears, fearing that he may be only building up false hopes. Their final pregnancy saw few sheets in the troubled bin, and they shared the joy of a healthy long-awaited son.

This is simply an example of the courage and resourcefulness of some couples who must face such periods of repeated loss and pain. We salute them, and sincerely hope that their needed courage will be forthcoming and that ultimately they will be rewarded for their efforts. What special parents their child will have, for they will be able to instil in their child a respect for effort and perseverance! They will be able to give them a real understanding and compassion for what it means to be 'kicked in the teeth' and 'down but not out'! Happily, the problem of repeated losses seems to be one problem in which perseverance is likely to pay off. Don't lose hope!

References
1. Gordon Bourne, *Pregnancy* (London: Pan Books, 1979), 285.

9 You and Your Relationship: The Parents — A Couple or Single

Throughout this book we have purposely discussed the problems of bearing a child in terms of effects on 'the couple'. This has been intentional for a number of reasons. Firstly, there is often inclined to be little recognition of the emotional needs of the male in situations such as these. He is seen by many as being strong and supportive. We wish to make it clear that these difficult situations happen to two people, who both experience their individual grief. Secondly, many of the couples who experience difficulties in bearing a child and would be reading a book such as this are intentionally trying to bear a full-term healthy child. Hence, most will try again to achieve this. This assumes some permanency of relationship, as occurs in marriage or long-term relationships. Thirdly, emotional reactions to these difficult situations are often profoundly affected by the character of the relationship of the couple.

In choosing to use the term 'the couple', we have had to overlook to some extent the group of single parents who face such difficulties alone. But we have not forgotten them, and apologize if it seems that we have not acknowledged them. It was difficult to make the decision to use the words 'the couple' rather than 'the parents'. Most of the feelings experienced by the individuals within relationships will be similar to those experienced by the single parent. Yet the single parent must deal with a range of problems unique to his/her situation, which add to its difficulty. Later in this chapter we shall look at their special problems, *not* as an afterthought, but in a section dedicated to them and the courage they have to find without the support of a partner.

Most couples enter a long-term relationship and marriage believing that they can discuss anything. This may be true of their hopes and dreams and the minor crises that occur in courtship and early marriage. Difficulty in bearing a child may be the first situation in their relationship over which they have little or no control, and which strikes at the very heart of their individual beings and their relationship. Many will develop the necessary skills to cope, and hence this crisis will forge a new strength in their bond. Unfortunately, other relationships do not have and will not develop these means of coping with such waves of torment, and they flounder. Most marriages or long-term relationships are not placed under the amount of strain that confronts the couple who face difficulties in bearing a child. The greater the strain a relationship must endure, the greater is the likelihood of cracks appearing in it. In fact, repeated difficulties in bearing a child substantially increase the chance of a complete breakdown of the relationship.

We shall now look more closely at the individuals involved in the relationship and then further at the relationship itself. Realizing the source of the problems can be the first important step in overcoming difficulties and rebuilding the relationship. It should be remembered that a relationship will be changed by crisis, no matter what its character before the crisis. Whether these changes are positive or negative will depend on the relationship and how the crisis is handled. Change is not to be feared, if it is handled appropriately.

The man

Unfortunately, the male is often overlooked when it comes to child-bearing difficulties. After a loss, he may be asked: 'How is your wife going?' Few question him about his own feelings. Many assume — incorrectly, of course — that he will be only slightly affected. At times, when he is confronted with such comments, he may feel like yelling: 'What about me? It's my baby too! Aren't I also entitled to be upset?'

In many cases, the male's own behaviour makes it more likely that his feelings will be ignored. He appears strong and in control of the situation. Often such a display simply hides his true emotions. Yet there are reasons why he may maintain a strong front. Even as little boys, males are generally not encouraged to display emotions openly: 'Little boys don't cry'. So the Australian male often learns to hold emotions within himself. His traditional role as the protector of his partner further reinforces this. The male often feels that he must remain strong and even unemotional to support his partner. This becomes more important to him if his partner is in pain or a highly emotional state. Unfortunately, his strength can be misinterpreted by his partner or others as a lack of caring. How unfair and sad it is for the male who has often had to find the courage to enter his partner's room without breaking down!

In many cases, the male will find it impossible to control his emotions. Males are often more able to express their anger at the situation than are females. He may pound his fist into a wall, kick a piece of furniture, or yell at the dog. Often his grief is expressed when he is alone, returning to an empty house from the hospital, outside in his workshop, or in his car. Few people realize that the husband may need the type of emotional support offered to the woman. Relatives and friends — particularly male friends — can provide some support through simple companionship, even when the male does not wish to discuss his feelings. In her physical and emotional state, his partner may not be able to provide him with the support he needs.

Any of the child-bearing difficulties dealt with in this book may leave the male feeling helpless. In infertility investigations, the woman generally has to undergo more physically demanding investigations than does the male. In situations of miscarriage, death, prematurity, and abnormality, his helpless position is even more obvious. His helplessness is further exaggerated when he is separated by distance from his partner. He may be torn between his grief at losing his child or potential child and seeing his beloved partner in physical and emotional discomfort. In some more serious cases, he may even fear for his partner's health and safety. But what can he do? Within the hospital or specialist clinics the medical staff are preoccupied with assisting his partner. He may feel as if he is in the way! Staff, and even the man himself, may discount the vital emotional support role he must play. Except in cases of medical emergency, this role may be the one of paramount importance.

The male may at times find it difficult to understand the intensity of his partner's reaction to their loss. In general, a man's self-image is not as intrinsically tied to child-bearing as is the woman's. His self-image may be more closely connected with his occupation, pastimes, and social habits. He may see his life-plan in terms of continuing in his occupation so as to support his wife and children. His partner may also have pursued a career, but many women see their role as working for a few years and then being at home, for some time at least, with their child or children. When the couple face difficulties having a first child, her perceived future is threatened. With any loss in child-bearing, her self-image as a woman and a mother is also shaken. The male must realize that her loss involves more than a beloved child; it also involves some of herself.

In cases of the loss of a baby, the male's knowledge of the child, in the early stages, is limited to his imagination. The woman is aware of the changes in her body, and bonding with her child begins at this early stage. But the first actual contact the male has with his child may be when movements can be felt. So the loss of a child due to miscarriage before this time may not be as devastating to him.

Life does not come to a halt when a couple are faced with a loss. Generally, the husband must continue to go to work, and even run the household if his wife is physically unable to do so. He does not have the luxury of time to experience his grief. His time may be filled with work, hospital visits, and household duties, leaving him physically as well as emotionally drained. He must confront people in the outside world who may be unable to communicate with him about his loss, or may be unaware of it. In dealing with colleagues or customers, he may need to slip into yet another role, that of the professional. This is difficult when he feels so sad, empty, and lethargic.

In some cases, the male, as protector, may take on all decisions to relieve his partner of any further pain. For example, he may make the funeral arrangements or discuss an ailing baby's progress with the specialist without consulting or informing his partner. Other practical decisions involving finances, home arrangements, or child minding he may take on himself. He may find it difficult to understand his partner's possible resentment of this type of decision-making.

There are other times when the male may be unable to understand his partner. For example, a woman whose life was to revolve around raising her own children, may be initially unable to accept her husband's suggestion of adoption. He, on the other hand, may see it as the practical solution. Of course, the situation may be reversed. In other instances, the male may not be able to understand his partner's preoccupation with a miscarriage. He may be relieved to see her out of physical pain, and may wish to look forward to a new pregnancy.

If time goes on and his partner does not seem to be recovering from her depression, the male may find it more and more difficult to be understanding. He may begin to resent her careless appearance, the untidy house, or the persistent crying. Some men may even react with anger. Others may react by staying out of the house more, often finding it difficult to continue supporting their partners.

The male may experience feelings of anger toward his partner, feelings for which he feels guilt. Such anger, part of his grief, may arise from the tendency to search for a reason for the loss. He may consciously or unconsciously blame his partner: 'She left child-bearing till it was too late.' 'She worked too hard.' 'She had that medicine early on when I urged her not to.' It is important that the male also be present when the facts of the loss are outlined by the doctor, so that he can be assured of his partner's innocence.

The male may desire that life return to some normality. This may include the area of sex. After the usual waiting period of six weeks, the male may wish to resume sexual relations. He may find his partner also willing, which may help both achieve some stability. But for other couples this is not the case. The woman may not wish to be reminded of how the baby was conceived, or of her failure to conceive. Both parents may fear another pregnancy. After a diagnosis of infertility, some may avoid sex, feeling: 'What's the use?' We shall look at sexual relations in more detail later.

If a pregnancy has been lost, the male may wish for a new one. Yet he may be torn by a wish not to see his partner face such pain and disappointment again. After all, her body must actually undergo the physical changes! The male may feel that he has no right to try to encourage a new pregnancy. When a new pregnancy is confirmed or fertility treatment begun, the male, unable to experience his partner's emotional and hormonal changes, may be bewildered by her changing moods. She may have appeared much more settled and confident for a period, allowing him to feel more relaxed. Then suddenly on a day when the pregnancy is concerning the woman, or a new treatment is due, she may return to deep depression. The smiling, reassuring woman he left in the morning may be replaced by an emotionally drained and crying one when he returns.

The strong desire to have children is often assumed by our society to be with the female. This is an erroneous assumption, for many men see their prospective role of father as a vital part of their lives. Much motivation for succeeding in his chosen career may come for such a man from his desire to provide well for his family. Therefore, many men are devastated when circumstances indicate that they may not fill their role of father, or may have difficulty doing so.

The woman

The woman's reactions in these situations are often more intense and longer lasting — although this is not always the case. There are two major reasons for this. Firstly, the woman may have to deal not only with her feelings, but also with the physical changes of her body or the medical treatments involved. Hormonal changes leading to normal post-partum depression ('baby blues') can complicate the emotional reactions of a woman who has lost a baby or delivered one with congenital difficulties. Some treatments for infertility also involve manipulation of hormones. Hence, emotional upheavals may also be expected in these cases.

Secondly, the woman's view of herself is tied closely to her child-bearing ability. A number of women today are choosing childlessness in favour of a career. In such cases, her self-image is tied more closely to this career, as has been the case with men in the past. But for the woman who has chosen to have a child or has found herself pregnant and decided to continue with the pregnancy, the loss of this child or an inability to conceive or bear a full-term healthy child can be devastating. Her image of herself as a woman can be severely tarnished.

Some women have resigned from their jobs as their pregnancies progressed. Other women, with the intention of making motherhood their career, may have taken jobs with no particular career opportunities. If then confronted with infertility or repeated losses, such a woman may lose interest in her job. Without career aspirations, and with her dreams shaken, this job may hold little meaning for her. For another woman, her career may have been important, and she may have delayed childbearing until she was older. If infertility or repeated losses then plague her, she may feel pressured as she sees her biological clock ticking away. She may experience some guilt for having been 'selfish' and waited so long.

Some women feel that their partner can never fully understand or share their grief. She carried the baby! She knew this baby better than he! These feelings may even turn to anger toward him if he becomes impatient with her continuing depression. In some ways she is correct in her feelings, for her bonding with the child before birth may be stronger than that of her partner. Yet to assume that therefore he cannot share her grief is unfair to her partner. Once the baby is born and contact made, his grief may be as intense as her own.

Unlike the male, it is the woman who must contemplate the thought of another pregnancy or the involved infertility testing required if her partner has been cleared of sterility fears. Her reactions to a loss can be affected by these added pressures. Pregnancy may serve to remind her continually of the child she has lost, while infertility testing may remind her of past and possible future failures. Combined with this may be the fear of pain and discomfort or future hospitalization. Women must cope with medical situations such as internal examinations; these may also be embarrassing and perplexing for some, since they may feel robbed of their dignity.

Generally, a woman is encouraged to discuss her feelings with others. She may find discussion with other women comforting, particularly others who have experienced a loss. Talking out feelings with her partner may be more difficult. Difficulties in understanding each other's ability or need to talk or not can heighten communication problems.

The woman may feel out of control of her body, her situation, and her future. She may feel angry and jealous toward those around her presently pregnant or with children. In fact, confused emotions may see her putting distance between herself and friends who normally would be important sources of support.

After a loss, she may have to face time alone at home, during which her depression may be weighing her down so strongly that she is unable to function. After a few weeks the sympathy of others may wane, and she feels, during those lonely hours, unwanted and useless. It may be a wonderful relief when her partner returns. Yet, in some cases, his patience may also begin to wear thin. She may find herself acting a role of coping, even for him.

The woman often experiences a very strong need to be pregnant to replace the lost child, to try again, to prove herself, to succeed. Attaining a successful pregnancy can almost become an obsession. It can become the focus of her life, excluding all other aspects. Involving herself in her job or other interests may be half-hearted attempts at something she feels she *should* do, rather than *wants* to do.

The relationship

We have seen that the individuals may have to cope with some intense emotions. Some are common. Others are more specific to the male or female. There is a belief that crises make a relationship stronger, and in some cases this may be true. But a crisis does not have some magical quality that enhances a relationship as long as the relationship simply survives it. A relationship that does survive, or is even enhanced by the crisis, is one that has been worked at by both partners during the crisis. Each individual must see the relationship as something worth salvaging. In some unions, the relationship may be more important to one individual than the other, which may lead to further complications.

Each individual must also be willing to accept responsibility for his/her behaviour and feelings. The crises of child-bearing often cause a breakdown of communication between partners. Even those relationships that are already strong and will inevitably endure may suffer some periods of trial. The longer and more severe the problem is, the more destructive the effects are likely to be.

Before we begin looking at rebuilding a relationship, let us look more carefully at the factors that can affect communication. Many of these have been mentioned before, but are worth specifying in this section.

1. The couple are bonded but not joined

Many marriage ceremonies use the phrase that 'two shall become one'. Yes, a permanent relationship does see built a strong bond of purpose and communication that links two individuals. But it is a bond built on shared experiences, understanding, and commitment, not subjugation of the individual. The man and woman are still individuals, with individual feelings, values, beliefs, and personality traits. Therefore their feelings and reactions may differ, as may their favoured means of coping with difficulties. Somehow these individuals must not only cope with their own emotions, but also with the emotions and behaviour of another.

2. Different rates of grieving

In each of the difficulties discussed, we have outlined the loss these couples may feel. They grieve, although the duration and the intensity of their grief may vary greatly. Individuals may also differ in the progress of their grief, reaching different stages of grief at different times. This is often a source of difficulty for the grieving couple.

3. Assumptions

Many misunderstandings occur because each individual partner assumes that he/she knows what the other is thinking, or why he/she is behaving in such a way. Often the assumption is incorrect. For example, a woman whose self-esteem is in tatters may misinterpret her husband's normal irritability after a hard day as relating to her loss of a much-wanted child. One partner may assume that a biological child is the only one acceptable to the other. Another woman may assume that her partner would be unwilling to undergo fertility tests, and hence not broach the subject with him. It is vital that couples clarify their real feelings in order to avoid such misunderstanding. That is, assumptions must be tested against reality.

4. The male and female roles

Even in this modern society, certain expectations are associated with the male and female in society. Child-bearing is still a very important part of a woman's role. Difficulties in this area can affect her adversely. Similarly, a man's self-concept may be affected by his infertility. Male and female roles may also affect the way a couple communicate. This can lead to difficulties when feelings are confused and raw. Faulty assumptions may be made according to these role expectations.

5. Other areas of difficulty in the marriage

A combination of stresses in a relationship can make a situation worse. Child-bearing difficulties are enough to cope with, without the pressure of added strains. Financial, communication, sexual, employment, familial, and social difficulties compound the strain the couple experience, making coming to terms with child-bearing more difficult.

6. Blaming and taking the blame

In most cases of child-bearing difficulties, one partner will have the medical problem. Generally, the partner with the problem will feel some guilt. Some may feel that they have failed their child and, perhaps more strongly, their partner. Feeling guilty as well as feeling a failure, they may try to make up for their apparent lack. Some may deny their right to feel or express negative emotions toward their 'blameless' partner. They may suppress genuine justified anger, and hold resentment within themselves. This may later show itself as depression or illness. The situation is worsened if the 'blameless' partner raises the problem within an argument as a means of hurting the 'guilty' partner. It is vital that couples see their problem as a shared one, irrespective of its source.

7. Differing reasons for wanting a child

Most people assume that a natural part of a marriage or a long-term relationship will be the birth of one or more children. Often the reasons for wanting a child are not even considered before the event. However, if child-bearing is difficult, these reasons may become important. If one partner is willing to have a child simply to fulfil the wishes of the other, the loss may not hold as much significance for him/her. If a family is seen as vital to the role one partner sees as desirable, he/she may have difficulty accepting a loss such as infertility. If a child who was conceived in the hope of 'saving' a relationship is later lost or born with a congenital abnormality, there will be more than grief to complicate the relationship. Generally, the importance of the role that the child

was to fulfil for each partner will affect the sense of loss that
he/she may experience.

8. The time-span of the difficulties

The longer a stressful situation lasts, the more likely it is to
cause serious difficulties within a relationship. Prolonged
infertility, repeated losses, and the birth of a handicapped child
are all situations which may produce prolonged stress. To cope
with such stress, the couple must develop highly effective
communication and maintain it. In some cases, the prolonged
stress becomes too much, and the couple part. Fortunately, most
couples will have their situation resolved within a reasonable
time period, through the birth of a live, mature, healthy child.

9. Inconsistencies in behaviour

People experiencing depression may sometimes behave
erratically in different situations. This may be due to the changing
moods of their depression. Unpredictable behaviour can make it
difficult for one's partner to cope.

The key to overcoming problems in relationships lies in
rebuilding or enhancing the communication shared by the couple.
However, for many couples, the question is 'How?'

Rebuilding or enhancing a relationship worn by crisis

Most couples are able to recognize when a relationship is
bending under pressure. The ease and security that they felt
within each other's company may slowly be replaced by more
frequent misunderstandings and withdrawals. They may find
themselves arguing instead of discussing, and find it difficult to
converse easily. An individual may find fault with even the
simplest things his/her partner does. Yet before, these same habits
were never a source of irritation. Allowed to fester, these sores in
a relationship may grow and cause an eventual breakdown. As we
mentioned, couples are often well aware of problems in their
relationship. Yet telling them to overcome these problems by
rebuilding their communication does not clarify the matter for
them.

Firstly, what is communication in a relationship? Communication is the ability of one individual to understand and respond appropriately to the feelings, actions, ideas, and values of his/her partner, accompanied by a security that his/her own feelings and needs are similarly fulfilled. Communication involves two aspects. The first is being able to express oneself openly in words and actions within an atmosphere of acceptance. The second is an intangible component of being 'tuned in' to the needs of one another, responding appropriately to an unexpressed need. Put simply, communication is being secure enough to be able to 'let it all hang out' and being willing to accept one's partner 'warts and all.'

What do we need to communicate?

Many couples are unsure of what they need to make known to each other. Therefore, before we look at how a couple may rebuild communication, we must look at what they need to communicate and why.

1. Feelings

A couple facing a crises in bearing a child are faced with many thoughts and emotions that may be confusing and even frightening to them. We have discussed in depth the feelings of failure, anger, depression, and helplessness engendered by such situations. We have also seen how feelings between males and females may differ and be hidden because of the roles they play. It is important that couples express their feelings honestly to each other, even when they seem irrational and perhaps shameful.

Some feelings, such as anger, may not be socially acceptable. Similarly, some expressions of emotion may not fit an arbitrary accepted social role. For example, it may not seem appropriate for the male to feel a need to sob. Forget society! Others may not understand, unless they too have faced a crisis.

A couple shouldn't feel threatened by their feelings. They should express them honestly as they occur. If each individual is to be honest with his/her feelings, it is vital that each is accepting and respecting of the other's unique expression of emotions. If one partner feels a need to withdraw for a time, then he/she should express this need simply. The other must then respect such a need.

Most often, anger is the feeling a grieving couple finds the most difficult to deal with. It is the feeling we as a whole society find difficult to cope with. At times, we cope with it incorrectly. We suppress it by sulking or playing the martyr. We let it simmer over time, keeping it bottled up with other simmering anger, only to explode suddenly one day. We collect annoyances and total them up, ready to use them as retaliation against another in a later argument. We behave badly toward others less powerful when the source of our anger is a superior. We let our anger be vented in physical or emotional abuse of those around us, or against ourselves in the form of depression. All of these expressions of anger are generally inappropriate. Many individuals fear that overt anger is a sign of a 'bad' relationship. Hence, they use these strategies we have mentioned to avoid an initial confrontation.

Anger is a feeling, an emotion, and in this is no different from other emotions. Anger is a natural part of grieving. The couple facing child-bearing difficulties must accept their angry feelings without guilt. They are angry. That's acceptable! Attacking one's partner over some trivial unrelated matter because of this anger is not acceptable. If the anger is to be resolved appropriately, the angry partner must first decide at whom or what he/she is angry. Is it really the dirty socks dropped beside the laundry basket, or is it that one resents his/her partner's apparent lack of concern about their lost child? Secondly, the angry partner must decide whether his/her anger is warranted. Is the partner's sloppiness reason enough to explode first before simply asking for socks to go into the laundry basket? Is the partner really unconcerned about the loss, or is he/she trying not to upset a loved one further? If one partner feels that he/she has a right to be angry, then this needs to be acted on. Yet always remember that enquiry should *always* precede explosion. Yelling or physical violence may help one vent anger, but it is only appropriate when the recipient of one's anger is an empty room or a pillow. A softened voice will communicate better to a grieving partner than will a yell. If the anger is not related to one's partner, but simply to grief, it is unfair to vent it on an innocent party. An inanimate object will recover faster after an outburst than will a grieving partner.

Whatever the feeling or emotion, express it freely to a partner. He/she will understand, for in most cases it is probably an emotion that lies within him/her. At times, feelings are so confused that a person is unsure of what he/she really is feeling. It may be difficult to verbalize the emotions stirred. When one tries to express it, it may sound irrational or completely different to what is actually felt. Partners need patience with each other. Each needs time to express himself/herself, to sort out the feelings in words. Being rushed by an impatient partner only leaves one feeling deprived, embarrassed, and rejected, especially if this partner has obviously misinterpreted the jumbled words. Expressing feelings is vital, but this communication needs time and patience on the part of both partners.

2. Support and caring

Grieving is a lonely business. Like the animal with a wounded paw, the individual with a broken heart can become self-centred, concerned only with his/her personal pain. This person doesn't feel that he/she has the resources and strength to cope with another's pain. Yet, support and caring expressed by one partner for the other can be vital in cushioning the pain of grief.

Support and caring can be expressed in many ways. They are founded on a feeling of love and concern for a partner, and a wish to share his/her pain. They can be expressed in words. The simplest and most effective words are 'I love you'. Others include 'I'm always ready to listen', 'I understand', 'It's all right to cry. You go ahead and get it out of your system.'

Where a couple find it difficult to express their support in words, actions can speak loudly. An arm around the shoulders or a cuddle when tears are flowing, a squeeze of the hand or a loving look, can provide support in difficult situations. Even simple close proximity can provide security, by conveying the unspoken support of 'I'm here. I understand it's not easy. We're in this together.'

The 'little things', too, can convey support, by helping a partner realize that the other has thought about him/her and what he/she may need. Cooking a meal, making a cup of coffee, a simple night out, a treat, anything that conveys to a grieving partner a feeling of being special, may give him/her support. The simplest act of displaying a willingness just to sit and listen will be viewed as of great importance by a thankful partner.

The thankful partner is as vital a part to a supportive relationship as is the partner who bestows the act or words of caring. Don't take each other for granted! Somewhere within one's depression it is vital still to be able to recognize and appreciate the effort involved in the words and actions of support offered by one's partner. A simple word of thanks, praise, or a reciprocal act of thoughtfulness can encourage a partner to continue such support. Without recognition or appreciation of the effort to provide support, an individual may tire and abandon his/her supportive role.

Support must be at least complementary, if not a complete two-way process. At times, one partner may be weighed down by grief more heavily than the other. He/she may therefore require more than an even share of support at this time. Neither partner should begrudge such support to the other in his/her time of need, for the other partner's time of grief may have been or may be yet to come. One shouldn't expect to receive support without giving some in return. No relationship can survive if one is expected to simply be a 'giver', while the other is a 'taker'.

3. The worth of the individual

As we noted, difficulties in child-bearing often bring intense feelings of failure, particularly for the partner who sees himself/herself to blame for the situation.

Self-worth should not be confined to one aspect of a person's life, for a loss in this area will be devastating. It can be important for a grieving partner to be encouraged to look to other areas of his/her life where there is evidence of success. One partner can help by encouraging the other in any pursuit, not related to reproduction, that the dejected partner may undertake. It may be difficult for a grieving partner to help the other in this way, but it is well worth the effort.

It is easy to lose sight of one's partner in your own depression. It may help to set aside time to list (perhaps on paper) some of a partner's good points, his/her abilities and successes. This may serve to remind each one that beyond the depression and little annoyances, his/her partner is a special person. Finally, each must be determined to remind the loved one of his/her special importance.

4. The meaning of marriage and family

Closely linked to the need to communicate to one's partner his/her importance, is the need to reassure the partner that it is the couple's marriage or relationship that is vital. Of course, any statement made must be honest. Hence, honesty with oneself is a vital first step. Did you really marry your partner primarily for himself/herself, or was it a family you primarily sought? Does it affect your feelings for your partner if he/she finds it difficult, or is unable, to parent your child? Would a life for just the two of you still be acceptable? Each individual must honestly answer these questions for himself/herself.

Some people find that a life without children, or the strain of losing children, is too much for them.

> We'd been trying for eight years to have a baby. They'd found at first that my wife wasn't ovulating. They fixed that, and still nothing. We found out that I was sterile. My wife wouldn't consider AID, and I too wasn't too pleased about it. She tried to tell me it would be all right, just the two of us. We were too old to adopt. Yet it hurt her deeply, and finally her need to be a mother was stronger than our marriage. She met another man and married him straight after our divorce. She has two children now, and is very happy.

If one partner honestly believes that it is the relationship with his/her partner that is vital, then he/she should tell his/her loved one this. This is particularly important if the loved one blames himself/herself for the child-bearing problem. Don't assume that a partner knows how you feel!

> I didn't marry you as a breeding machine. I married you for you. We'll work this out together.

> Yes, I'm hurting too because our baby died, but you will always be my number-one concern.

> We're a family now. It's going to be a lot of work. What's happened has happened. You didn't do anything on purpose. How were you to know about a faulty gene or be able to stop it? I love you, and together we'll do a darn good job as parents.

5. A willingness to change and to make an effort

A couple may realize that they are behaving in ways that are damaging their relationship. Such behaviour will continue its destructive work unless the cycle is broken. To do this successfully, the individual partners must be willing to change. The effort must be sustained to effect real long-lasting changes, rather than short-term truces.

At times, one partner is not willing to make such an effort. This does not mean that the situation is doomed. If the other partner changes, the reluctant partner may find situations altered, generally for the best. Such changes in a relationship may even cause a reciprocal change in the once-reluctant partner. For example, it is very difficult to build up into a full-scale argument when one partner no longer enters the ring ready to retaliate with unrelated issues.

One important point to remember in any relationship is that miracles don't happen immediately. Real change takes time and effort. Hence, a determined willingness to change is a vital component of the process.

6. Space

In highly emotional situations, such as those involving child-bearing difficulties, there is often a need for each grieving parent to spend some time alone. During this time they can sort through their own thoughts and feelings. Grieving is a very personal experience. Sharing is important, but privacy also plays a role. A couple must recognize this need in each other. If one's partner needs time alone but can't express this need, it is important that the other does not take the subsequent withdrawal as a personal rejection.

7. Decisions about the present and the future

As we have seen, there is often a large number of decisions involved with difficulties in bearing a child. Such decisions include medical treatments for infertility, autopsies and funeral arrangements, and the timing and advisability of a later pregnancy, to name but a few. Ideally, decision-making should involve the collecting of information and the weighing of options, followed by a seeking of a consensus on the action to be taken. Both partners should be involved in making important decisions. Unemotional discussion is the most appropriate; to ensure this, it may be necessary for both partners to have moved some distance toward resolving their grief.

At times some difficult decisions will have to be made with no guarantee that the decision will bring the most desirable consequences. Deciding to institutionalize a severely disabled child, to try for another baby when there is an increased risk of miscarriage or abnormality, or to undergo microsurgery or *in-vitro* fertilization, provide no certainties of a favourable outcome. No decision ever comes with such a guarantee!

Some decisions concerning the future may force the couple to confront eventualities that they would rather not consider. For example, some couples may have to face the possibility of a future without children. To the couple's certain relief, this does not eventuate in most cases. But in facing the possibility of the worst that can happen and preparing for it, the couple may be, at worst, prepared and content, and, at best, pleasantly surprised by the birth of a full-term, healthy baby.

How can couples improve communication?

We have looked at some of the topics and emotions that couples may need to communicate about. Yet when communication is ailing, many couples are unsure of how to go about soothing the wounds and healing the rifts. There are no hard-and-fast rules, no sure prescriptions, no magic cures. Generally, improved communication occurs when two people make an effort to change by looking into themselves, at each other, and at their relationship. We shall simply discuss some techniques that may help improve the chances of more effective communication between partners. Individual couples will find their own particular means of achieving this aim.

When looking to improve communication, many couples wrongly assume that the process will be shared equally. Few, if any, relationships are shared evenly in all aspects. Generally, one of the partners is more verbal or demonstrative. His/her prior life-experiences will influence this. Some families encourage discussion of feeling; others don't. Some argue quite vehemently, while others seem to discourage anger. What was considered normal in a person's family is seen as desirable behaviour when he/she later enters new relationships. Encouraging a person who is not used to talking to tell of his/her feelings will take time and patience, and a grieving partner may have little of such patience. Finding the patience requires deciding that the relationship is worth the effort.

Before communication will improve, each individual must be prepared to look closely at himself/herself and decide to take certain actions. Firstly, each must be prepared to 'own' his/her own problems. Neither should try to blame the other for his/her loss or feelings. Similarly, neither should accept the blame for those of the partner. If one feels depressed and isolated, he/she shouldn't blame his/her partner and expect him/her to overcome such isolation. Rather, the isolated partner may need to get out on his/her own. Similarly, don't feel responsible for causing your partner's anger when you know that you have done nothing to cause such feelings.

Secondly, each must look carefully at his/her different moods and their effects on a partner. For one day, or preferably longer, take a notebook and put down your moods as they change. Beside them, note the moods and mood changes of your partner. Compare them. For example, is your depression changing the more relaxed mood of your partner into one of depression or anger?

Thirdly, remember that even in strong relationships the partners do not become mind readers. One partner cannot know what the other is thinking or feeling unless he/she is told! Some individuals feel angry at their partner because 'they don't understand', yet they have simply assumed that their partner knows what was troubling them. No one can really understand a problem unless he/she knows what the real problem is. Unfortunately, these situations are further complicated when the individuals are themselves unaware of the origins of their feelings. Grief can cause feelings that seem to surface with no rhyme or reason. A person knows that he/she is upset but can't pinpoint any particular incident that caused the upset. He/she is simply upset! This confusion about one's feelings may need to be expressed to a partner, so that the partner can understand these feelings and also the confusion.

A. The words you use

Words are our prime means of communicating, yet they can so easily be misinterpreted, leading to further communication breakdown. Words should be used to express feelings, not to blame another. The behaviour of one's partner may make one feel upset or isolated, but it is important to voice feelings rather than accuse the partner of unacceptable behaviour. Many arguments begin 'You do . . .' 'Why can't you . . .?' Such statements are an attack on one's partner.

> You never listen to me. You always walk away.
> Why can't you stay and listen to me sometimes?

The offending partner simply defends himself/herself, often by attacking or withdrawing further into depression.

> Well, you can talk! What about you? You're so busy feeling sorry for yourself you couldn't care about me!

To prevent such situations, each must honestly express his/her anger by replacing the statement 'You ...' with 'I feel ...'

I feel upset when you walk away from me.
I feel rejected when you don't return my cuddles.

When feelings are expressed in this way, the offending partner is inclined to be less defensive, as he/she is not the target of an assault. Secondly, by using such statements, the individual is taking responsibility for his/her own emotions.

Communication is enhanced when positive things are said. Telling one's partner how special he/she is, thanking him or her for any assistance offered, and being able to laugh with him/her makes the partner feel content and warm. Concentrate on the good things a partner does. Where possible, ignore the irritating ones, remembering that we all have our faults.

At times, it will be necessary to let a partner know that there is something he/she does or says that causes the other pain or considerable irritation. It is important to create an accepting atmosphere before broaching the painful subject. It has been suggested that an effective way of doing this is to avoid a full frontal attack of bluntly stating a complaint. Rather, use the rule 'Three positives, a negative, a positive'. This means, say three good things about your partner, then state the complaint using 'I feel ...', and finally finish with another good point. An example is given below.

> I know you work so hard darling [positive], and are usually there when I need you [positive], but sometimes I feel so lonely at night when lying in bed and you won't speak to me [negative]. I'm sure you will understand how I feel [positive].

Such an approach may seem strange at first, but when one realizes that the aim is to support a grieving partner while seeking some changes to fulfil one's own needs, the benefit will be obvious. Don't expect the change from 'You do this ...' to 'I feel ...' to occur immediately or automatically. It requires practice.

Start by determining to use it once a day, and gradually build up to it becoming normal usage.

False assumptions often lie at the base of many communication breakdowns. A wife who feels a failure may assume that her husband's irritability after work has to do with some anger directed at her. She may feel rejected, and so withdraw. This leaves the husband, who has simply had a bad day at work, wondering why she is behaving in this way. He may then assume that he has done something wrong, and two people who need each other are separated through misinterpretations. Neither partner should assume that he/she understands the other's feelings. If one partner seems disturbed and the other is unsure what is the cause of this, ask! Don't assume!

> Honey, you seem a bit down tonight. Is there anything wrong? Have I done something to upset you?

Sometimes one partner wants to discuss something with the other but feels uncomfortable or embarrassed, unable to find the words to broach the subject. He/she may be afraid of being rebuked, or simply feel uncomfortable about discussing feelings or problems. Unfortunately, there is no magic cure for such uneasiness except practice. One may have to face disconcerting responses from a partner at first, but don't be put off by these. Once again, honesty with one's feelings is important.

> Honey, there is something I would like to talk over with you. Could we turn off the TV after this and talk for a little while? I'm a bit unsure of what I want to say, but I know talking would mean a great deal to me.

Be firm. Don't beg for time, but don't be demanding or uncompromising. This highlights another aspect of communication.

B. The timing of your communication

Deciding on the appropriate time to open up communication may be difficult. Physical support, such as cuddles and loving looks, should be given often, particularly while one's partner is experiencing some socially difficult situation or expressing his/her emotions. In fact, spontaneous displays of affection and support can warm a depressed person at nearly any time.

Similarly, words of encouragement are vital at any time, but particularly when emotions are obvious. Words need not be many in number. Stroking a partner's hand and saying 'I'm here' as he/she cries may be all that is necessary.

At times, the couple may need to discuss a subject in depth. Here, timing is vital. Trying to communicate about sensitive issues when either or both are tired, tense, or irritable is doomed to failure. Confronting each other as one partner arrives home from work after a long day and tense travelling is unfair. Both partners need to have had time to relax and unwind before emotional subjects are broached. A time when interruptions are likely is best avoided. After children are in bed is preferable to the hectic pace experienced before that time. It may even be necessary to make time for communication. Busy people often find it difficult to find time to relax. This may be even worse with those people who seek to avoid grief by becoming 'hyperactive'. A couple may even need to make an 'appointment' with each other. There is nothing wrong with doing this!

> I know you're busy tonight, but tomorrow night neither of us has anything planned. I would really like to have some time then to talk with you about something.

The timing of your communication is often closely involved with the setting.

C. The setting of your communication

A noisy, bustling atmosphere is not conducive to two people being able to express their thoughts and emotions freely and fully. The daily routine may harbour little irritations that intrude on attempts to communicate. It may be best to set aside time in a favourable setting out of the normal environment or cycle of events. Take a long walk in the park or even around the neighbourhood. If necessary, find a babysitter for the children to allow you time to do this.

Romance and closeness will often help relaxation and hence communication. A couple may need to try to rekindle those days of courtship and marriage before the crisis. Why not treat yourselves to a candlelight dinner? It doesn't matter if the dinner consists of gourmet delights or take-aways. It is the atmosphere of relaxation and togetherness that is important. Perhaps there often used to be activities that you participated in and enjoyed as a couple; take time to do them again. Simply enjoy each other's company. That is part of communication. Talking will come with patience and relaxation. One can take a renewed interest in things that are important to one's partner. Not only will this make a partner feel important, but it may help to re-establish the closeness the couple once felt. Communication may then follow more easily.

The list of possible settings for renewed communication is limited only by the couple's imagination. Here are a few examples. Take a drive and park beside the river or in a park. Have dinner out under a tree in a backyard, picnic-style. Go to the beach or a restaurant. Turn off all the lights in the house except one, and play soft music as you relax in lounge chairs. Indulge in mutual massage, or take a holiday. The list goes on. Relax first! Discuss later! A couple shouldn't make a definite decision that they *must* talk seriously and then try to force themselves to do it. Firstly, relax and discuss any topic that is not threatening, and then gently lead into a discussion of feelings. Perhaps open questions such as 'How are you feeling?' or 'I feel . . .' statements may help you begin. If you still feel uneasy, say so.

> I don't know how to start. I do know that lately we are upsetting each other, and we need to talk. I don't know why I behave so strangely sometimes . . .

Some couples may initially find it impossible to sit and discuss their feelings face to face. They may feel that discussion is useless because 'it always ends up in an argument'. Others may feel too embarrassed to discuss feelings. Such situations can be eased by allowing a time-gap between the expression of the feelings and discussion of them. This may be important, particularly if feelings are negative. The time-gap can provide a 'cooling-off' period. One way to accomplish this is by means of a notepad or letter. Some people are better able to express all their thoughts on paper without fear of being 'cut off' in mid-sentence. A letter may allow this. It is important that such a letter is written with 'I feel . . .' statements, combined with positive points about one's partner. The letter may be left for a partner to read while the other is out or he/she is relaxed. It may include a final written suggestion that they don't discuss its contents until after a certain period of time.

Another way of opening communication may be for a notebook to be kept somewhere in the house, drawn up into headings such as: Time, Feeling, Incident, Preceding Feeling (if any), and Behaviour of Partner at Time (if relevant). Each partner may then jot down important feelings as they arise, allowing the other to read and understand them more fully.

There are many other ways individual couples may reopen communication. Yet once again we emphasize that success depends largely on the willingness of each individual partner to make an effort to foster honesty and express his/her feelings in a non-accusatory manner.

Some couples find that they are unable to avoid confrontation and rebuild communication alone. If this is the case, a third party may help to clarify feelings and defuse emotional issues. Often, couples who are tied up in their individual pain are unable to look beyond themselves. They may misinterpret their partner's words and actions, and attack in defence, basing such an attack on false assumptions. A third party can sometimes provide a medium through which messages can be disentangled and honest feelings probed and explored. In some cases, the third party may be a friend or relative who listens to one partner and is able to interpret an incident from a different perspective, allowing the partner to see that perhaps the other was not really behaving thoughtlessly. Many women have found that a woman friend who tries to be objective, rather than one simply willing to participate in a 'howl down your partner' session, can give her new insights. Unfortunately, men do not discuss situations in a similar way with other men quite so often.

Perhaps the most effective third party comes in the form of a counsellor. Such a person is trained to encourage honest communication through a fair hearing for each partner, combined with an encouragement of each to look carefully at how his/her behaviour and words affect the other. Marriage guidance counsellors are most skilled in dealing with couples with communication breakdowns. Other assistance may be obtained from clergy, psychologists, social workers, and doctors trained in counselling. Once again, success is most likely when both partners are willing to attend each session. The counselling setting can often provide an atmosphere away from the home, the scene of most misunderstandings.

D. Learning to listen

Perhaps the most vital component in rebuilding communication is not the ability to talk but the ability to listen, *really* listen. The word 'listen' means much more than just hearing the words a partner speaks. It means hearing the unspoken words and understanding the feelings behind those words. Unfortunately, very few people are good listeners. We simply think we listen to other people. Let's look at some of the ways we fail to listen.

You don't listen when:

You assume that you know what the other is going to say *before* it is said.

You think you know what 'their problem' is immediately.

You are planning what you are going to say next while the other is speaking.

You cut the other off while he/she is still speaking.

Your attention is focused somewhere else in the room or on some other matter.

You tell the other about something that happened to you that was worse, hence making him/her feel that his/her experiences are not important.

You offer advice immediately.

You criticize the other's clumsiness with words.

You hear only the words and ignore the tone of voice and the facial and bodily expressions.

You assume that the other is always blaming you.

You 'know' you're innocent of all fault.

You accuse the other of trying to 'psychoanalyze' you.

If we look honestly at these statements, we know that all of us are guilty of not listening. A couple within a permanent relationship can become so familiar with one another that they begin to assume that they know each other's thoughts. Hence they fail to really listen to what is said.

Listening is a process that requires a great deal of concentration. How can someone improve his/her listening? Below are a few guidelines that might set you on the right path when they are combined with plenty of practice and patience.

1. Attend to your partner.

Effective listening begins with a clearing of our minds of other matters and fixing our senses on our partner. Look at him/her, and concentrate on his/her face and hear the tone of the voice and the words spoken. Don't allow yourself to be distracted from your partner as he/she speaks. Without making him/her uncomfortable, move reasonably close, as sometimes distance can destroy intimacy.

2. Make sure you understand what has been said.

Often in conversations it is obvious what has been said, particularly if the communication is a simple request or question. But when couples discuss feelings, the real meaning may not always be so clear. A partner may have difficulty expressing himself/herself, leaving the other confused. It is important for each partner to be sure that he/she understands what was actually meant by the words expressed. One way to do this is to listen carefully and then rephrase what you believe was said. This belief is then tested out on the partner. 'Yes, that's right' or a similar response tells you that you are on the right track. For example:

Husband:
I sometimes feel as if the baby is more important. I know he has a handicap and I shouldn't feel ... Well, sometimes it would be nice if you'd take some notice of me alone. I am your husband, after all.

Wife:
You mean, you sometimes resent all the attention I give the baby, leaving you to feel that I don't love you as much.

Husband:
Well, yes, I suppose that's right.

In understanding what has been said, you need to note the feeling underlying the words as much as the actual words themselves. Are the words said with anger, a sense of sadness, frustration, hopelessness, or confusion? These feelings, too, must be compared with reality; for example: 'You seem angry. Are you?'

In making such attempts to listen effectively, you can let your partner know you really are interested in what he/she has to say. In such an accepting atmosphere, there is a security for both partners that will encourage healthy discussion.

3. Don't take everything said as a personal slight.

Many cruel things are said out of pain and hurt, and directed toward those whom we care most about. So one partner must not assume that every angry word or criticism is based on a lack of feeling that his/her partner may have for him/her. Many of these feelings and angry words are the result of grief. Try to listen for the pain behind the harsh words, and respond to the distressed person inside rather than the anger expressed.

If honest criticism is made during a discussion, it will not help if one partner retaliates with a list of the other's bad points. We must accept that we all have aspects of our behaviour and personality that may need changing. At these crisis times in a couple's life, when their self-esteem may be low, this is difficult to accept. But real listening includes a risk of hearing something which one would prefer not to be confronted with.

4. Be comfortable with silence.

At times, one partner may find great difficulty in expressing himself/herself. He/she may begin and stop or fumble. There may be a long silence, or there may be tears. Often a person jumps in to fill the silence, so preventing his/her partner from fully expressing his/her feelings. Generally the silence is filled because one is uncomfortable with silence. If you don't really have anything to say in the silence, don't try to say anything. A simple expression of support, such as a hug or the stroking of a hand, may say much more.

5. Don't jump in too soon with advice or solutions.

In some relationships, one partner makes most of the decisions. He/she may lack the patience to listen to a partner. Every person has the right to be heard and express an opinion. One must not be tempted to interrupt the other with advice, criticism, or solutions. The best way to resolve feelings is to be allowed to express them and work them out for oneself. The grieving individual needs to own his/her problems and feelings and find his/her own solutions. Most will, if they are provided with a listening ear.

E. Arguing constructively

Perhaps this section is better entitled: 'Learning to negotiate'. At times tempers become frayed and an argument ensues. Arguments do not have to destroy a relationship. Arguing can be constructive; it can release built-up tension. But most importantly, it must not end on a negative note. The issues underlying the outburst must be brought out and discussed once the heat of the moment has dissipated. Avoiding an argument is difficult when emotions are raw.

In working to avoid arguments, the first step is to look at the arguments the couple have and try to identify what the circumstances surrounding them are. Is there one particular issue that causes intense irritation in one partner? Do tempers flare at a particular time each day or in some particular social situation? Are there certain issues that can never be discussed civilly by the couple? If the couple can identify such explosive circumstances, they are on their way to overcoming continued trouble by consciously avoiding such situations or modifying behaviour in these situations.

For many couples, arguing has developed into a habit. The cycle is always the same. Some people harp on a subject that they know will annoy their partner. They may always remind the partner of a past incident that they know will hurt him/her. This is particularly painful if the incident relates to the couple's child-bearing difficulties. The offended partner may then respond to such attacks with his/her own sets of complaints about the other. Other people may blatantly refuse to discuss an issue, or avoid it by continually changing the subject.

Arguing constructively occurs when a couple are able to forgive an outburst and begin to look carefully at their argument. This may only occur after a 'cooling off' period and when each individual is prepared to accept some fault. The couple must look at what they have in common and then at their individual feelings, expressing them in ways we have already discussed. Most importantly, both must listen and then come to some agreement after weighing all options. A piece of paper on which the pros and cons of each option can be noted is a useful tool.

At times, the couple may devise a signal that is given by either partner when the beginning of an argument is recognized. It may simply be a statement such as 'We're doing it again' or a physical act such as a whistle or an umpire's time-out signal. This may precede the partners going off by themselves to calm down for some minutes. In this way, the couple may be able to break the argument cycle.

Finally, the couple have the best chance of breaking the cycle when neither feels the need to win every dispute. Individuals may need to look closely at themselves to determine if they have such a need. Do they always have to have the last word? Do they need to have their point of view accepted in full as a solution? Must their partner always be the one who first apologizes? Do they ever apologize? Arguments don't produce winners and losers, only misunderstandings and bruised egos. If one partner must always win arguments, constructive arguing in which compromise can be reached will not occur.

F. Build up, don't punish

The aim of any effective communication is to build the feelings of security and understanding of oneself and one's partner. Behaviours that aim to punish some perceived wrong in a partner are not communication.

A couple facing child-bearing difficulties may have low self-esteem. Either or both partners may feel unworthy of love and attention. If one partner blames himself/herself for the situation, this partner may even feel a need to be 'punished'. At times, to achieve such punishment, such partners may deliberately cause arguments to arouse the other's anger. Yet they will not retaliate, for they feel that their partner's anger is justified against such a 'useless person' as themselves.

Others may resist any attempts to be encouraged or refuse to pamper themselves, due to this same self-directed anger. Similarly, if they unconsciously blame their partner for the loss, they may not be blatantly hostile but instead may refuse their partner the little luxuries of life.

It is vital to recognize those nagging feelings of anger within oneself and be able to talk them out. Anger is not to be feared unless it remains trapped inside and only shows itself in ways that punish both partners. Even if the feelings are vague and not readily understood, they need voicing.

Neither partner should punish himself/herself or his/her partner. This is only destructive. In the majority of cases, no one is to blame for a couple's child-bearing problems. The past is simply that — past. To allow it to destroy a relationship gives a painful incident the power to hurt twice. Be gentle with each other. Even splurge a bit. Enjoy time and a few pleasures together. If a couple are then able to relax, they may see their communication build.

Communication in a delicate area

The sexual side of a relationship can be adversely affected when couples have difficulty bearing a child. In general, couples who are facing communication difficulties also often experience some faltering in their sexual relationship. This may improve as overall communication improves.

Unfortunately, there is an added dimension of possible misunderstanding in the sexual relationship of the couple experiencing child-bearing difficulties. For in their case sexual intercourse has been directly involved in their crisis.

We are pleased to point out that for many couples intercourse after a loss is fulfilling and even enhanced. It is found by such couples to be a vital part of helping to heal the wounds. It provides the most intimate expression of their love and support. This closeness and security in each other is in some small measure able to compensate indirectly for their overwhelming loss. For those able to conceive, it can also remind the couple that a later happier ending has a chance of occurring, thereby providing hope for the future.

On the other hand, for other couples intercourse is difficult, for it is tied closely to memories or feelings that are painful. For the infertile couple who desperately want a child, the sexual act may be a reminder of failure. It may simply become a means to an end. Sex may become a mechanical act, dictated by mucus changes, temperature rises, and fertile days. It may become a performance activity, in which ejaculation is classified as success. Intercourse can become anxiety-provoking for both partners, interfering with the spontaneity of the act. In fact, physiological processes may be interrupted. There may be less lubrication, and erection and ejaculation may be more difficult to achieve. This may further increase feelings of failure and unsatisfactory outcomes. If intercourse is so disrupted during the fertile days, another chance of pregnancy is lost and depression may result. The achievement of a pregnancy can be all-consuming, and intercourse as an expression of love may become lost in its role as the mode of precreation. This may happen not only for the infertile couple, but also for the couple who lost a child and wish to try for a new one as soon as possible.

For the couple who have lost a pregnancy in its early weeks or whose child has died, intercourse may trigger other feelings. Some may fear another pregnancy and the possibility of a loss recurring. Intercourse, being the cause of pregnancy, may then be rejected.

For others, intercourse is interrupted by a loss of self-confidence. One partner may feel so undesirable that he/she cannot understand how the other would want to be near him/her, and hence may reject any advances.

Others may feel guilt: 'How can we try to find pleasure when our baby is facing such a crisis?' If intercourse has been suspected by the couple of causing the loss, even when this belief is unfounded, it may be rejected: 'How can we have sex? We couldn't control ourselves before, and look what happened.' In cases of death before delivery, a male may even feel a sense of fear about his partner's body.

One of the most common symptoms of depression is a lowered sex-drive. This may be complicated by the extreme fatigue experienced by the parents of a premature or abnormal child. The lowered sex-drive worries couples, but it must be remembered that this problem will generally ease as grief is resolved. The mind seems to be so preoccupied with its pain that it is unable to concentrate on feelings of closeness. An act such as intercourse that holds reminders of how a lost or ill baby was conceived, may deepen depression and hence is avoided.

Individual feelings of partners may differ due to differences in grieving as well as physiological differences. Often after a loss of a pregnancy, the woman is more depressed. Her male partner may wish to resume sexual relations before she is ready. This she may resent.

Overcoming such problems within sexual relations may require time and patience. It also requires one vital component, that of being concerned foremost with the needs of one's partner, and being willing to adapt to these needs. In many cases, the more willing partner may have to make sacrifices during the initial period, and wait until his/her partner feels comfortable with the resumption of intercourse. Such a sacrifice will be rewarded later. If there is pressure on the unwilling partner, he/she may feel rushed and resentful, and may be left with long-term difficulties.

If couples can express their feelings, fears, and misunderstandings about sex, some problems may be overcome.

Unfortunately, discussing sex is often difficult for couples who feel embarrassed about such intimate subjects. If couples find it impossible to talk together, perhaps they could read together one of the fine books written on the subject. Such reading may help to make the subject less threatening, and hence open it up for discussion.

It is important for the couple to allow themselves time to overcome difficulties. Don't try to rush a solution. Each partner must be given time to work through his/her emotions and fears. If pregnancy is feared by either partner, a method of contraception that is highly effective should be employed. The partner may feel differently, and wish to achieve a new pregnancy as soon as possible. But this is not advisable until both partners have become comfortable with such an idea. Respect for a partner's wishes must be an integral part of any communication. Other fears, such as that of another loss, should be discussed with a doctor, who will be able to provide an informed opinion of the risks involved. This may relieve some tension.

To renew confidence and revitalize a sex life, the couple need to try to divorce sex from reproduction. They need to re-experience intercourse simply as an act of intimacy. This may be extremely difficult during the fertile days, when conception may be uppermost in the mind. The couple should therefore concentrate on the other weeks of the cycle, when conception is not expected. They may spend such time trying to reintroduce romance into their relationship.

Sex needs to become more than a physical act. It needs to be a gradual build-up of caring and emotion, which is finally expressed in complete intimacy. The environment is important in making the couple feel relaxed. Why not begin dating each other again? A candlelight dinner (even of fish and chips); a quiet evening, listening to music and dancing around the lounge room; a picnic; a moonlight stroll; a glass of wine on the patio in the cool; walking in the rain and drying off in front of the fireplace or in a warm kitchen; so many situations can become romantic when daily distractions and routine are removed. If there are other children, find a baby-sitter for an evening every now and then, and spend time alone. It is not necessary for romance to be expensive. Romance is born in closeness and the attitude of the participants.

Romance should not be limited to an evening specially set aside for it. Little actions unrelated to sex can rebuild those feelings of love. Surprise each other! Leaving a little loving note in his lunch box; giving an unexpected hug; doing that job your partner has been harping about, without his/her knowing; preparing a favourite meal; cooking a tasty treat by the one who is not normally the cook; preparing a bubble-bath for a tired worker, when he/she comes home; an interest shown in a partner's hobby, even if the other may feel that his/her time could be better spent; bringing home a flower or his favourite magazine (expense is not necessary); offering to take the kids out so that a partner can rest; the special surprises are limited only by one's imagination. The importance of such acts of romance lies in recognizing and appreciating one's partner. If one partner does something special, the other must accept it gracefully in the way it was intended. One must resist the tendency to suspect that the other simply wants something from him/her, or is 'buttering them up' as a prelude to 'falling into bed'. Of course, the bestower of the gift must be sure that he/she does not have an ulterior motive. In general, try to accept each loving act as having the best of intentions. These acts and words of romance help to build the confidence of each individual, which is vital to re-establishing an intimate sharing. Each should make a determined effort to treat his/her partner as someone special — he as a mixture of Superman and the world's greatest lover, she as Miss World and Wonder Woman.

When intercourse is feared or causes distress, it may be best to rediscover other ways of intimately sharing affection. If a reluctant partner is reassured that he/she will not be pressured into intercourse, this person may be able to relax more easily in the caresses and gentle close contact of a partner. The gentle kisses, stroking, and holding close may provide a deep security and reduce the feeling of being threatened, by increasing a person's confidence in his/her desirability. As the couple relax in these intimate surroundings, their need for the greater intimacy of intercourse may come as a natural progression, although this progression may take considerable time.

For other couples, intercourse is not interrupted but has lost its passion. Romance may help revitalize its fire. For many, it is the loss of spontaneity that has affected it. It has become habit. Sometimes simple changes may help alleviate the loss. Vary the timing and environment. Why not use a different bed or place or position or time of day? Why not dress up as if homecoming and dinner were a special occasion? Change the environment. A messy room or an unmade bed may be less conducive to relaxation and intimacy than clean crisp sheets in an immaculate room with low lights, soft music, and fresh flowers. Two clean cool bodies, after perhaps a shared shower, invite a mutual massage and increased intimacy.

In some cases, a couple may find that the problem seems to remain an obstacle they find difficult to overcome. In these cases, it is important that the couple seek professional help early. Marriage-guidance counsellors or sex therapists are trained to assist couples to deal with these difficulties. Doctors are usually able to refer couples to such individuals. In some cases, sexual difficulties may reflect deep unresolved problems being experienced by one partner or within the interactions of the couple.

There is one situation in which couples have to employ immense self-control. In general, doctors advise that intercourse can be continued during pregnancy without fear of harming the baby. But in some cases of repeated miscarriage or premature labour, intercourse may be advised against throughout the entire pregnancy, or at least during some 'danger' period. Where hospitalization is involved, the situation seems more final. For couples denied intercourse, their task is to maintain intimacy and overcome any frustration. It is vital in such circumstances that both partners realize the importance of abstinence and are committed to the child whose future the advice is intended to protect. Close bodily contact and foreplay activities may still provide some intimacy when couples are at home. Within the hospital setting, simple actions are important, the hug, the hand-holding, the kiss, and even the cuddle when either partner is depressed.

Sexual relations can be interrupted when couples face child-bearing difficulties. Sex is closely tied with the crisis. Overcoming these difficulties will require patience, tender caring, and respect for the fears and feelings of one's partner.

The single parent

In discussing the single parent, we must consider a varied group of people. There are those women who have been left single through divorce or the break-up of a de facto or long-term relationship. Then there are single teenagers, and career women who have made a conscious decision to have a child. The widow or widower has a second major loss to add to his/her grief. The single father may also experience feelings of grief for a lost child if his relationship with the child's mother has come to an end.

The single parent will experience many of the same feelings as other parents facing child-bearing difficulties. But there are also added pressures on them, caused by their particular situation. Perhaps the greatest strain on the single parent is the lack of the strong, involved support of a partner who shares the crisis. They don't have that one person who is fully involved with the loss of this particular child. Others may provide support, but the single parent may still feel very alone. There is not the loving partner to hold them in bed at night when the tears flow, to share the anger and frustration, or to make the lonely visits to the hospital to see their child. Often relatives and friends are unable to understand the depths of their emotions.

> When I had the toxaemia, I had to come to Brisbane because I didn't have anyone to look after me. That was when I felt the absence of a husband.

When there has been a breakdown in relationship, the woman must deal with the grief of the separation while having to face the prospect of a life by herself with the baby. The fear of financial difficulties and the social problems of raising a child alone, particularly if that child suffers from some abnormality, may then be combined with grief. There may be the trauma of reconciliations and further breakdowns, and the difficulty of making the final decision to end this relationship. Many struggle with the decision of whether or not to end the pain, only to replace it with an even more uncertain situation. For many, the pregnancy may provide a reason to plan for a future. Others may resent the child, particularly if there is a feeling that the pregnancy in some way disrupted the relationship. If the child is later lost, feelings of futility or guilt may then emerge even more strongly.

The pregnant teenager or the woman not expecting the pregnancy may face the disapproval of those around her, the sadness of rejection by the male involved, and the fear of the future.

> When I fell pregnant it was a big shock. It was totally unexpected. I told the father. Even then, he wanted me to have an abortion. I'd already decided I wouldn't have an abortion. I'd never do that. It was hard telling him. It was a very casual relationship. I had no intention of marrying him, but I was happy to tell him that he was the father and that he could see the child. He couldn't cope with that, and I never saw him again after that. That was hard for the first couple of days and weeks. He said other things, such as that I couldn't cope with it, my whole life would be wrecked, and I would never manage. He said that I was too young. I was angry with this reaction.

Some teenagers may have become pregnant in the hope that a baby may help them resolve problems. They may feel that a baby will have to love them, when others around don't seem to. The young teenager who feels a failure in so many areas may be attracted by the attention and success afforded a woman when she is able to produce a child. If the baby is lost, the problems she sought to escape will return, made more intense by a new sense of failure. Some may then wish to become pregnant again as soon as possible to obliterate this new failure. Grief may not be resolved, and the internal conflicts may deepen.

For the single teenager or the woman who did not wish to be pregnant, there may be feelings of relief if a miscarriage occurs. Yet such women may feel guilt for such feelings, and be unable to accept such conflicting emotions. Teenagers who suffer a loss are not only faced with intense grief, but are also expected to cope with this grief at a time in their lives when their emotions, values, and feelings are already confused. The teenager may have to cope without the approval and support offered to an adult couple. It is little wonder, then, that these young women often never fully resolve their grief.

In more recent years, there is a growing number of women making a conscious decision to have a child. Often they are women in their late twenties or early thirties who have established themselves in a career. They find themselves without a long-term relationship, either through choice or circumstance, yet they feel able to care for a child. The lead up to the pregnancy is usually well planned. For some, their dream may be shattered when there appears to be some period of infertility. They continue with their career, but the loss of their dream of a child may have tarnished the attraction of their career. The desire to be a mother may make other aspects of their life that used to have such significance, pale slightly.

For the woman who does attain a pregnancy, there may be some social misunderstanding and disapproval of her actions. She must learn to cope with such misunderstandings, which may lead to some changes in her relationships with friends and family. Her relationship with the baby's father may also have to be considered, and may cause some difficulties. To have overcome such difficulties and then to lose the child, can leave the woman feeling hopeless and introduce a sense of failure she may have never before experienced in her previously successful life. At times, she may even feel that she is being punished for having done something that is not socially acceptable. Her loss may be treated less sensitively and compassionately than that of a married couple. There may be some feeling among relatives and friends that perhaps 'it was for the best', although this may not be openly expressed.

> I went out to lunch with this guy. I'd said something to someone about how I'd just like to be pregnant again. I thought she'd understood what I meant. But it had got back to this guy that I had an urgent need to rush out and become pregnant again immediately, that I was actually planning to do that. So he gave me a big talk on how next time I'd better make sure it was someone who loves me, that I had a permanent relationship, and that it would be foolish to go out and get pregnant now. I was amazed. He said that it's wrong to say that it's a blessing, because it's so hard to be a single mother; it's better it happened this way. But I'm no different from a married woman; I love my baby just as much. I want it just as much. Maybe I've even gone through more to have it. I have just as much grief as someone else.

One of the deepest pains of all must be that felt by the widow who has been unable to bear a child or who loses the child of her beloved husband. In some rare instances, a husband may lose either his wife or child, and then face the loss of the other through severe complications. Grief upon grief! That such people are able to cope at all seems hard to believe. If there are no other children from this relationship, there is the loss of a permanent reminder of the loved one. These people require a great deal of support. The severe strain often causes physical illness in such people. The problem in such a situation is so immense that it is beyond the scope of this book. Professional help may be required.

For many couples, the final resolution of their loss often comes after the later birth of a live, healthy, mature baby. They may seek to become pregnant as soon as possible, and there is then a feeling of compensating for their loss in some way. But this is often an option not available to the single parent. So there is a further loss — the loss of being able to hope for a happier outcome in the near future. Some single women still feel a strong need to have another child and plan to do so, but face practical difficulties. Friends and family may find it difficult to understand such a need, and discourage such plans. If the need is overpowering, relationships with males may be affected. Any relationship which is entered into for only one reason is likely to face real difficulties, and is unlikely to develop on a long-term basis.

> I find the need to have a baby very hard. I remember saying to one of the nurses: 'What am I supposed to do now? Get married so that I can have a baby?' You do cling to the idea of having another baby. It's a lot harder for me. If I do it, I'll have to plan it this time. It won't be an accident, and I may not get as much support from people as I did this time. Mum and Dad are terrified that I might do it again.

The single father is generally forgotten. After the breakdown of a relationship, many males disappear from the life of the woman. Others remain tied to some degree to the woman through the child that is expected. If the relationship has not been one of marital commitment, the father's role and rights may be unclear. If the child is lost or is born with an abnormality, he may also suffer all the pain of grief but may be denied the right to grieve by those around him. If the relationship has ended quite amicably, he may feel deeply pained for his ex-partner, sharing her grief, yet being unsure of whether or not expression of this concern is appropriate.

As we can see, single parents must face grief, but often without a great deal of support and with added complications from other problems that affect them because of their particular circumstances. Single parents may need to seek out those people able to accept their grief and understand the courage that they must find.

Conclusion

The relationship a grieving parent may find himself/herself in may change when faced with child-bearing difficulties. In some cases, changes will see the relationship enhanced. Unfortunately, in other cases there will be a breakdown of the relationship and the loss of much support. An ailing relationship may be rebuilt with much patience, care, and a willingness on the part of both partners to change their individual behaviours and their interaction. An acceptance of one's partner's basic humanness and his/her pain, and a rediscovery of the fine points of character of the other that one fell in love with, are vital to rebuilding a life together. The single parent must find the strength to cope alone, and must be provided with caring support to assist him/her.

10 The Reactions of Others

This chapter is dedicated particularly to our families, to our obstetrician, Dr A. Neil Astill, and the staff of the Mater Misericordiae Mothers Hospital, Brisbane, all of whom gave us confidence and security through their expert knowledge, caring, and basic understanding of our needs.

The reactions of other people can have a significant effect on the grieving couple. We are social beings, with many of our attitudes about ourselves and society being shaped early in life. We constantly seek acceptance and understanding from those around us. If others seem unable to understand our feelings, we feel alone and isolated.

The ability of others to respond to a grieving couple in such a way as to provide real support may be affected by a number of factors. Firstly, the personalities of individuals can differ greatly. Some are relaxed and self-confident, finding it relatively easy to be open and friendly toward most people. Others are more reserved, finding conversation difficult. Secondly, each individual has a role to play, whether it be that of a mother, father, doctor, nurse, priest, child, grandparent, or friend. Each different role has some expected behaviours. For example, a grandmother may be expected to be nurturing, loving, patient, and moderate in her habits. The grandmother who rides high-powered motorcycles and swears profusely may not appear to fit the role as expected. Often, people react according to the behaviour they believe is expected of their role, rather than reacting to their feelings. Thirdly, those who are often most capable of dealing with another's crisis are the persons who have experienced a similar situation or have met and dealt with some other difficulty. These people are more able to respond to the feelings of another, having themselves experienced such feelings first-hand. Others may only be able to theorize about what the grieving couple must be experiencing. Finally, some people, through prior experiences or training, have developed skills that allow them to communicate caring, and react appropriately to people in crisis. Others are not so readily able to do so.

If we realize just how varied are the abilities of people to relate to others in crisis, it is not difficult to understand that at times some people will say or do things that hurt the grieving couple. The couple have a right to feel hurt, but in connection with hurtful remarks we wish to make one important comment: The vast majority of those who make hurtful comments or act inappropriately will do so out of ignorance rather than malice. People are generally uneasy with crisis, not knowing what to say or do. They may find themselves relying on clichés and platitudes, not realizing the possible inappropriateness of these. It is important to remember that without an intimate knowledge of the couple, the situation, and one's own feelings, people are liable to make mistakes. However, the grieving couple may find it difficult to accept such human error when anger or depression are their constant companions.

At the same time, other people can be a positive force in the life of the grieving couple when those around are sensitive and know something about the crisis, and when the couple are able to view the occasional inappropriate comment as due to human error rather than malice or thoughtlessness.

Doctors

Patients and doctors may unknowingly set the stage for problems within their relationship. Many of us as patients have looked on the doctor, the 'expert', as almost god-like. Most doctors deserve a great deal of respect, but they are not omnipotent. Many patients suffering a medical condition expect a cure from their doctor, and are discouraged and even angered when the cure, to the extent they expected, is not forthcoming. Some doctors, too, have encouraged such thinking in patients by playing the 'expert' role, showing the attitude: 'I know what is best for you, so don't you worry'. Such paternalism further reinforces the belief in the patient that the doctor must be able to produce a cure or solution.

This belief is further strengthened within this age of modern medicine. This is the era of *in vitro* fertilization, transplants, and other medical 'miracles'. Diseases that in the not-so-distant past would have spelt death are now curable. The loss of a baby through birth difficulties and complications is now a fairly rare event. When failure does occur, it is often difficult for both doctor and patient to accept. There is an expectation among patients that there is little that the doctor cannot explain, treat, and eventually cure.

Unfortunately, although there is great progress in medicine, doctors don't have all the answers. In the area of gynaecology and obstetrics there are large gaps in their knowledge. Theories abound, but finding a definite cause and a sure cure for a condition may yet be some time in the future or may never eventuate. Why is it that a couple whose tests show no abnormal functioning are still unable to conceive? Why does a group of women continuously begin to labour prematurely? Why do some apparently perfect babies suddenly die in the uterus? What causes some abnormalities that seem to have no genetic component? What causes actual labour to begin? The list of unanswered questions goes on. Even specialists in this area will admit that, irrespective of all the research and sophistication, there is still a lot to be learnt. Therefore, it is unfair for doctors to be expected to have the answers for all problems in all situations. It can be expected that they keep up with modern developments and research, as does any other professional. It is often difficult for patients and even doctors to accept that there is not always an answer. Patients, in desperation, plead with the expert: 'But you're a doctor, can't you do something?' Patients often want a doctor to be all-powerful, for the alternative of accepting that at times a situation is out of all human control is too painful to contemplate.

The doctor is not infallible, although most are highly professional and mistakes are rare. They are not gifted with the power of predicting the future, so are at times faced with extremely difficult decisions. In hindsight, some of these decisions are found to be incorrect, and doctors themselves will be the first to agonize over such a decision. They may blame themselves and fear the reactions of patients. Fearful of possible anger or personal recriminations, they may withdraw from the patient physically and emotionally as quickly as possible. If a grieving parent turns his/her anger upon the doctor, the situation is made even more difficult. Of course, this is not to deny that in some rare instances doctors have been negligent and anger is justified. Fortunately, such cases are extremely rare.

Doctors are skilled technicians, having great knowledge of the human body and its workings. But they remain human! Doctors will be the first to admit this. Being human, they suffer from the same frailties, insecurities, and fears as the rest of us. Unfortunately, our view of doctors and what we have come to expect from them often prevents them from relating to patients on a more human basis. At times, patients complain that their doctor is 'cold' and 'doesn't understand'. Some doctors in their role of expert may be afraid that becoming involved with a patient or expressing emotion over a loss will be received by patients as unprofessional, as weakness, or as appearing to admit some guilt over an incident. In some cases this feeling is justified, for some patients do feel confidence in a doctor who appears as the aloof, unemotional expert. Unfortunately, others feel alienated by such behaviour.

Most specialists in the area of gynaecology and obstetrics are males. It is not surprising, then, that at times it is difficult for these specialists to understand fully the feelings of the women with whom they are dealing. Their information is based on books, their female loved ones, acquaintances, and other patients — all second-hand experience. In noting this, we are not implying that male specialists are unable to understand or that women specialists are necessarily better qualified to work in such an area. A male doctor with a respect for his patients and their intimate connection with their body and baby, combined with a willingness to listen, is superbly qualified to deal with child-bearing difficulties. Women doctors may have first-hand knowledge of pregnancy in general, but unless they themselves have faced child-bearing difficulties they may also be unable to understand fully the problems of such couples.

Doctors, like most other people, may not have come to terms with their own feelings about certain issues. One issue comes to light when a baby is born with a severe abnormality. The doctor may feel strongly about the injustice of such children being born to parents who have taken such care throughout pregnancy, or who have suffered prior difficulties. They themselves may be unable to visualize their own reactions to such a child, and hence are unable to offer much moral support. For many doctors, the death of a child is difficult to accept. Like so many of us, they have not come to terms with their own mortality or that of their loved ones. There is a fear of death, a fear of this finality being out of one's control. Many are unable to cope with death emotionally or feel comfortable with those who are close to it. In this way, many doctors are no different from the rest of us. They fumble for words or withdraw from the situation.

Problems in the doctor-patient relationship

In the medical model there are two major roles — that of the doctor and that of the patient. The relationship between these two people is often dictated, not by personalities, but by what one expects from the other. If a patient wants the reassurance of being told what to do without question by an expert who views the patient as someone to be given such advice, the traditional relationship may work well for both parties. There is nothing wrong with the relationship of traditional expert and passive patient if both parties feel that their needs are met by such a partnership.

In many other instances, patients are uncomfortable with remaining passive. They see a highly professional manner of a doctor as aloofness. Such feelings arise when doctors are unable or unwilling to discuss openly with a patient the causes of a condition and the treatments to be carried out. The 'expert' attitude of a doctor makes many couples feel discouraged to ask questions. Some patients feel shy about asking questions for fear that they may be considered ignorant or that the doctor may react unfavourably. A few doctors do react to questions as if they are an attack on their knowledge or as if they indicate a lack of confidence on the part of the patient in their ability.

Unfortunately, many patients are unnecessarily afraid to ask questions. Their doctor may be quite willing to answer their questions, but if they fail to ask them, information is not ventured independently by the doctor. At times, there may be an assumption on the part of the doctor that a patient may not be able to understand an explanation. This may be the case where there is an excessive use of medical jargon. Some patients are content

without an explanation, but many others feel more secure w
some explanation given at their level of comprehension.

It is important, then, that each doctor-patient relationship be
viewed independently. The doctor needs to be able to
individualize his/her approach to suit the needs of each patient.
Difficulty in doing so, and hence the use of a standard approach for
all patients, may leave many patients feeling resentful or
alienated. When contact is made only through a few short
consultations, it requires a great deal of sensitivity on the part of
the doctor to be able to relate successfully to the individual needs
of every patient. This is an almost impossible task for any person,
even a doctor.

Couples facing child-bearing difficulties are experiencing a
very emotional time in their lives. In many cases it preoccupies
their minds. On the other hand, the doctor may see such
circumstances occurring much more commonly. He/she may
realize through experience that in many cases the incident is
unlikely to recur. The doctor may therefore find it difficult to
understand the intense emotions of the patient. This may happen
in such cases as when patients seek help in the early months of
finding difficulty in conceiving, or in early miscarriage. Patients
don't have the doctor's knowledge of such events, and are also
living each day with their grief and fears. A doctor who does not
understand this may see intense emotional reactions as being
symptoms of something more serious, or as being an unnecessary
overreaction to a situation. If this attitude is communicated to the
patient by a doctor's manner, the patient may begin to feel
'neurotic', to feel that most of the problem is 'in their heads'. This
feeling can further complicate the couple's already low opinion of
themselves and the sense of failure the grieving parents may
already be experiencing. Being labelled 'neurotic' may lead a
patient to ignore signs or become hesitant about reporting fears in
a later pregnancy.

Another difficulty can arise for a couple after the birth of a
premature baby or one with an abnormality. During the months of
pregnancy, the couple, particularly the woman, may have built up
a close relationship with her obstetrician. After the birth of the
baby, this support may be lost too soon when she leaves hospital
and the baby's care is relegated to other professionals.

Overcoming difficulties

The couple can help build a satisfying relationship with their doctor by being aware that he/she is a person first, a doctor second. Doctors deserve respect and acceptance for having limitations as do other humans.

As in any communication, it is important that a patient does not expect the doctor to be able to read his/her mind. If there are questions a couple want answered, they should ask them. If a couple feel nervous when in the doctor's office and forget what they wish to ask, they may write down their questions beforehand as they come to their minds and take them to their doctor's appointment. If something worries them about the situation, or if they want anything in particular, they should ask their doctor. He/she may feel relieved by being given some concrete way of helping in a situation in which the doctor himself/herself may feel powerless.

Doctors, too, by their actions can help to build strong two-way relationships with patients experiencing child-bearing difficulties. They can provide support to their female patients by encouraging their partners to be fully involved in discussions and appointments where possible. It may be necessary to arrange appointment times to allow a couple with difficulties to attend together. The couple need to feel that they are involved in making any decisions about testing and the future. Honesty is vital. Straightforward discussion on a level suitable to the understanding of the couple is necessary. Treatments and their effects should be fully explained.

It is important that doctors realize that pregnancies following a loss will be accompanied by fears of a further loss. Such fears must be treated with understanding, and much can be done to alleviate some of them. If the patient wants and can afford it, the doctor may suggest more regular appointments. Practical reassurance at each visit, such as the amplification of the foetal heartbeat and full examination and explanation of the progress of the pregnancy, can be vital. Such women may be more aware of their bodily changes and the activity of pregnancy. They may be concerned unnecessarily, but such concern must be treated with patience and understanding. Simply saying 'That's normal. Lots of women have that' is not as reassuring for a woman as having her doctor examine her carefully to rule out any possible problems. Some doctors are concerned that if they look worried their patient will be unnecessarily upset. Hence they adopt a highly optimistic, even jovial, appearance, feeling that this may relieve the patient's worries. However, generally a patient will not be upset by a doctor's appearance of concern, and if the doctor follows this concern by an examination and reassurance on the grounds of this examination, the woman will be comforted. The patient is more likely to see the doctor's concern as a willingness to take seriously what she says. Hence, she may be reassured of his/her concern and be able to relax more effectively. Even more importantly, it must be remembered that some women *will* experience repeated losses, and their seemingly innocent symptoms may actually signal a possible problem.

Women who have suffered repeated losses may be reassured by knowing that they can ring their doctor at any time if they are uneasy. A doctor may even set aside a special time each week during which time the patient, when she feels the need, is encouraged to contact her doctor to simply report on her progress and receive reassurance and encouragement. Such patients may also feel more at ease when treated as an old friend rather than a nervous patient. Since the patient may feel shy about seeking such considerations from the doctor, it will most likely be the doctor who will have to offer such reassurances to his/her patient.

Some child-bearing situations require very careful handling. The failure of an *in vitro* fertilization attempt, the onset of miscarriage, premature birth, death, or the discovery of an abnormality are all accompanied by strong emotions. A doctor can be most effective in such instances when he/she has some understanding of grieving. The couple's emotions will then be more predictable, and responses to them more easily shaped. An angry or withdrawn reaction may then not be viewed by the doctor as some attack on him/herself. Therefore, the doctor may be less likely to withdraw from such patients when he/she may be needed most. The doctor may help in grieving by preparing his/her patients honestly for events that may occur. Understanding an event can remove some of the fear from it.

It is a very difficult time for doctors when they must deliver sad news. As human beings they feel pain and suffer some difficulty in finding the right words. Bad news should be given to parents together in a place conducive to the expressing of their emotions. It may be a private room set aside for such a purpose, or, if in a labour ward, one where others will not interrupt the discussion. The couple will be initially shrouded in shock, and hence a detailed explanation of the event may not be appropriate at this time. Many of the details may be forgotten or denied as the realization of what has happened sinks in. Therefore the initial discussion must be gentle and compassionate, providing the basic facts stated in a simple straightforward manner. At such times a gesture of compassion, such as a hand on the shoulder or a squeeze of the hand, may be reassuring for the couple. Some doctors may be embarrassed by such a gesture, and fear it may be misinterpreted by the grieving parents. Generally, this will not happen. Rather, such a gesture can create a special bond between doctor and parents. A more detailed discussion of the loss should be arranged with the parents at a later date, when the initial shock has subsided and their minds are full of questions. Some hospitals arrange a conference six to eight weeks after the death of a child. This is conducted by a senior neonatologist, and may include other personnel such as nursing supervisors, social workers, or pastoral-care workers.

In many cases, the first contact a couple has with a doctor after a loss is the six-weekly visit after a birth. In cases of miscarriage, there may not be a follow-up visit at all. Many women feel that six weeks is a long time to wait to get answers to their important questions. A woman may therefore be offered an additional earlier appointment, during which time she can simply ask the questions that may plague her. Her six-weekly check-up may then be devoted simply to physical examination and other questions she may like to ask after considering the information provided at the earlier visit. Her appointments may be organized for a time when she is least likely to encounter many other pregnant women. They should not be hurried, and staff should be informed of the visit so that antenatal checks are not erroneously attempted, causing the patient unnecessary distress.

> After I lost the baby I went back for my six-weekly check. I still looked pregnant. It was hard, going into the doctor's office and seeing all those pregnant women. I was still upset, but coping

> pretty well. Then the doctor's receptionist called me over to the side room. I wasn't sure what she wanted. She told me to stand on the scales and asked if I had brought a urine sample. She thought I was still pregnant, and wanted to do normal antenatal checks. I just went to pieces. She wasn't very understanding.

It may be extremely difficult for the doctor at the time of the loss to see his/her patient displaying such intense emotions. He/she may prescribe sedation in an attempt to ease obvious pain. Unfortunately, sedation may serve only to dull the emotions and senses, and simply delay grief. Grief must be experienced, and sedation will not overcome it. Perhaps it may be more appropriate to prescribe that someone is available at night to listen if the woman finds herself unable to sleep and wishes to talk. In some cases, limited sedation may be effective.

Many doctors are able to build a strong two-way relationship with their patients, providing them with information, support, and expert treatment. We applaud such doctors. The comments made above are not ones of criticism of the medical profession as such. They are made in the realization that doctors may have limited first-hand experience of child-bearing difficulties, and hence may be unaware of how their behaviour may be viewed by a couple experiencing such difficulties.

Choosing a doctor

It is not unusual for a couple who have experienced a loss to want to remove all memories of the loss in later pregnancies or when further testing is required. This may mean wanting a change of doctor, which is an understandable reaction. Yet in one way a doctor may find it difficult. After having experienced a loss with the couple, it may be difficult for him/her to see a colleague sharing with the couple the joy of a later successful pregnancy.

Some couples feel guilt on changing doctors or seeking out a second opinion. Such guilt is unnecessary, for in many relationships there may come a time when the needs of one party are not being met. Parting is then the best alternative. Patients pay for the services of a doctor, and if they are not satisfied they have a right to look elsewhere. Unfortunately, some patients continually change doctors in the hope that they will receive the news they wish to hear rather than face an unpleasant truth. In general, though, a change of doctor comes about when a patient perceives a breakdown in communication with his/her doctor.

Couples experiencing child-bearing difficulties require not only a doctor with medical expertise but also one who is willing and able to provide the emotional support they require. A doctor who elicits confidence and a relaxed feeling in a patient is able to provide the best atmosphere for open communication. Different doctors will suit different patients, but in general most patients are able to relax in an atmosphere where the doctor appears concerned, confident, efficient, open, and welcoming. A doctor who recognizes the vital part played by the emotions of couples with child-bearing difficulties is one who is on the way to providing the psychological support which, for such couples, is as important as medical expertise.

Patients within the public hospital system may not be afforded the constant supervision of one doctor. Difficulties may then arise in recounting past history and receiving consistent medical treatment and psychological support. For this reason, inservice training of doctors to alert them to the emotional aspects of pregnancy and child-bearing difficulties may be necessary to ensure that all patients receive appropriate care.

Often patients are unsure of how to choose a doctor. Doctors vary in many aspects: age, personality, sex, patient involvement, training, specialities, hospital connections, partnerships, and general medical beliefs. Patients generally are referred to a specialist by their local general practitioner (GP). Few patients who are not happy with this specialist feel comfortable about returning to their GP for a referral to another specialist in the same field. A GP can be guided in his/her referrals by seeking out information from patients on the type of specialist with whom they would feel comfortable, and by noting patient reaction to prior referrals. GPs therefore should not confine themselves to referrals to only one specialist, but rather refer to a number who have the necessary expertise but differ on their personal approaches.

A patient may also receive information about doctors from other patients, remembering, of course, that a non-professional judgment must be considered carefully in case there has been a personality clash between the doctor and this particular patient.

Often, women who have experienced similar difficulties, particularly repeated losses, have had time to build up relationships with doctors and hence have more informed opinions.

Finally, patients may actually 'test the waters' by making one visit to a particular specialist. During such a visit they may simply discuss their past history, ask questions, and seek out doctors' opinions on their cases. During such an appointment, the patient may then be able to formulate some impression as to whether or not she would feel confident with this doctor's particular approach.

Doctors are skilled persons, with in-depth knowledge in the field of medicine. But they are not miracle workers. They are limited by the realm of human knowledge and their medical and personal experiences. Difficulties can arise when we as patients fail to accept that they do not have the final control over birth and death. In giving doctors respect for their expertise, acceptance of their human personalities, and guidance as to our own expectations, we are able to encourage a relationship with them in which our needs will be served. Yet, as patients, we must accept that at times there may be a breakdown in communication with a doctor, which is best remedied by seeking out a second opinion or another doctor whose approach is better suited to our particular personality and needs.

Hospital nursing staff

Hospitalization of a woman for child-bearing difficulties can be an emotional and trying time for both patient and nursing staff alike. The nursing staff at this time will have more direct contact with the grieving patient than will her doctor. It is they who may see the tears and experience the brunt of the shock and anger, and it is they who are around the patient in the long night hours.

As with the general population, nursing staff may feel at a loss for what to say to grieving patients. They may retreat behind inappropriate clichés, or simply avoid the subject altogether. Without first-hand experience of loss themselves, nursing staff may find the intensity of emotions expressed by patients confusing and sometimes exaggerated.

Actual daily care of the patient may fall to the nurses who are usually at the bottom of the power hierarchy of the hospital. Such nurses may be unsure of whether or not they may be breaking some unwritten hospital code by attempting to comfort the grieving parents in some particular way. They may also feel quite inadequate to meet the needs of this situation, due to their inexperience. Therefore they may simply make 'small talk', take their observations, and leave the patient. In fact, patients experiencing child-bearing difficulties may find themselves left alone more often than other patients, due to staff uneasiness, adding further to their feelings of isolation and alienation.

Problems in the relationship with hospital nursing staff

As we have noted, the grieving patient may feel isolated and unacceptable. Staff are often unsure of how best to deal with patients threatening to lose, who have experienced a loss, or are undergoing testing or treatment for infertility. False cheerfulness is often seen by patients as insincerity or flippancy, and continual reassurance that all will be well when facts speak otherwise may later be resented. Staff may therefore decide to adopt a professional attitude involving a certain degree of detachment. There are a number of other reasons that such an approach is adopted.

Firstly, staff may fear that a show of emotion by them may lead to further distress for the patient. As with many others, there is a feeling that somehow the pain of grief will be lessened if the couple do not dwell on their loss too much, and so staff make attempts to behave normally and cheerfully. Secondly, a professional approach provides the situation with some structure, which removes some uncertainty as to how one should behave. He/she acts 'professionally'. Thirdly, staff fear that becoming involved with such patients on a regular basis may lead to their becoming emotionally drained or suffering 'burnout'. This may be more pronounced in high-pressured areas such as the Intensive-Care Nursery, where staff can become attached to babies who later die. In the wards, the pressure may be distributed more evenly among staff, since such patients are in the minority.

'Burnout' is a problem that must be considered, but emotional care of a grieving patient need not lead to this end. The adoption of a detached professional approach may guard against this, but then the patient may suffer. Staff can learn the skills of providing a listening ear and be made aware of the words and actions to avoid. By realizing that the problem belongs to the couple and that no one else can prevent the pain, staff may be able to provide support without becoming emotionally drained themselves.

Staff may have built up a relationship with a couple who experience a loss. This may occur when couples have been involved in such procedures as an infertility program, long hospitalization, or intensive care of their premature infant. When the loss then occurs, staff may also grieve. They may experience some of the shock, anger, and depression felt by the couple. At times, staff's grief may be directed at parents. For example, when a prematurely delivered infant dies, there may be anger directed at the heroin-addicted mother, the mother who smoked heavily, or the parent who failed to visit regularly. Staff's pain may be camouflaged by their remaining 'professional'.

Unfortunately, staff fail to realize that rather than seeing an emotional display as distressing, most couples will find such honest expressions comforting, showing that someone is able to share their grief in some small measure. Leith's daughter Rebecca had died before delivery due to a massive haemorrhage:

> After the caesarean, the doctor had me returned to a different ward, which was better. Yet a lot of the nurses I had had before came to visit me there. They were wonderful. It was really nice to know they felt it too.

Del's son Anthony died after birth due to an infection:

> The staff were really good. They said 'We're really sorry about your baby'. It helped me that they said that. They didn't just ignore it.

Trying to force cheerfulness or optimism from a couple may hinder the resolution of grief in that couple. They need to grieve, and staff need to facilitate, not deny, this need.

> After I had the miscarriage at 18 weeks I was devastated. A few hours later I felt the need to know if the baby had been a boy or a girl. I asked one of the nurses. She looked horrified and fumbled out 'I'll just get Matron'. The Matron came down and asked me what the problem was. I simply said to her again that I

wanted to know if the baby had been a boy or a girl. She looked horrified too, and her exact words will stay with me for life. She said: 'Don't be so morbid! Go home and forget about it!' I was so embarrassed and upset, yet I needed to know and so pressed her. She begrudgingly told me it was a boy. I'm sure she and the nurse later discussed my 'sick' behaviour.

In the anger of grief a couple may strike out at anyone around them, including medical staff. They may be irritable, unfriendly, sullen, or seem to overreact angrily to a seemingly innocent comment. Staff need to realize that it is the pain of grief causing such reactions, rather than an individual's normal pattern of behaviour. No one, including medical staff, likes to be near someone who is irritable. Yet staff who understand grief may be more inclined to continue close contact with the couple, recognizing that their pain is not a personal slight or a criticism of the care being offered.

Unfortunately, a breakdown in communication within hospitals can create unnecessary pain for a grieving couple, particularly the mother. Allocating a woman who has lost or is threatening to lose a child to a room with newly delivered mothers and their babies serves only to remind the woman of her problems and her failure, further intensifying her grief. Similarly, if staff are unaware of the particular situation of the woman, they can make hurtful blunders.

> The physiotherapist came in on Tuesday, and was telling me the usual about sit-ups and so on. Then she said: 'And when you are bathing baby ...' I just burst into tears. She was very apologetic, but that stuck in my mind.

> They finally were to induce me to bring on the baby, as natural labour had not started within two weeks of the baby dying. I was admitted the night before. After I was settled in bed, a nurse came in to do observations. She produced a pendopler, and went to listen for the baby's heart. I broke down, but couldn't tell her anything, as I was so upset. Suddenly she realized that I was the IUFD. She was very embarrassed.

Rooming rounds in which nurses look for dirty baby linen and nappies can also cause unnecessary upset for women who have lost a child.

In general, staff do not have sufficient time to spend with a grieving patient. Hospitals are generally tightly staffed, leaving time only for basic nursing duties. Patients suffering a loss are also often discharged from the hospital as soon as possible. Hence, staff may have little time to develop a relationship with the couple, and may be forced to deal with patients while they are in a state of shock and numbness. In large maternity hospitals, nursing staff may see a steady progression of couples who have experienced a loss or are threatening to lose. Over time, it is possible that staff become unable to see beyond the clinical description of the patient's condition to the grieving individual. They may begin to act automatically to patients. This may be particularly apparent in staff who have lost some of the motivation they once felt for their job, as happens to nearly all workers at some stage. Staff can become complacent about such patients, and treat them more as a condition rather than a person. Fortunately, these types of reactions are uncommon.

In situations of threatened miscarriage and threatened premature labour particularly, staff often realize that most patients will go on to normal full-term deliveries. They may therefore find it difficult to understand the fear and anxiety of the individual patient. This patient may be aware of every bodily twinge, even being fearful of innocent happenings. Nursing staff, having a more in-depth knowledge of the danger signs, may give the patient the impression that she is overreacting.

> When I went into hospital in prem. labour I knew the pains were contractions. They hurt. After they had stopped the labour and I was back down in the ward, I got so confused. The nurses would ask me if I was having any contractions. I would say Yes, and then they'd ask if I was sure they were contractions and not just tightenings. Everybody was always trying to tell me they were only tightenings that everyone had. Soon I felt so confused and neurotic that I started not reporting them any more.

Overcoming difficulties

Couples experiencing hospitalization concerned with child-bearing difficulties can be greatly assisted, not only by appropriate reactions of hospital staff, but also by carefully considered hospital policies.

Nursing staff who are able to provide honesty of words and emotion, combined with a listening ear and an open manner, can be vital sources of support for couples during such difficult times. Staff should never feel ashamed to be open with their emotions. A tear, a gentle touch, a squeeze of the hand, a caring look: all can be openings into the isolation of the patient. Being willing and able to listen to the patient is vital. She may need to talk over and over about her loss, or may not wish to talk much at all. The staff need to be aware of the particular needs of the patient. Awareness comes most accurately from asking what the patient wants and needs. At times, the need to talk comes at night, and without a chance to talk, the patient can become extremely lonely during the long night hours. Patients should not be discouraged from talking at night by staff determinedly suggesting sleep, or even medication.

Staff need to be open to patients' questions, ready to answer them with honesty and compassion. Often questions will be of a more practical nature, about such topics as the physical after-effects of birth or miscarriage, any further testing for infertility and the procedures, where to get help for their handicapped child, or what will happen to their stillborn child. Other questions may involve looking for reasons for the loss, how long to wait for another pregnancy, or what a new procedure such as a D and C will be like. Where possible, staff should answer questions within the range of their knowledge. If questions are beyond their knowledge, they should take it upon themselves to find someone able to discuss the matter knowledgeably and arrange for the patient a visit by such a person. Where questions should be directed to the patient's doctor, staff may help overcome any possible doctor-patient communication difficulties by alerting the doctor to the fact that the patient has asked such a question. At times, a patient may feel more comfortable asking questions of nursing staff, whom they see as closer to their status level, than asking their doctor, whom they see as an 'expert'. If nursing staff have some prior idea of the type of information patients may wish to know, they can be readied with reliable accurate information. If patients' fears, complaints, or questions appear to be taken seriously by staff, they may receive some reassurance, feeling that others around are concerned and hence will be willing to watch them carefully. Keeping patients informed of what is being done for them can also help. For example, if injections are ordered, patients should be told why they were ordered and what will be their likely effects.

Nursing staff, not knowing how to help, may deliberately avoid the grieving patients. Privacy for such patients is vital, but this must be balanced against a tendency to isolate them. At times, when the father is not able to be present, a woman can feel very isolated and look forward to some human contact. If it appears that she welcomes nursing staff, she may feel further isolated if such company is denied her. Staff must be guided by each individual and her needs. Some need company, while others prefer solitude. Sensitivity on the part of the staff will help to distinguish the needs.

Beyond the actual personalities of nursing staff, some hospital policies and practices concerning couples with child-bearing difficulties can provide means of overcoming problems that may arise. All nursing staff who are to have any dealings with the patient should be informed of the situation. Such information may be provided during change of shift reporting and on patient boards in nurses' stations.

Some hospitals attach a symbol to the door of the room where there is a grieving patient. Such a device alerts all staff to a loss, and this can be beneficial, but it may also have some drawbacks. The woman may feel marked as a failure by the outside world. Staff may avoid such rooms, or may feel obliged to make some comments which may be inappropriate. There can be difficulties in deciding who will be told of the loss. Respect for the patient's privacy and confidentiality must be considered against the risk of hurtful comments being made. Whether or not domestic staff are informed of the loss requires careful consideration.

Deciding where the mother will be accommodated after the loss can also be important. Some hospitals provide a ward away from the obstetric units for women who have experienced a loss. Others provide a private single room as far as possible from the nursery or as close as possible to the Intensive-Care Nursery if the baby requires special care. Visiting hours for partners should be less restricted, and the care of such patients allocated to experienced nursing staff. Most women will be relieved to be able to close the door of their room to the sounds of crying babies. However, others may be comforted by the sight of a baby, and may even secretly wish for a walk to the nursery. Rather than assume how a patient may feel, staff should seek clarification from the patient as to her needs and wishes, and these should be respected.

Parents whose baby is within the Intensive-Care Nursery should be encouraged to visit their child often. Most units allow parents to visit at all hours of the day or night. By having free access, parents, during and after hospitalization, may feel closer to their baby and be able to visit together. Where visits are not possible, it can be reassuring to parents if they are encouraged to phone at any time, even after the premature baby goes home.

Where parents lose a child through death or miscarriage, well-thought-out hospital procedures can help ease grieving. Such procedures must never be inflexible, to be strictly adhered to under all conditions. Rather, they should act as guidelines, based on common reactions to grief. After a stillbirth, parents may be encouraged to hold their baby. This is generally beneficial, but it must never be forced on a couple. Some hospitals routinely take photographs of the dead child, take foot and hand prints, and keep hospital identification bracelets. Some even keep a lock of hair for the couple. These tangible memories are offered to the parents. If the parents initially reject the collected items, they are tagged and filed away. This is because couples often reconsider their initial refusal, even months after the tragedy.

Where a child is or was severely deformed, staff may wrap the child in such a way as to mask the deformity, while leaving perfect parts of the body visible. Parents may then be encouraged to hold their child. In cases of miscarriage, some women are assisted in grieving by seeing the foetus. Such an encounter needs to be handled carefully, and should not be forced on a woman.

Once again, it is important that hospital procedures are not binding on couples, forcing them to do something they are not prepared for. Neither should they be denied the right to be comforted through some unusual individual action. Couples should be asked about their wishes, and perhaps given a variety of options.

Some hospitals applaud the concept of community support for grieving couples in the form of support groups. Others are sceptical of such groups. A close liaison between a hospital and such groups can clarify the expectations of each. Information about groups, or a visit or phone call from a group member, may be offered to the patients non-threateningly, leaving the decision of whether or not to take up the offer to the couple themselves.

In some hospitals some staff are specifically trained to deal with the care of grieving patients. Besides social workers and psychologists, hospitals may also allocate such responsibility to nursing supervisors, or in hospitals with religious affiliations, to hospital chaplains and pastoral-care workers. Such persons must be trained to cope with difficult situations. In many instances, even training is not sufficient; such persons require an open, caring personality, able to empathize with those in crisis. Such staff have to deal with difficult practical subjects such as funerals, autopsies, and financial arrangements, as well as be able to provide caring and compassion.

Education in midwifery should involve not only the theoretical aspects of fertilization, birth, and pregnancy loss, but some knowledge of the positive and negative reactions to pregnancy and the complexity of emotions of those couples experiencing the types of losses we have discussed. Nursing staff can then more effectively care for the whole patient, rather than simply the physical needs.

Nursing staff provide a vital service in their support of the grieving couples in the initial difficult days of grief. By allowing couples to experience their grief in a supportive atmosphere, they can provide total care of their patient and her grieving partner. A little knowledge and some thoughtful procedures can go a long way toward removing fear and overcoming misunderstandings.

Children

Even at a very young age, children will realize that there is something wrong in a situation. They may not be aware of the actual problem, but may be alerted to the difficulties by changes in the behaviour of their parents. Parents experiencing child-bearing difficulties must deal with intense emotions. It is often difficult for them to concentrate on their own feelings, as well as those of their children. Even if parents try to hide feelings from a child, they are usually unsuccessful.

Children are self-centred individuals. One result of this is that they often interpret events around them as having been caused by them. A change in attitude or behaviour of a parent may be viewed by the child as some reflection on him/her. If Mummy is crying, a child often assumes that he/she has done something to cause this. If children are not relieved of this burden by reassurance, it can cause problems. Where parents feel that they are unable to discuss the full situation with the child, they must still reassure him/her.

> Mummy is sad. Sometimes things make Mummy sad, and she cries. It's all right if Mummy is sad, just as you are sometimes. You haven't made Mummy sad. She loves you and is very proud of you.

Children may have a limited grasp of a subject or a limited vocabulary. Yet they can understand many situations that are explained to them on a level adapted to their age and comprehension ability. Their comments or questions can sometimes cause some distress for their grieving parents, but these questions help them make sense of the situation and also give parents some idea of how well they have understood an explanation.

Children and infertility

In some cases a couple are unable to add to their family, although they may dearly love to do just this. Generally, children are unaware of the difficulties that parents are experiencing. They may become a bit concerned that Mummy seems to be visiting the doctor so often or cries more than usual.

When parents realize that there may not be another child, their relationship with the child or children they already have may change in character. Some may become more protective of the child. Others may become more demanding of this child, as all their dreams about their children's future may now have to be achieved through this child. They may put more emphasis on the child, and more time into him/her, perhaps even curtailing their child's time with others. Such extreme reactions can cause difficulties for the child. Other parents provide a great deal of time for their child, without 'smothering' him/her. Some even seek out ways other than childbirth to complete a family.

There may be times when children ask the difficult question of 'Why don't I have any brothers or sisters?' or 'When are you going to have another baby, Mummy?' Often these questions arise when school-mates or kindergarten pals are discussing new brothers and sisters, or a relative or friend has a baby whom the child finds fascinating. The feelings may come from loneliness, but they can also arise from the child wanting to be like his/her friends, to have a baby to make *him/her* the centre of attention.

Leith was advised against ever having any other children after a stillbirth:

> People think that you're just feeling sorry for yourself. They don't realize that you're grieving for the child. Also they're not aware of the feelings of the other children. After we lost Rebecca both neighbours got pregnant, and Melissa and Kirsty had to watch the other people's children fussing over the new baby. I longed for someone to say to them: 'You have a nurse of the baby'. Let them fuss around a bit. Perhaps that's worse because I can't have any more. I grieved a lot. I couldn't give them this baby they'd looked forward to for nine months.

Parents who provide opportunities for their child to be closely involved with other children of all ages, particularly those in the extended family, can help overcome difficulties of loneliness. A close relative or friend who is having a first child may also help by allowing a couple's child to be involved with her pregnancy and be a substitute big brother or sister to the new baby. They may explain that 'Our baby doesn't have a big brother or sister to help, so we'll need someone like you'.

If pregnancy is unlikely ever to occur, parents may wish to explain to a child on a level that he/she can understand that sometimes people are not able to have any more children. The degree of explanation as to why this occurs will vary with the age of the child. Children may find it difficult to understand that Mummy and Daddy, who solve all the child's 'big' problems, are not in control of a situation. Why don't they change things so that they can have more children? Parents may need a great deal of patience and understanding in explaining this, and may even have to wait for the child to mature further before the explanation is fully accepted.

Children and premature deliveries

The premature delivery of a baby brother or sister can be very confusing for a child. Children are aware that a baby is due, and may have become comfortable with Mummy's expanding figure, knowing that inside her is 'our baby'. Even without a good concept of time, children are able to realize that it may be a long time before the baby is born. Parents have often decided how they will cope with mother's absence while in hospital after the birth. They may have plans to familiarize the child with being cared for by someone else as the time for delivery draws nearer. Suddenly everyone around the child is looking concerned and even panicky. With the onset of premature labour the mother may be taken immediately to hospital, and the child placed in the care of relatives or friends. Initially, everyone may be so concerned about the event that there is little time available to explain to the child what is happening. If the mother is in pain, the child may become frightened, particularly if father returns home without her.

If labour is able to be delayed, the mother may be required to spend some time in hospital. Such premature separation of mother and child before adequate preparation is made can be traumatic for both. This is particularly apparent when mother has to be transferred to a larger hospital some distance away. In such cases it may be very difficult for the child to visit his/her mother. Reassurances from those around the child that Mummy is safe and well may not be sufficient. Where possible, the child should be able to visit mother or at least speak to her on the phone to be reassured that she really is all right, will come home, and still loves him/her very much. During prolonged hospitalization, the child may begin to wonder if Mummy is ever coming home. The longer a younger child spends with other caregivers, the more he/she adapts to this new situation. It may be difficult for a mother who is hospitalized when her young child seems settled with another caregiver, and does not seem to miss her. Yet, children are affected by mother's absence, although this may not show until the child is threatened with a later separation.

> Brendan seemed to cope well with my hospitalizations until later. After the last baby died and I had to go into hospital again for a week, he became really upset and he wouldn't go to kindy.

When a pre-term baby has been delivered, particularly one of less than 30 weeks' gestation, parents may be concerned about this baby's well-being. They may be unsure of what to tell their children. Suddenly this happy event of having a little brother or sister is clouded by fear and doubt. People around the child don't look happy, which confuses the child. He/she may know there is a baby, and yet not understand why he/she cannot see the baby straight away. Children may sense their parents' concern, but are often left ignorant. Yet the situation can and should be explained to even young children:

> You have a lovely brother. Sometimes babies come too soon, as our baby has. He needs to be looked after very carefully by some special doctors and nurses. He is very small, and at the hospital they have a special place that will look after him for us until he gets stronger. We will all see him soon.

Photographs of the premature baby may help the child to realize that there really is a baby to look forward to.

If the situation is more serious, the parents can help prepare other children for any eventual outcome by telling them the facts:

> Our baby was born too soon. She is a lovely baby, but she is very small and weak. She is a sick little baby. They are trying hard to help her get better at the hospital. She is trying hard, too.

If death then occurs, the child is not frightened by the suddenness of the event.

Staff of Intensive-Care Nurseries realize the importance of other children in the family having contact with their younger brother or sister. When the premature baby is well enough, other children may be allowed to see and even touch their younger sibling. Careful preparation is required before such a visit. A child may be frightened by the equipment in the nursery. It needs to be explained that the baby is in a special place surrounded by machines that are helping to care for him/her, and so there is no need to be afraid of them. Favourable reactions of parents to the premature baby and the machinery help to overcome children's fears.

Once home, premature babies require a great deal of care. Sometimes other children can become resentful of the amount of time and attention their parents spend with this new addition. Parents needs to take special care to find time each day specifically set aside for each of the other children in the family.

Children and abnormality

The reaction of a child to a baby born with an abnormality will depend largely on the severity of the abnormality. In situations where the abnormality is fairly minor or easily corrected, other children in the family may be told that their sibling has a little problem but that the doctors will make him/her well very soon. After correction, life then returns to normal.

In cases of severe abnormalities that will affect the child throughout life, other children must be prepared carefully. Parental reactions to the baby and the situation are of vital importance here. Parents grieving the loss of their 'perfect' child may find explanations difficult and fear the reactions of their other children. It is important to remember that children are often more accepting of differences and disabilities than are adults. Where the abnormality is obvious, a simple explanation to other children — including what the baby looks like, that the baby will need care from the whole family, and that the baby is loved just as they are — will generally suffice. The child, seeing the baby with an abnormality, is usually satisfied by such a simple explanation of why the baby is different.

Where the abnormality is not obvious, such as occurs in mental retardation, the child may find it more difficult to understand that this baby, who looks just like any other baby, has a problem. The child will need an explanation that sometimes problems are inside, although this may not be necessary immediately.

> Peter is a beautiful baby, but he is a special baby who has a problem. I know he looks like other babies. We can't see his problem because it is inside his body. He will need lots of love from us all. I know he is very lucky though, because he has a big brother who is going to help him so much.

In some cases, parents have had to make the difficult decision to institutionalize their severely handicapped child or have him/her fostered. Other children in the family can make such a decision even more difficult, as they try to understand why their new sibling is not staying at home. In the world of such children, families all live together. Their baby, whom they knew lived inside their mother's body and whom they expected with excitement, is suddenly not to come home. Parents will need great patience in explaining the situation. It is not easy to get across the idea to a child that parents do still love the baby, but that sometimes babies are born with problems which mean that families are not able to care for them properly, and that there are people and places who know what is best done for their baby and can do it. Regular contact visits by other children are vital to their accepting the affected sibling. Suddenly seeing their mother's body return to normal and being told that there is a baby, yet never seeing him/her, can be frightening to a child.

In some cases, abnormalities are so severe that the baby will not be able to live. Preparing children for an inevitable death is difficult for both child and parents. A child's grief is usually more easily resolved when he/she has some contact with a dying sibling. Once again, prior preparation is vital. The reactions of parents to the impending loss will play a vital role in helping children cope. Being excluded from the loss by being sent to relatives and remaining ignorant of what is happening is frightening for the child, who is made aware of some problem by the reactions of those around.

Children and death

Many couples postpone telling their children of a pregnancy until they are into their fourth month or further. This is generally a good idea, for, as we have seen, early miscarriage is not an uncommon occurrence. Children can become quite distressed when the baby they expected is suddenly not going to come. Without the expanding figure of their mother to indicate the pregnancy, the child can become confused about this baby that was there and now has suddenly disappeared. Although the situation is distressing to the parents, many couples feel that in cases of early miscarriage it is unnecessary to burden or confuse children with the details of the loss. Reassuring them that their parents' sadness is not their fault may suffice.

In cases of late miscarriage, stillbirth, or neonatal death, there is a need to discuss death with the children. Contrary to what many adults feel, death is not a subject to be avoided with children. Even very young children have their own concepts of death. Their thought-processes differ from those of adults, but explanations tailored to their level of understanding can build a solid foundation on which they can come to terms with the death of a sibling, and death in general.

Surviving children can be greatly affected by parental reactions to the death of a sibling. Conflicts about the death can be reflected in parents' behaviour toward their other children.[1] Some parents feel unable to discuss the death with their children. This may be because they feel in some way guilty of causing the death. There may also be denial of the death, and hence 'blocked' grief. For others, there may be some fear of 'upsetting' the other children. The surviving children in such a situation soon learn that there is an unspoken rule that the subject must not be broached. The event can take on the character of a fearful mystery, which can cause intense confusion. The child, in trying to make some sense of the situation, may then blame himself/herself for the death.

In other cases, parents may become intensely protective of surviving children for fear something may also happen to them. This may be particularly evident in situations where there has been a child born after a number of losses. After the birth, the parents may be so fearful of losing this child to cot death or other disasters that they may purchase all kinds of protective equipment. If the child is to be an only child, this protectiveness may continue throughout life. This may also occur with a sibling of an infant who dies; the child, who before the death was quite independent, may find much of his/her freedom curtailed due to parental fears and attempts to prevent further losses. The child may become fearful rather than outgoing, and be stifled in his/her necessary exploration of the world. Paradoxically, with this overprotectiveness can come some unconscious rejection of the child by the parents. Fearing the possible death of another child, they may withdraw emotionally from this child to some extent. Although the parents' reaction is understandable, it can be damaging to the child.

Some families try to replace the dead infant with another child, usually through another pregnancy. The new child may be accepted not for himself/herself but according to how well he/she displays the attributes of the dead child, whether these attributes were known or were simply the fantasy of parents. At other times, the parents attempt to find a replacement by adoption or fostering. One of the surviving children may also be chosen to play the role. Generally, parents hold an idealized picture of the lost infant, and it is virtually impossible for any other child to measure up to the required standard. The child can become depressed through his/her constant failure to meet these standards of excellence, and hence may decide to settle for negative attention or withdrawal.

From the above, we can see that the most vital component in helping a child come to terms with death is that parents are made aware of the effects of their behaviour and reactions to death on their children. In cases where parents are paralysed emotionally by their loss, close relatives or friends may provide a vital link in helping children understand what is happening around them.

Care must be taken in the words used to explain death to children, for even commonly accepted adult explanations can be frightening to them. Children who are brought up to believe that heaven is for good people, and are then told their baby brother or sister has gone to heaven, may become concerned about their own lives. If good children die and go to heaven, they may reason that if they are bad they will be saved from a similar fate. Similarly, explanations that angels took the baby can instil in them some fear that they too may be 'kidnapped'. Sleep disturbances are common in children to whom death is explained as 'going to sleep' or 'gone to sleep'. They don't want to go to sleep ever again if that's what happens to you! If death is explained as the baby's having 'gone away', a child may naturally assume that he/she is coming back. Children, being self-centred, may also wonder what they did to make their baby go away. In other explanations, the word 'death' is replaced by the word 'loss' in statements such as 'we lost our baby'. This is a common statement when adults discuss the death of a child, and in fact we have used it in this book. This is appropriate for adults, who are able to understand the symbolic use of words, but a child is not able to do this. If the baby is talked about as lost rather than dead, children may not understand the permanency of death. They may become extremely fearful if separated from their parent in a supermarket or some other place; they fear being 'lost' too.

Some children may have developed a concept of death as punishment. Perhaps they have heard of a dog that was killed after biting someone, or understand something of capital punishment. They may then become overly compliant to avoid such an outcome for themselves.

Following the death of a sibling, other children may fear their own death and become very confused. Explanation to children and reassurance of them are vital. In explaining death to children successfully, it is important that the explanation be tailored to suit the stage of development of the child.[2] Children younger than the age of three or four generally have no concept of the permanency of death. To them, death means an 'absence'. When told a baby is dead, they may appear to accept the situation, only to ask at a later time when he/she is coming back. Parents may have to repeat the explanation many times, which can be very painful for them. At times, parents may feel intense frustration with the child, but they must realize that this is a necessary part of grieving for the young child. Such very young children are usually unable to understand much of the detailed explanations given to them. Hence, simple statements with little detail are best. These children do respond to the feelings of those around them. They can be very confused and frightened by the intensity of emotion expressed by their parents and others close to them. They are comforted by reassurances of their parents' love for them through words and actions. Such close, reassuring warmth must be directed toward helping them realize that they have not caused the changes in the people around them, and that they are still loved and treasured.

Slightly older children, from about ages four to nine, have had some experience of death. They have seen plants and insects die, and perhaps have even buried a pet. In books and on television they have been exposed to death as a concept. Unfortunately, the 'death' of cartoon characters is often short-lived, which does not assist them in grasping the idea that death is a permanent state. They can accept that they are separated from whatever has died, but may still expect a later return. In explaining the death of a sibling to children of this age-group, it is best, where possible, to relate it to their own limited experience.

> You remember Guppy, your goldfish? Do you know what happened to him? . . .
> Yes, he died. He was no longer swimming around. He did not breathe or move any more. He wasn't alive. Well, our baby died too. Nobody did anything to hurt him. Goldfish die and people die too. Even babies die sometimes. We will remember our baby

just as we remember Guppy. We will always love them, just as Mummy and Daddy love you.

Somewhere between the ages of seven and ten, children realize that death is final and will eventually happen to us all. It can be quite frightening to a child to be so closely confronted by death. They may fear their own death, and need reassurance that their death and that of their parents is a long way off. Children at this age are also aware of specific causes of death, such as illness, accident, or old age. They are more able to accept spiritual aspects of death. Therefore, such reassurances can be included in explanations to children of this age, while also relating to their own experience.

> You know Melissa was a sick little baby when she was born. Well, she was too sick to live, and she died today. Sometimes sick babies die. Remember when Rover died. He was very sick too. It is going to be hard for us all, because we all loved her and will miss her. At least we know she'll be with Jesus and he will take care of her for us. One day we will die, but for you and Petey and Johnny, and even Mummy and Daddy, that's a long long time away. Sometimes we will all be sad about Melissa and may cry. It helps to cry when you're sad, so you won't be frightened if you see Mummy or Daddy cry, will you? Now, you won't forget that Mummy and Daddy love you very much, just as we will always love Melissa even though she is dead.

Older children and teenagers are aware of death and its permanency. Some may even have experienced the death of a friend, increasing their awareness of the power of death. Realizing that it must eventually happen to all can be quite disconcerting for older children. The death of a baby can leave them wondering about the meaning of life itself. These older children are more able to deal with abstract concepts like death, life, and goals, particularly in teenage years. A greater awareness of the pain their parents are feeling can bring new depths of understanding about others around them. They are able to share their parents' grief and provide some support, as well as being supported themselves. Being able to help their parents may actually assist their own grieving. They may wish to discuss the confusion and futility they may feel. Parents who can provide the opportunity and understanding to do this according to the age of the child, are providing their children with a solid basis on which to accept and resolve later grief surrounding other life-situations.

Even after well-considered explanations are given, a child may not have fully understood the situation. Being egocentric and slightly 'magical' thinkers when young, children may concentrate on one statement made by parents and distort it into an inappropriate explanation. By asking children to retell what has been explained to them, parents can find out what the child has understood and correct any misconceptions.

Parents often feel that they should not express their grief in front of their children. It is true that a complete breakdown of those they love would be frightening for children. But they should not be shielded from the normal crying and grieving of their parents. They should be encouraged to share grief, their own and that of their parents. In doing so, they are permitted to see that such emotions are normal and acceptable, and that these emotions too can be expressions of love both for the dead child and those remaining.

Children should never be made to feel guilty for being cheerful and happy after the death of a child. In their depression, parents may not be able to feel the same enjoyment of life, but they must never discourage their children. Close relatives and friends may be able to provide some breathing space for parents and children when there are differences in the ability of each to enjoy life during grieving. Such people may also help by being aware of the child's grief, and being willing to listen or discuss the subject of death at times when parents are unwilling or unable to broach this subject.

Children are often denied the opportunity to attend the funeral of a sibling. As we have seen, children under the age of seven do not have a concept of the permanency of death, and hence may be frightened and confused when the body is buried. But children over the age of seven may actually be comforted by attendance at the funeral. If the child is well prepared, attendance may help to remove some of the fear and mystery of death. They too are then able to see that death is a permanent state, and are able to share in the grief of those around them. Hence, they may understand it better.

Grandparents

Grandparents or prospective grandparents often have a special role and special difficulties to face. Not only must they grieve for the loss of their awaited grandchild, but they may also hurt to see their own child and his/her partner in such emotional or physical pain.

Through infertility or repeated losses, some grandparents may have to face the fact that their role of doting grandparent may not eventuate or at best will be delayed. Their future, as they have fantasized it to be, may not come to pass. They may need to grieve their loss too. Where there are other grandchildren, this problem may not arise.

Grandparents may often look into their own past to try to find some reason why these events have occurred. If an abnormality is of a genetic nature, or repeated losses have been linked to outside agents in their own pregnancies such as DES, the grandparents may experience guilt. They may fear rejection from their children, and hence withdraw when their children need them most.

As their children grew, these prospective grandparents had the prime responsibility of comforting their pain. Now they must temper the urge to be prime comforter with the realization that this role now belongs to their child's partner, and that as adults their children must make their own decisions. Grandparents may think that they can ease pain by removing some of the responsibilities, such as arranging a funeral. To avoid problems, they should wait to be asked by the couple or wait for the couple to accept their offer of help before doing anything.

In most cases of child-bearing difficulties, grandparents have provided an important source of support. In times of grief, their adult 'child' may need the warmth and reassurance he/she felt as a child. Staff of hospitals often realize the importance of grandparents, and hence encourage them to have some contact with a premature baby, stillborn infant, or handicapped child. If death follows birth, grandparents then have actual memories of their grandchild.

The later acknowledgment of their lost grandchild can be very important to the grieving parents.

> Mum won't use Anthony's name. No one will bring it up. I talk about it, but they'd rather I forget it. I feel it's really important that grandparents are able to accept that the child existed.

> Mum and Dad were wonderful. They asked us to get a copy of Kate's photograph for them. Mum has it in her photo album with all the photos of my niece. We told them how important it was to us that they didn't forget her. They haven't. On the first anniversary of her death we made a donation to the hospital, and when they found this out, they did the same thing.

In fact, when there are other grandchildren, grieving parents who still feel strongly about the limited life of their child may feel resentful when the grandparents fail to acknowledge him/her also as a grandchild.

> To this day I don't think my family would remember that her birthday is coming up this month, and I doubt whether they'd know how old she'd be. They may have felt something themselves, but weren't game to say it to me in case I cried.

Grandparents feel extremely powerless. Some may even feel the injustice of a little baby dying, while they continue to live. The sense of powerlessness is further intensified if they are separated from their children and the situation by distance. Open expression of their feelings, and words and actions of support, are the best means of assisting the grieving couple. These can be offered over a long distance by telephone and even by letter.

In very close families, brothers and sisters may also feel the intense pain of their sibling and the loss of his/her child. Along with grandparents, they may provide a strong close network of support vital to the grieving couple.

Other relatives, friends, and strangers

There are no hard and fast rules for predicting how others will react to the couple experiencing child-bearing difficulties. Some will be wonderfully supportive, while others will be clumsy with their words and actions or may even withdraw completely. The appropriateness of reactions may depend on a person's relationship with the grieving couple, and his/her experiences and ability to cope with crisis.

It is important for a grieving couple to realize that most people will be unable to understand the intensity of the feelings they are experiencing. Many will be embarrassed by the situation and may fumble, eventually saying the wrong thing. Others will avoid contact with the couple because they 'don't know what to say' or don't feel comfortable around people who are 'down'. Some will contact the couple only through other relatives, and then wonder why the couple are not comforted by this second-hand support. Even if the message is delivered, the couple still feel isolated and ostracized, as if they were carrying a deadly disease. If others have children, they may avoid the couple for fear of upsetting them, or may tell the couple how lucky they are to be childless or at least free of a new baby. They may send flowers or a note, but never visit themselves.

Many will find it difficult to realize that this is a major tragedy in the couple's life. They may play down the event, or become impatient when the couple don't seem to be getting better after a few weeks or are living a life alternating between hope and despair.

Many people are not comfortable with emotional incidents, and seek to avoid them. They may avoid the touchy topic, under the guise of not wanting to upset the couple. Confusion about their own feelings may occur, as the loss of the grieving couple brings to the surface old inner conflicts they had hoped were put to rest. Others simply lack effective communication skills to help them deal appropriately with grief.

A couple may find that changes will occur in their relationships with others, depending on the reaction of others to the crisis situation. There may be feelings of alienation and even resentment toward those who withdraw or make thoughtless comments, thereby affecting a once apparently-close relationship. There may be others willing to discuss the subject only briefly if it is raised by the grieving person. Their obvious discomfort often appears a signal to the person in pain that the discussion is not really welcome, simply tolerated. A relationship that cannot share personal pain is bound to change. Another group will encourage discussion of the loss frequently, but will do so as they see the grieving person 'in great need of my help' or as a source of gossip. This patronizing attitude may be resented later by the grieving person, who needs to be seen and valued as a person, not just because he/she makes others feel righteous about themselves and their willingness to help.

There is one group of people who will be of immense support, through their willingness to talk and listen, and their acceptance of the grieving person as a whole real thinking person, whose time of need is presently here. Such people realize that everyone has a time of need, and that their own time may soon come. The basis of such a relationship is mutual trust and deep caring, mixed with humility and real compassion.

How do I help?

If we assume that most people are genuinely concerned about a person who is in crisis, we must assume that they also wish to help. Most of the comments made, even the hurtful ones, are made with the underlying intention of comforting the grieving couple. But intentions are often clouded by the inappropriateness of statements, or actions born of ignorance.

In this section we are going to attempt to help the helper. It may be useful to start by looking at the statements and actions that are not helpful, so that they can be avoided. Then we can look at more appropriate ways of helping that can fill the void.

Non-helpful reactions

Surprisingly, many of the comments commonly made to people who are grieving are essentially not helpful, particularly in the early stages of grief. Let us look at such comments and why they often do more harm than good.

Comments are not helpful when they:

1. Deny the reality and seriousness of the situation

The loss of a dream of a family or of a perfect baby is a tragedy for a couple. It is not something from which they will necessarily recover quickly. Those not directly involved may find it difficult to accept that this situation can cause such distress. They try to get the couple to 'look on the bright side', not realizing that in their grief the couple can initially see no bright side. Instead, they may see these comments as denying their right to feel sad about their tragedy.

The following are some comments in this category:

> You can always have another baby.

> Children really tie you down. Look at me. At least you'll be able to do all those things I couldn't.

> You shouldn't keep talking about it. It'll only upset you, and you'll never get over it.

> Don't cry. It won't help.

> Lots of people have a miscarriage.

> You're not the only one this has ever happened to, you know.

> I really think you're overreacting a bit.

> Cheer up! It could be worse. At least your baby is alive.

> I can remember another girl, doing what she thought was best, talked about everything else. When I came home, she was bright and breezy. 'Welcome home! How are you? Great to have you home.' I thought she was crazy.

> When they say 'It's all for the best. He was too weak to survive', it's more as if they're trying to convince themselves that there is a reason for it, that it's not as tragic as it seems.

2. Attempt to force a solution

One of the most common techniques people use to try to overcome a crisis is to encourage the couple to find a solution to the problem. Generally this problem-solving is forced on the couple too soon. As grief is resolved, the couple themselves may seek a solution and will welcome assistance. But early in their grief, advice-giving may be seen more as trying to force the couple to forget their loss. They may see this as others wishing to restore normality by ignoring their feelings.

Comments may include:

> You mustn't dwell on it. It will only make it worse.

> It's past now. Put it behind you, and get on with your life.

> It happened to a friend of mine, and they got pregnant right away. They're so happy now. Just think, in a year's time this will all be just a memory.

> Of course you'll put your names down for adoption now.

You mustn't be upset. The baby will pick that up, and he'll be distressed too.

You know you should really take a holiday. Get away! Forget about it!

Get busy! The only way to get over it is to help people who are worse off than yourself.

3. Rationalize or moralize

Some people believe that grief is an intellectual phenomenon that can be dissipated by thinking rationally. Others feel that grief displays a lack of faith or a weakness that can be remedied by words of comfort. However, grief is usually a highly irrational process, based on feelings. Rationalizing or moralizing simply denies the right of the couple to feel distressed.

Common comments include:

It is God's will. He has a plan, and he knows best.

Your baby is in heaven. He will never feel pain again.

You ought to be thankful that your baby is alive.

At least it's a problem that can be fixed.

He's in eternal rest.

It's probably for the best. Most miscarriages are due to some deformity.

At least you have one child.

Some people aren't meant to have children.

There are others a lot worse off than you. At least you have each other.

You mustn't forget that God knows what is best for you.

Children should only be part of your life, anyway.

4. Deny or fail to accept the expression of grief

Grief must be allowed to be expressed and accepted as normal and natural if it is to be resolved. Denial of it will only lead to later problems. The uncomfortable silences when someone cries or the halting of a conversation when the grieving person joins the group indicate others' uneasiness with grief. Avoidance of the couple also indicates this. If others view grief as morbid, they leave the couple feeling ashamed of their normal healthy reactions. Non-helpful comments include:

> You really should forget it. You should be over it by now.

> You mustn't cry. Think of the children. You're only upsetting them all over again.

> People are beginning to avoid us because you cry all the time, and I don't blame them.

> You mustn't be angry. That doesn't help anyone.

> You don't really mean that.

> There are others a lot worse off than you, and they don't go on like this.

> You must feel better now that you know what the problem is.

> After I came home, I met a neighbour. You know how you tell it from your own experience, and I was talking as if it had happened only to me. This neighbour later said to my husband: 'Leith should realize that it isn't only she who lost a baby. It's you too!' That hurt and embarrassed me. It made me feel guilty for feelings I didn't have. I knew only too well Darryl's loss: I'd only been home a couple of days as well. She couldn't really understand. There was no one more aware of Darryl's loss than I.

5. Are a means of avoiding the issue

Rather than confront a possible painful situation, people may avoid the issue of the loss altogether. They may stop the couple talking about it by changing the subject or pretending a statement was never made. When general conversation drifts around to children, there may be a distinct silence, following by frenzied activity to change the subject. The grieving person is soon aware that he/she is making everyone else feel uncomfortable, which may add to his/her sense of failure and alienation.

Typical comments include:

> When Johnny was born . . . (Silence) . . . You know, I haven't seen Mandy for so long, have you?

> Griever: I still feel so down at times.
> Companion: Yes, I know. Sometimes I feel so exhausted, what with running a house and working as well. You really need to be superwoman these days.

Griever: I think of the baby all the time.
Companion: Another cup of tea, honey? Do try these new biscuits I made. I've never used this recipe before.

I think it is best we avoid that. It will only upset us both. Let's talk about something happy.

6. Assume that understanding of the couple's problem is quite simple

It is very difficult for someone to understand the feelings of another, unless that person has himself/herself had a similar experience. Even then, the assumption that everyone feels and reacts in the same way is incorrect. Grief is a very personal thing. Others can empathize and understand similar feelings, but to assume understanding of feelings that are so raw and recent is dangerous. Over time, as the crisis is resolved, the feelings ease in intensity, and it can be difficult even for couples who have had a similar tragedy to rekindle the same emotions.

The most common comment that fallaciously assumes an understanding is:

I know how you feel.

After I lost the baby I went back to Uni where I was doing a couple of Psychology subjects. While in hospital, I had missed handing in one of my assignments. I went to this senior tutor to clear up the matter. He pressed me about why it was late. I tried to avoid it, but finally said: 'I've just lost a baby'. He immediately said — and I'll never forget it — 'I know exactly how you feel. My cat died on the weekend.'

Helpful reactions

Many of the comments mentioned above are not always harmful. If said in the context of a sharing relationship or as grief is being resolved, some may be appropriate. But in general, if used in the early stages of grief, they will cause more pain for the already grieving couple. What, then, can one do to help the couple experiencing child-bearing difficulties? Below are a few hints that may help the person who wants to be a real source of comfort.

1. Accept their grief; allow and encourage them to express it and talk it out

Learning about grief allows one to understand it. Understanding it removes much of its mystery and fear. The reactions of the grieving couple are then more predictable. Seemingly illogical and unreasonable behaviour is then more easily accepted and understood.

Don't assume that the couple will not want to discuss a painful subject. On the contrary, most will feel a strong need to discuss it, and will welcome a willing listener. When discussing the subject, be prepared to be honest with your own feelings, and encourage the couple to be honest with theirs. Be prepared for tears or other outward signs of emotion. Rest assured that you are not hurting the person further if they begin to cry. Tears are due to the situation, not people talking about it. Tears that are able to be released are healing. Therefore, don't feel guilty if through your willingness to listen, the grieving persons cry. You are not 'upsetting' them. Provide what comfort seems appropriate for the particular persons. If you feel that an arm around the shoulder or a squeeze of the hand would help them, then comfort them in this way. Offer a tissue if appropriate. If you sense that they need to be alone for a while, then go and make a cup of tea, but *always* return! Reassure them that you are comfortable with them and that emotions are acceptable. Be guided by your own feelings of what they need. If you are unsure of the needs of a grieving person, ask him/her:

> Would you like me to stay, or leave you alone for a while? I want to do what is best for you, but I'm not sure what you want.

Many people are unsure of how to begin a conversation about grief. When a grieving person comes to visit, do you keep up the initial small talk or begin a deeper conversation about grief? How do you get over this transition? Open questions such as 'And how are you feeling inside?' or 'Do you want to talk about anything? I'm willing to listen' are helpful. Other statements such as 'I don't want to upset you, but I don't want to avoid the subject of the baby. Do you need to talk at all?' are also useful. Even a simple question accompanied by a knowing and caring look or a squeeze of the arm conveys your meaning without words. Don't force the grieving person to talk about it. Offer him/her the option, but leave the decision on whether or not to take up your offer to the grieving person. Sometimes he/she is talked out and simply needs your company.

If a baby has died or is separated from its parents, the acknowledgment by others of the existence of the baby is comforting to parents. The parents will often be encouraged by someone willing to use the baby's name and share the photographs and other memorabilia.

Grief does not confine itself to a specific time-period or time of day. A friend who is available and ready to listen whenever a grieving person needs comfort is important. Such a friend may have to listen to the details of the loss many times over as grief progresses, but patience to do just this is necessary. If those who are grieving find it difficult to contact others, a comforting friend should contact them: 'Hi! I was just thinking of you and wondering how you are.'

As time goes on and grief is being resolved, the grieving person may wish to look to the future. He/she may wish to seek out more information about future possible pregnancies. A comforting helper will be ready to help and encourage the grieving person to seek out informed opinion, even accompanying him/her to doctor's appointments if the person so wishes.

2. Listen effectively

Allowing someone to talk is ineffective unless the helper listens. Listening involves hearing not only the words but also the feelings behind both the words spoken and those unspoken. Give the grieving person plenty of time to say what is on his/her mind. Don't interrupt. If he/she seems to fumble over words, do not rush in with lots of verbiage. Accept silence while the grieving person gathers his/her thoughts. Let the thoughts be expressed fully. Don't prevent it by offering lots of advice or using some of the non-helpful comments already mentioned. Rather, restate in your own words what the person has said or the feelings he/she has expressed. If you do this, he/she knows that you have really heard and understood what has been said.

If the grieving person is able to talk, his/her conversation can be encouraged by moving close, nodding, and offering encouragement through obvious attention. More details about effective listening are given in Chapter 9.

3. Don't feel that you are responsible for other people's feelings, or have to have the answers to all their problems

Many people feel inadequate in crisis. They avoid the subject because they are afraid they won't know what to say. When the couple don't seem to be getting better, they feel helpless and withdraw. Others must accept that they are not responsible for the feelings and problems of another. People must find their own solutions, and generally do. All others can do is be willing to listen and act as a 'sounding-board' for the thoughts of the one in crisis. You do not have to have the answers to the problem. You can help people in crisis find their answers by responding to their feelings and words with compassion and understanding.

It may be necessary to realize that at times relationships may change when one person in that relationship faces a crisis. These changes need not be negative. When two people are able to share times of crisis openly and accept the resulting change in each other, relationships may even be enhanced.

4. Assure them of their worth, even if the crisis takes time to be resolved

Couples experiencing child-bearing difficulties often feel a deep sense of failure. Their feelings of self-worth can be shattered. When others avoid or patronize them, these feelings are intensified. Remind them that they are cared about and thought of often. A simple phone call may be all that it takes. Grieving can be a long process, and a couple need this reassurance not just initially but throughout the long hard times. Too often, support disappears within a couple of weeks or a month. Life goes on around them, yet the couple still grieve. When others forget, they feel isolated. Gestures of caring such as hugs and even knowing looks convey continued support.

Helpers must be sensitive to the needs of the grieving persons. They must know when to provide closeness and when to give them space. If closeness seems to elicit a negative reaction, don't take that as a personal slight, but rather as a signal to put some breathing space between you and those grieving. Never desert them! Leave the situation settle for a while before attempting a new approach.

At times, the grieving couple may avoid friends and acquaintances who have children or are pregnant. This is difficult if such friends want desperately to help the couple. Such prospective helpers may find it difficult to understand why their grieving friends are behaving so negatively toward them. In some cases, helping a grieving couple may mean allowing them to withdraw and the relationship to 'cool' until the couple are able to cope with it again. It is difficult for friends to accept this, and they may feel rejected and hurt. Assuring a couple of their worth may mean accepting their withdrawal while leaving the door of friendship open for a later re-entry.

We all have our own defences against pain. Some grieving persons reject other people for fear of being hurt further. Some wish company, while others seek solitude. Some deny the situation. Others feel and display anger. Some become lethargic, others active. We must never assume that one approach to grief is superior and the only one acceptable. A person's defences must be respected, for even inappropriate ones may initially be the only means the person has of coping.

Sometimes words hurt. Concentrate not on the words spoken in grief, but on the relationship. First and foremost, remember that these are persons for whom you care a great deal. They are in crisis. At times, weighed down by grief, they may behave badly toward you. Reject the behaviour, not the person!

As time goes on, the couple may need to feel valuable as persons again. They may resent being continually treated as 'emotional invalids', or only viewed according to their crisis. A person in crisis is still a person first. Encourage such people in other areas of their life, while supporting them when the going is tough.

5. Be aware of them in social situations

Venturing back into society can be difficult for the grieving person, particularly when he/she must face thoughtless comments and behaviour. When emotions are still raw, situations in which outward displays of pain are not really acceptable can be difficult. The couple don't wish to be smothered or hovered over. Yet a sensitive friend who is able to convey by a small word or gesture the feeling 'I'm here. You're not alone. You're understood' when needed, is invaluable. A grieving person doesn't want you to fight his/her battles. The effective helper is simply there in the backlines ready with the supplies and support when called upon.

6. Provide any practical help that may be needed

Support doesn't come only in the form of words. Many who feel that they are unable to find the appropriate words can show their caring in more practical ways. If the woman has required hospitalization or further testing, she may appreciate a hot meal, the shopping done, a clean house, or errands run. Some people may simply appreciate company, even if the subject of the loss is never discussed. An offer to help acknowledge bereavement letters in writing may help to make a difficult job easier. Breaking the news of the loss to other friends may also relieve some pressure. It is vital to remember that even simple acts of help must never be forced upon a couple, but offered in such a way that the couple will not feel that they have hurt you by rejecting your offer.

> I was wondering if perhaps you could use some lamb casserole. I made too much, and thought that you might not feel up to cooking. Please don't feel that you have to say yes. I won't be offended. I'd like to help more if I could. Please feel free to ask for anything you need. You mean so much to us.

7. Be humble

An effective helper is one who is able to realize that the grieving couple are facing a real crisis, and deserve respect for their attempt to cope with it. Even if at times you feel that they are overreacting or behaving badly, respect them. It is so easy to criticize when standing on the outside looking in. From your secure state you may be tempted to silently criticize their coping and feel superior. Don't! Be humble and thankful that you have been provided with an opportunity to comfort another human being, for one day you may also need such support. Offer what you have to give, not out of pity but out of real caring.

Coping with thoughtless comments

When confronted by hurtful comments, the grieving couple may recoil. Like an animal with a wounded paw, they need to protect the wound. Some may withdraw to cry alone. Others may strike out in anger, alienating those around them who are unable to understand their grief.

If someone makes a comment which a couple disagree with, it is best for them not to argue. Instead, they should simply state clearly and directly their feelings on the matter. They should be assertive, recognizing their right to feel the way they do.

> Companion: You can always have other children. You mustn't feel too bad. Lots of people have one miscarriage.
> Griever: I realize that a miscarriage is quite common. But this was my child, and this child has a right to be cried over. I don't want to forget this child. There may be other children, but I loved this particular child.

> One girlfriend said: 'This may sound cruel, but my mother always says it's harder to lose them later on. You probably won't agree with that.' I said: 'No, I don't'. I don't know why she had to say it.

If others are abused by a grieving person following an inappropriate comment, it is easy for them to blame the grieving person for the attack. Instead of recognizing the fault in his/her own statement, the person can explain away the grieving person's reaction by thinking: 'I suppose he/she is upset. After all, I was only trying to help. I'll have to excuse him/her.'

If the grieving person decides that the comment was made out of ignorance or discomfort, he/she needs to accept this and give the person another chance. The great majority of people are like this; they do care, but they are only human. But if the couple's honest belief is that the comments were made to keep them feeling inferior or to patronize them, then perhaps they have found out something about the deep insecurities of another person around them who needs to feel superior to others.

Conclusion
Honesty — the key

We don't live in a world isolated from others. In situations of child-bearing difficulties, the grieving couple must still maintain their relationships with others. Their roles as patients, parents, children, brothers, sisters, friends, and acquaintances must all continue.

For both the couple and those they come in contact with, the key to overcoming difficulties and providing meaningful support is honesty. An honest relationship between medical personnel and a patient helps to build confidence, and fulfils the needs of the couple for information and understanding. Honesty with children on their own level of comprehension removes their insecurities and their need to resort to incorrect explanations of the event. Honesty with family and friends conveys genuine feelings of support. Even when the right words don't seem to be there, an honest expression of feelings of helplessness spoken by any person wishing to comfort a grieving couple can convey the necessary message:

> I really don't know what to say. I'm afraid of saying the wrong thing and upsetting you. All I know is that I'm so very sorry and I do care. If I can help I truly want to. I've got a willing listening ear and two willing hands.

You can't go wrong when your words and actions are based on a genuine concern and caring for the couple in crisis, and are backed by a bit of sound knowledge and a willingness to really communicate.

References

1. Robert Krell and Leslie Rabkin, 'The Effects of Sibling Death on the Surviving Child: A Family Perspective', *Family Process*, 18 (1979), 471–477.
2. B. Richardson, 'Children's Reactions to the Death of a Sibling', Newsletter of SANDS (QLD) Inc., No. 7 (June 1984).

11 The Final Solution — You
General Crisis-Coping

Difficulties in bearing a live, mature, healthy child are just one set of problems that may arise in the lives of ordinary people. Other crises, such as the loss of a spouse, unemployment, family illness, and work pressures, can also produce strain on the coping skills of the individual. Although others may be able to help through caring and understanding, each crisis is personal. Your feelings about, and reactions to, the crisis situation are uniquely yours. In the final analysis, the problem is yours alone, and within you lies its solution. This is a hard fact to accept.

As children, we took our pains to our parents to soothe. As adults, our pains are our own. In many cases, time and the support of others will cushion our time of crisis, and eventually it will pass. Grief is like this. Sometimes, though, we are able to assist our own crisis-resolution by positive action. Such action, if fostered in one crisis, may later hold us in good stead when we are faced with other crises.

Our individual means of coping with crises are as varied as are people. Generally, our favoured means of coping are ones that have served us well in past crises. The decision to cope in one particular way is unconscious, and we are generally unaware of its appropriateness or inappropriateness. Some people withdraw from the situation and from others. They refuse to confront the problem, feeling that if they ignore it long enough it will go away. Others accept the facts of the crisis, but repress their feelings about it. These feelings may surface later in related physical illness or during a later difficult time. Yet others become extremely hostile toward the situation and those around them, looking for someone or something to blame. Such people often see the crisis as out of their control. There are other groups who attempt to find solutions through sound reasoning, often denying their right to feel upset. In contrast, some people let their emotions show freely in crying, or while talking with others.

Depression

The most common and the longest-lasting reaction to a loss in the area of child bearing is some period of depression. We commonly hear of people being depressed; everyone feels depressed at some time, but such depression is generally short-lived. Some depression is precipitated by a particular event. People suffering from such depression usually do come out of it, although the healing period can vary from days to months, depending on the type of loss. In contrast, some depression appears to have no obvious immediate cause. It builds up over time. It is thought that it may have some biochemical basis, although this is disputed.[1] Professionals also recognize **Postpartum** depression, which occurs in many women in the first week after giving birth. In some cases it fails to lift, and prolonged depression results. Some women do not experience the onset of this depression until some time after birth, usually within the first six months. Where there has been a loss of pregnancy or the birth of an abnormal or premature child, this normal hormonal-related depression may be complicated by the depression of grief.

How do we recognize depression? Depression can display itself in many different ways in different individuals. There are general feelings of unhappiness and hopelessness, a feeling that life is a burden that must be endured. The depressed person may lose interest in all activities or decision-making, and may find concentrating difficult. There may be absentmindedness and frequent mood swings. Sleeping patterns may change, with some depressed people sleeping a great deal, and others suffering from insomnia. The temper may be short, weeping compulsive, and thoughts disordered. There may also be a loss of sexual interest. The close link between mind and body is seen within the many physical symptoms that may present themselves in the depressed person. Symptoms include headaches and muscular tension, a loss of taste, chronic constipation or diarrhoea, and increased or decreased appetite, to name but some. There may also be a weakening in the response of the immune system for a period during severe depression. The depressed person may notice this when he/she seems to fall prey to every cold or flu virus that seems to be around. Some women also notice that during times of depression they are more susceptible to yeast infections, such as thrush. Most people appear to have a 'weak spot' in the body, where they usually notice a reaction to stress. Hands may become cold and clammy. The head may ache, and vision becomes blurred. The bowel or bladder may become irritable, leading to an increased frequency of urination or motions. Acid may arise from the stomach. The heart may suffer from palpitations, or there may be nasal congestion.

A person's ability to cope with depression depends on many factors, such as the success in coping and resolving past crises, the amount of support available, and the personality characteristics of the person. People who have resolved past losses successfully may suffer from a period of depression after the loss, but find that it is overcome with time. For others, a child-bearing loss may rekindle old unresolved insecurities, serving only to complicate and deepen the grief surrounding this most recent loss. Where loss is prolonged or never fully resolved, depression may be longer lasting. This may be the case in situations of infertility, repeated losses, or rearing a handicapped child. In such cases where some hope still remains, the final impact of the loss may not be fully felt, and hence grieving may be delayed.

A depressed person may not be able to change the situation that precipitated the depression. Similarly, they cannot banish their depression simply by making a conscious decision to do so. Yet, there are things that can be done to assist the healing process. At times, a depressed person is his/her own worst enemy, actually deepening the depression by engaging in negative behaviours and thoughts that could be controlled.

Coping with a crisis and its depression

The most outstanding feature of depression is often a feeling of lethargy and hopelessness. Motivation to do even the simplest task is difficult to find. Feelings of failure can then be deepened, as the person feels that he/she is losing control of life in general. Being able to feel that you are doing something to help yourself can help raise the spirits of the depressed person to some extent.

Diet

Depressed persons often become haphazard about their diet. Inappropriate eating habits and the resulting physical changes can actually accentuate depression. Overeating can lead to weight problems that further erode self-esteem. Eating irregularly or consuming the wrong foods can lead to fluctuating levels of blood sugar. The loss of some essential vitamins and amino acids can affect emotional well-being. The depressed person can help, rather than hinder, his/her recovery by following a sensible healthy diet and a few simple hints.

1. Make sure you eat regular meals. Three meals a day is most common, but some people actually find that they feel healthier eating five or six smaller meals in one day.

2. Eat a good breakfast. People expend most energy during the day, and need sufficient fuel from a hearty breakfast to maintain blood sugar levels. The fuel from a heavy evening meal may not be used by the resting body. In fact, some people experience sleeping problems following such a meal.

3. Eat to satisfy hunger, not for solace. Many depressed people find solace in food. Avoid the kitchen except during meal-times. When feeling particularly depressed, find some other activity besides eating to occupy your mind. If you are unable to do so, keep the fridge stocked with only low-kilojoule foods, such as raw vegetables or fruit. If you have a weakness, don't keep high-kilojoule food like cakes or biscuits in the house at all.

4. Avoid alcohol and tranquillizing drugs. Alcohol and many prescription drugs are depressants, which means that they slow down (or make more tranquil) the body systems. Hence, such drugs may actually add to depression.

5. Plan your diet weekly. Not only will planning ensure that you have available in your home healthy foods, but it may also give you a sense of having some control over your life.

6. Eat foods rich in complex carbohydrates and B vitamins. Food containing complex carbohydrates help to maintain the levels of blood sugar for longer periods. Food containing B vitamins help replace stores of vitamins thought to be concerned with enhancing emotional well-being. Such

important foods include whole-grain breads and cereals, fish, green vegetables, fruit, and eggs.

7. Avoid highly sugared, salted, processed, or greasy food. Not only will too much of these foods be detrimental to your health, but they can also aggravate weight and skin problems, further demoralizing you. A small treat every now and then won't hurt, as long as your usual diet is composed of foods more suited to maintaining health.

8. Make the effort to eat regularly, even when you don't feel like it. Often depressed persons lose their appetite, and find that food loses its taste. The effort required to prepare tasty foods is often beyond them. But appetizing food doesn't have to be difficult to prepare. Fresh fruit can be eaten immediately. Whole-grain bread can be topped with tomato, shallots, or herbs and cheese, and then grilled for a tasty treat. Use garlic and herbs to add flavour to bland-tasting dishes. A variety of fruit can be blended for an appetizing drink that serves as a healthy light meal. A salad sandwich is also good health value. Seek help from a friend or a cookbook for simple, healthy meal ideas that take only minimal preparation. Write the recipes down and leave them in your kitchen for those times when your motivation is running very low and you may be tempted to snack on foods that are less desirable.

9. Drink tea and coffee only in moderation. Excess quantities of tea or coffee can lead to palpitations and headaches, which make a depressed person feel even worse. The stimulating effects of the caffeine are only short-lived. Drink more water flavoured with lemon juice, if need be.

10. Make sure you have adequate fibre in your diet. Fibre enhances the efficiency of the digestive system by acting as bulk, which encourages the movement of food through the intestines. It is a natural means, when combined with drinking lots of water, of relieving constipation, which may accompany depression and can cause further distress due to its inconvenience and associated feelings of ill-health.

What constitutes a healthy diet is hotly debated. Hundreds of books have been written on the subject. We do not intend to try to provide in-depth dietary knowledge. For such information, choose a book that is based on sound medical knowledge and includes a wide range of foods and a great deal of flexibility. Here, we simply intend to look at the basic foods that should be included in a healthy diet and how they may easily be included daily.

a) Whole-grain products — 4 serves daily. Eat wholemeal or grained bread instead of white. Eat porridge for breakfast. Bake with wholemeal rather than plain flour. Use brown or converted rice. Make your own muesli from such ingredients as rolled oats, unprocessed bran, wheatgerm, dried fruits, and nuts.

b) Fruit and vegetables — at least 4 serves daily. Eat them raw as snacks. Don't peel vegetables, but scrub and steam, microwave, or only partially boil. Eat potatoes wrapped in alfoil and baked, and then topped with herbs. Use fruit on top of muesli or as a dessert. Try baked apples filled with dried fruits covered with skim-milk custard. Eat plenty of salads.

c) Protein foods in limited amounts — 1 to 2 serves daily. Eat chicken, fish, eggs, legumes such as soya beans and peanuts, or limited amounts of red meat. Try peanut butter on wholemeal bread or eggs on toast. Omelettes are simple to prepare and tasty.

d) Milk products — 1 to 2 serves daily. Use skim milk for cooking and drinking. For main-course accompaniments, use white or cheese sauce. For dessert, try baked puddings and custard. Cheese on toast is easy to prepare and is nutritious, as are personal packs of yoghurt.

e) Fats — use sparingly. Some fats are necessary in our diet, as certain vitamins and minerals are fat-soluble. Unfortunately, we generally eat more fat than is necessary. Try lightly buttered toast, or stir fried vegetables.

Exercise

Exercise is known to help improve the functioning of a depressed person. It is not fully understood how this happens, but it is believed that exercise may cause hormonal changes in the body; may increase the beta-endorphins, the mood-affecting chemicals of the brain; and may improve the functioning of the autonomic nervous system. Its benefit may also come from the feeling of taking some control of your life and the diversion from depressing thoughts which exercise offers. Exercise also enhances the circulatory system, the skin, the hair, and the physique, which helps to bolster self-esteem.

It is important to have a full medical check-up before beginning any exercise program. This is sound advice, not only to check for circulatory problems, but also because such an examination may uncover some underlying conditions, such as a thyroid dysfunction, which may be contributing to prolonged depression.

Exercise may be broadly divided into stretching and aerobic exercises. Stretching exercises are important in warming up, to avoid damage to tendons and ligaments while exercising. Exercise best able to assist in relieving depression is regular, pulse-raising, and enjoyable. Aerobic exercise such as swimming, aerobic dancing, skipping, cycling, jogging, or rapid walking performed for a period of 15 to 20 minutes at least three times a week is favoured by many. Other exercise performed in a social setting, such as tennis, netball, hockey, football, or other sports, may help the depressed person by making him/her feel involved, while obtaining the physical benefits of exercise. Before undertaking any aerobic — that is, continuous pulse-raising exercise — get advice from a recognized instructor concerning a sensible program suited to your individual needs, age, and level of fitness, to avoid possible damage from excessive, badly-designed exercises.

General exercise that concentrates on the areas of the body most prone to stress can relieve tension. Exercises for the facial, neck, shoulder, and lower-back muscles are of particular importance.

Relaxation and sleep

When a person is depressed, sleep is often disrupted, and daylight hours are often accompanied by feelings of tension in the mind and the muscles of the body. To overcome such problems, many depressed persons and even doctors have come to rely on prescribed drugs. Unfortunately, rather than relieve depression, these simply treat a symptom, and should never be considered as a long-term solution for depression.

Relaxation techniques can be learnt, and will be discussed within this section. Firstly, let us look at sleep and a few simple suggestions that may make it possible to avoid sleeping pills.

To encourage sleep:
1. Eat an early dinner rather than one later at night, when your body will require energy to digest this food.
2. Stop worrying about falling asleep. Worry will more likely prevent sleep. Adopt the attitude that if you don't sleep tonight there is always tomorrow.
3. Take a lukewarm bath before retiring. Don't shower, but bathe in lukewarm rather than hot water. Soak and enjoy the relaxing warmth.
4. Drink a glass of warm milk. Avoid coffee, tea, hot chocolate, or cola drinks. Milk contains an amino acid called trytophan, which acts as a sedative, and whose activity is increased by heat. The caffeine in coffee and other beverages stimulates the system and can hinder sleep in some people.
5. Make sure your bedroom is quiet, darkened, and well ventilated. Having fresh bed-linen and a tidy, fresh-smelling bedroom can also assist sleep.
6. Take alcohol sparingly. Although alcohol is a depressant and hence may make you feel drowsy, too much may cause you to wake after only a little sleep.
7. If worry is keeping you awake, write down your worries on a pad close to your bed or speak into a portable cassette recorder. Then determine to forget these worries until morning.
8. Entertain yourself with a dull activity before bed. Watch a boring television show, read a dull book or magazine, or listen to gentle soothing music with the lights down low. Avoid anything that stimulates your imagination. For example, don't read a gripping whodunnit and find yourself awake trying to find the answer.
9. Practise a relaxation technique on retiring. Relaxation techniques are not confined to one type. There are methods of relaxation involving biofeedback techniques, self-hypnosis, autogenic training, yoga, and other eastern practices. All are beneficial, and the chosen method is determined by the particular needs of the individual. All techniques depend on the person undertaking them creating an environment of peace and tranquility. A darkened, quiet, well-ventilated room, comfortable in temperature, is best. Also of vital

importance is a relaxed attitude on the part of the person. It is important that you be open to the relaxation experience. Try not to think about other things. Blank out your mind to worries. If you do find yourself concentrating on a thought, focus on it and then let it go naturally. Sometimes imagining a word like 'relax' or 'blank' in your mind's eye will help abolish other thoughts. For in-depth work on relaxation you could contact the Community Health Centres, Relaxation Centres, some General Practitioners, or individual psychological professionals within your State.

In this section, we will simply outline a simple relaxation technique that can be performed anywhere at any time without special training, and may help the depressed person in the initial stages of grief before he/she may feel able or willing to seek outside help.

1. Allow approximately 20 uninterrupted minutes for relaxation. Ask your partner to mind the children if necessary. Putting aside a special time each day for relaxation will help it become a habit, which will be of most benefit.

2. Darken the room and block off as much outside noise as possible. Lie down with only one low soft pillow under your head, feet about 25 centimetres apart, toes rested and pointing outwards, and arms by your side with the palms up. Alternatively, sit in a comfortable high-backed chair, with your head resting gently on a small pillow. Put your feet gently on the floor so that pressure from the chair is not felt on the back of the knees or lower thighs. Rest your arms gently on the chair arms or on the thighs, palms up. Close your eyes.

3. Allow your body to flop like a rag doll. Feel yourself sinking into the bed or chair with each breath out.

4. Concentrate only on your breathing. Imagine you are the air coming into your lungs and going out. Try to blank your mind to all but imagining the journey of air into and out of your lungs. Do this for at least ten breaths.

5. Focus your attention on your individual arms and legs. Tell yourself they are heavy and warm. Simply say in your mind that 'My right arm is heavy, very heavy. My right arm is

heavy. My right arm is warm, very warm', and so on for each limb. Repeat these statements a number of times.

6. Return to your breathing. This time, with each breath in, visualize in your mind the words 'I am . . .', and, with each breath out, visualize '. . . relaxed'. Continue this for another ten to 20 breaths.

7. Focus on each set of muscles in your body individually. Imagine some soft fingertips gently stroking and massaging the muscles. Begin with the muscles of the forehead and temples, followed by the cheeks, the eyelids, the front of the neck, the back of the neck, the shoulders, the shoulder blades, the collar bone, the middle back, the lower back, the abdomen, the upper arms, the lower arms, the hands, the thighs, the calves, and finally the feet.

8. Imagine yourself in this position in a tranquil spot, such as on a deserted beach or floating in the middle of a lake early on a warm summer's day. Listen for the gentle sounds of the sea or lake, the birds overhead, or the splash of fish jumping. Allow yourself a minute or so of complete peace in this environment.

9. Return to your breathing for five to ten breaths, visualizing the words 'I am relaxed'. Concentrate now on your heart for about a minute. You may even be able to feel a pulse-beat in some parts of your body. Tell yourself that your heartbeat is strong and regular. Now return to your breathing.

10. Imagine now that you have a hole in the top of your head and a thick soothing blue or green liquid is passing through you from head to foot removing any left-over tension. Visualize its journey into every nook and cranny of your body, soothing and removing the tension as it leaves your body through your feet.

11. Return finally to your breathing for another five breaths.

12. Return slowly from your relaxation. Move your fingers and toes gently, and feel the energy coming back into your body. Finally, open your eyes and sit or lie quietly for a moment before rising.[2]

Don't expect to feel miraculously revitalized when you first begin relaxation. It takes time and patience and practice before you will be able to recognize the way your own body enters a relaxed state. Relaxation is not something to be achieved, but rather to be experienced. Don't aim to be the 'most relaxed person in the world'. Aim rather to experience what you can, becoming more at ease as you discover your own individual path to relaxation.

Relaxation through mutual massage is one of the most effective techniques, for not only are muscles relaxed, but there is also a bond between the couple as one provides warmth and caring for the other. A warm bath followed by a massage with warm hands and oil, talc, or body lotion is probably one of the best sleep-inducers for the depressed person.

Relaxation techniques can also be used to help you cope with difficult situations. The process is known as systematic desensitization.[3] If you must attend a social function which you know is likely to cause you distress, you can use relaxation to ease the burden. Firstly, write down a list of the sources of stress in the situation, noting them in ascending order, from that which would cause you least difficulty to that which would cause greatest distress. For example, if you must attend a baptism of someone else's child, your list might read:

> Getting dressed to go out
> Getting to the church
> Meeting the family outside without the baby
> Seeing the family with the baby
> Going up to meet the family with the baby
> Going into church with the family
> Holding the baby during the ceremony

Now undertake the relaxation techniques already outlined up to stage 9. Continue your breathing and using the words 'I am relaxed'. Visualize the first stressful situation on your list. You may find yourself tensing. Try to maintain your regular breathing, while holding the image. Return to your 'I am relaxed' breathing. If you feel able, work your way through the list, always returning to your relaxed breathing between steps. Only imagine a new stress situation from your list when you can imagine the previous one while still maintaining a relaxed state.

Rethinking — asking yourself some important questions

Child-bearing problems are difficult enough in themselves. Yet their effects are compounded when they disrupt our perceived dreams, future roles, and image of ourselves. The sense of failure can grow out of proportion, affecting the whole life of the individual. Perhaps the greatest difficulties arise when the problems actually affect our view of the future by threatening to deprive the couple of the number or type of children they desired or by depriving them of children altogether. During the time of child-bearing difficulties, the attaining of the goal of a live, healthy, mature infant can become the focus of life for the couple or an individual partner. In fact, it can almost become an obsession. Failure in this area then affects the general functioning of the individual, and depression deepens.

At times, the depressed person's thoughts are his/her worst enemies, sinking him/her further and further into feelings of hopelessness. Of course, the couple facing a single loss that is resolved on a second attempt or by a favourable outcome such as may occur in single cases of miscarriage, death, or premature delivery, may not be as deeply affected as those facing infertility, repeated losses, or the raising of a severely handicapped child.

Most of us have a romanticized view of life in general. If our ideal includes a family, we visualize an ideal number of perfectly healthy, well-behaved, emotionally stable children, who came into the world naturally, and with whom early bonding was a joy and privilege. Child-bearing difficulties tarnish our view, and may even destroy our dream completely. Yet, many continue to hold on to that dream, putting themselves through their own version of hell on earth. How the couple cope with these situations may be affected by their ability to accept reality and what moulds our reality. Reality may be difficult to face. We often have to ask ourselves questions and rethink our situation.

The first question you may need to think about is: How much is your attitude to your situation affected by what other people think? Is your wish for a family one you have considered right for your life, or is it something you assumed necessary for happiness because that is what everyone else sees as necessary? Is your child's handicap distasteful, or is it simply that others are narrow-minded? Do you feel inferior to others who have children without problems? Can you visualize a life without children or with a handicapped child, and still see yourself as 'fitting in' with your friends and family? Is comparing yourself with others adding to your depression? Unfortunately, overcoming societal pressure is very difficult. People's status in our society is still tied with being part of a pair and being a parent. The worst part of failure is what you think others will think of you. Mix this with disappointment and doubts about yourself, and it is easy to see why depression can set in. Accepting yourself is difficult at this time, but vital. What right do others have to make you feel inferior? There is a wonderful verse of Scripture that we need to consider, even if perhaps we have no religious beliefs. It says: 'What is man that thou art mindful of him?' It has a point! You are no less a person for having child-bearing difficulties.

Secondly, are you living in the future rather than in the present? Is your happiness dependent on the future outcome of a live, healthy child? Is the present simply something to be endured until the future day? Many people find it difficult to accept a change in their perceived future life-plan, and fight desperately against it. They have inflated expectations of the future, which keep them going in the present. They find it difficult to accept that no matter how hard you work at it there are no guarantees that the future will arrange itself as you desire. You must accept that you have some choices, and accept change. Change is the way in which the future comes into our lives. Your actual future may not be any better or worse than your perceived future, only different. It cannot be better if we won't allow ourselves to investigate the options, and instead cling stubbornly to our tarnished dreams, even when the facts signify the futility of this. This is not to say that the future may not turn out as you desire, or that you should give up after one setback. It simply means that it is vital to look at all the options that the future may hold, so that your decisions about your future will offer you hope and security. In the meantime, a view of the future as worthwhile, whatever it may hold, allows you to enjoy the present without dread of possible future outcomes. Many people feel that facing the worst and developing plans to cope with such an outcome help a great deal. If the worst then occurs, they are ready to deal with it. In contrast, if a more favourable outcome occurs, they will be pleasantly surprised. For example, some couples face up to the problem of 'What will we do if we can't have children?' They then make moves toward a future for themselves, perhaps looking into a change in occupation or situation, travel or adoption. If they are then able to have a child, they are even more thrilled. Believing there is a future one can look forward to, goes a long way toward relieving the distress of a depressed person.

Thirdly, are you trying to force answers to unanswerable questions? Looking for reassurances and causes is a part of grieving, but if they begin to preoccupy us, we are only hurting ourselves. Some questions don't have answers, and we must accept this. Every grieving couple asks 'Why us?' There is no answer, except in accepting that life isn't fair. As children, we believed that good children are rewarded and bad ones punished. To make sense of the 'Why us?' question we may look for something we did that caused our loss, and so berate ourselves. We need someone or something to blame, so that the whole mess makes sense. In some cases, a cause may be found that can be attributed to our partner or another person. Guilt and anger may then become intense. Forgiveness is very difficult to achieve in such situations, until one can accept the fallibility of mankind. Where no cause can be found, the depressed person may invent one as a means of making the loss appear rational. Don't blame yourself or others. Rather, accept that the joys of life are not distributed on merit. There is no such rational basis for what happens in the world. 'Why us?' may be replaced by 'Well, why not us?'

Another unanswerable question is 'If I try again, will the same thing happen?' Others may quote statistics that indicate your chances of a recurrence of the problem or of resolving the problem. Generally, such figures are encouraging. But to a grieving couple statistics don't seem to mean a great deal. When you've been a statistic *once*, you can't see why you may not be again! Such couples may refer to statistics to help them make a decision, but finally they have only one decision to make: Do we try again or don't we? If they decide against a new attempt, then the fear of a recurrence does not arise. If they do decide to try again, that is the only decision that they have to make. They can't decide to try again on the proviso that they are sure it won't happen again. Trying again does mean taking a risk. There are never certainties about the future. Hence, the decision to try again requires courage. It also requires an attempt to be optimistic, to anticipate success. It means believing that the bad times will pass. A series of losses can destroy optimism about the future, but consciously trying to rekindle some spark of hope amid the darkness can help. Don't set yourself long-term goals. With each new pregnancy, take one day at a time. Let the future take care of itself. Worrying about the final outcome won't change the present or the outcome itself.

Fourthly, a final question involves the effect my depression is having on those I love. Am I making their lives more difficult by my prolonged depression? Can I pull myself out of it for a while to tend to their needs? When weighed down by depression, we are often unable to consider the needs of those around us. Although we need not feel guilty about being depressed, we do need to try to find some time when we put aside our feelings and realize how fortunate we are to have people around us who hurt for us too. They may need our support, and finding the strength to assist them at some time can actually also ease our own pain.

Rethinking our situation is often difficult when we are depressed, but can actually help us to develop a new perspective. But thinking alone may not help you find the new direction. You can act!

Medication

Commonly, doctors prescribe antidepressant medication for persons experiencing depression. Research[4] shows that such drugs are often useful for relieving depression in the short term at least. What must be avoided is the tendency to prescribe such drugs indiscriminantly without knowledge of the needs and circumstances of the patient and discussion of possible long-term effects.

Taking action to help overcome depression
1. Be assertive

Persons who feel depressed may not have the confidence to make the changes that they feel are desirable. Being assertive begins by realizing that you have a right to express yourself. Ask for what you need. Be honest. Make your own decisions. If you state your requests honestly and without demanding, most people will be happy to listen. If they react negatively, that is their problem, not yours.

2. Find a support group

People who have experienced a similar loss are often best able to understand the feelings of depression. Such people generally have a great deal of patience with others who are struggling with a difficult situation similar to one which they have endured. It can be very reassuring to a depressed person not to have to explain his/her feelings to another, but rather to be understood implicitly. See the end of this book for lists of support groups. Other groups may be located by contacting social workers of community health centres or major hospitals.

3. Seek out new friendships and experiences

A person facing a crisis is often changed by this situation. Relationships can change. Some are enhanced; others become strained. There will be people unable to understand or accept the changes in you. You may need to seek out others who are able to fulfil your needs. However, relationships need not break down when friends are sensitive and honest with each other. Never feel guilty if over time your feelings for a friend or acquaintance change. Life brings changes, and at times we must move on.

A depressed person may also need to discover other areas or new areas of life in which they are able to feel worthwhile. Success in some activity, feeling useful, and enjoying oneself, can help raise the self-image. Join a social sporting club or exercise group; begin an educational or hobby course; volunteer for charitable work or a political cause; start a neighbourhood morning-tea group; or seek out new avenues in your job or a new job altogether. The list goes on. At the very least, becoming immersed in some other activity may help you forget your problem for a little while. At best, success in a new activity may provide some new direction in your life, some feelings of value, and new friendships.

4. Enrich your relationship with your partner and other children

One's partner and children are those most affected by the moods of the depressed person. Think of their needs. Their appreciation and love, combined with your concern, may actually bring new light into the darkness of your depression.

5. Learn to recognize the difficult times

Sometimes depression is deepened. Such times may be connected with events that remind the depressed person of the loss, or may occur during particular times of the day. For example, you may find depression deepened at the sight of pregnant women and babies, at anniversaries of a loss, in the early morning when temperature charts are made and hence infertility highlighted, at bedtime when the night seems to stretch ahead forebiddingly and sleep seems unlikely, during a sudden lull in a busy day, or when you see a particular newspaper story. Being aware of these times may allow you a chance to prepare for them, using the relaxation techniques already discussed. Changes to your routine to avoid such difficult times may also be possible.

Be gentle with yourself

Depression is a normal occurrence following a loss. It is nothing to be ashamed of. You are not weak because you are depressed about your situation. You have a right to feel this way. You should feel proud that you are making moves to relieve your depression, but don't try to *force* yourself to get over it too quickly. Grief is a slow process. Even if you have a positive outlook, don't expect too much too soon. For a while you will have to accept a lower level of functioning. It is important to live only one day, perhaps even one hour, at a time. Set yourself small goals. You may decide that today you will phone around to find out about some outside activity, or will buy a book on exercise and diet. You may decide to take your children to the park, simply to enjoy it with them. In the first days of depression be content to set yourself only half an hour in which to do something to relieve your depression, and be proud of accomplishing small goals. Larger ones will follow.

Pamper yourself a little. Soak in a relaxing warm bath. Go to see that movie. Buy take-aways for tea when you can't face cooking. Enjoy a walk while having the children baby-sat. Read a book. Cry. Laugh. Generally, be gentle with yourself, for you are convalescing, recovering from your loss, and hence deserve such consideration. Soon you will find your old energy returning, better equipping you to cope with the day-to-day pressures. The house won't fall down or the children suffer from malnutrition as you take this time of healing for yourself.

How do you know when you need outside help?

At times some people find their grief overwhelming, and are unable to cope. In some cases, present grief may be complicated by past losses or problems that have never been resolved. In others, grief may become 'stuck'. A lack of support or other difficulties may see the grieving person fixed in a particular stage of grief, such as denial, anger, or depression. He/she seems unable to move through to a resolution of his/her grief. Recognizing a person whose grief is abnormal (or pathological) is often difficult for others; but recognizing it within yourself is even more difficult. However, there are some behaviours that point to difficulties in resolving grief.[5]

1. Absence of grief

The person does not display any of the characteristics of grief. He/she carries on as if nothing has happened. In fact, some become overactive while others react blandly, showing no ups or downs.

2. Extreme anger

Although anger is a normal part of grief, at times it is extreme, accompanied by little sadness. The griever cannot be comforted and is unable to accept rational argument. Anger that is intense and prolonged may indicate difficulties.

3. Extreme guilt

At times the griever's anger may be directed toward himself/herself in the form of guilt. This is particularly likely where the griever has decided, rightly or wrongly, that some action of his/hers has caused the loss. Such people may hate themselves, and their self-esteem is extremely low. In extreme cases such guilt may lead to self-destructive behaviour, such as attempted suicide. This behaviour is based on the belief: 'I have caused this. I don't deserve to live.'

4. Acquisition of the symptoms of the deceased

In rare cases, if death has occurred due to prematurity or abnormality, the griever may take on the symptoms of the deceased, such as breathing difficulties when the baby died of lung failure. An intense fear of one's own death or that of a partner or children may also be present.

5. Extreme and prolonged depression

Depression is normal, but at times it shows no sign of being resolved even after many months. It interferes with the ability of the depressed person to lead a normal life. His/her home life and work may suffer considerably, as even relatively simple tasks are difficult to carry out.

6. Denial of the loss

In some cases grief does not seem to be coming to an end because unconsciously the person has denied the permanency of the loss. The thoughts may run: 'If I keep my grief alive, the one lost may come back'. Some actions, such as refusing to dismantle a nursery or using contraceptive measures after a hysterectomy or expecting normal milestones from a mentally retarded child, may indicate such a denial. In fact, if the grieving person begins to feel better, he/she may feel guilty for denying the baby they subconsciously believe will return.

7. Changes in relationships

Crises can bring about changes in certain relationships, according to the level of support communicated during the crisis. This is normal. At times, though, the griever may withdraw from all relationships and become reclusive. This is generally a gradual process. The person's reasons may be understandable, and may include not wishing to make it difficult for himself/herself or uncomfortable for others. However, reclusive behaviour will interfere with his/her ability to function normally, and will deeply affect those, such as partners and children, from whom withdrawal is impossible without final separation.

8. The appearance of medical disorders with a strong psychological link

At times feelings are repressed and the person appears to be coping well with the situation. The strain remains hidden until a later time, when it is displayed in some physical disorder. Many disorders, such as ulcers, some skin disorders, spastic colons, and severe headaches, can be linked to underlying strain.[6] Such disorders may in some cases — not all — indicate that grief has not been resolved. Such symptoms may have a physiological cause, and must be referred to a doctor, not assumed to be due to grief alone.

9. Heavy use of alcohol or prescribed drugs

The general warning signs of abnormal grieving are extreme behaviours that are prolonged, a prolonged interference with normal life, behaviour that does not appear to alter with time, or behaviour that changes suddenly.

Accepting another's concern or one's own concern over grieving problems can be extremely difficult. Our society has a frightening attitude toward mental health. If physically ill, we quickly seek out help. Where illness involves our mental or emotional functioning, we often deny ourselves help for fear of being labelled a 'looney' or 'sick in the head'. The stigma surrounding mental illness in our society is prominent, yet unfounded. Anyone can suffer from emotional problems, particularly those who have suffered a severe loss, such as occurs in some child-bearing difficulties. Yet we like to feel that we have everything under control, that we are tough, and that nothing 'gets under our skin'. We try hard to keep up a front to fool each other, and we don't do a very good job. Addictions to drugs, food, and gambling are rampant in our society. The coronary death rate is extremely high. It is not a person alone who has caused his/her own emotional pain, but the situation in which he/she is placed. If others try to appear superior to such persons because they have sought professional help for emotional problems, it is the others who have the problem, not the distressed persons.

Many people are unsure of where help may be obtained. City areas are much more fortunate than country areas in having greater access to facilities that provide the necessary help. Yet help is available in most areas. Below are some places where help may be sought. If you are afraid to go alone or contact a centre, ask your partner or an understanding friend to accompany you until you feel more at ease.

Help may be obtained from:
1. **One's family**. Some family members are well equipped to assist their loved ones, since they have also suffered and survived crises of their own.
2. **Local clergy, churches, and the associated caring groups.**
3. **Local General Practitioners**. These may be able to provide support or refer a person to another who may help. A person

needs to seek out a GP with whom he/she feels comfortable, and who appears willing to listen rather than simply wish to speed an exit by immediately providing a prescription for some drugs. It is important to remember that GPs are not trained counsellors, and so may not always be able to provide the necessary support themselves.

4. **Lifeline or Crisis Line Services**. These generally operate 24 hours a day, providing a willing listener, information, back-up counselling, and practical services. They are generally noted in the front of the local telephone book.

5. **Social workers and/or chaplains attached to the local hospital**. If the hospital is not large enough to have a resident social worker, it may be served by social workers who travel even into remote areas of Australia. Such people may be happy to talk with you. They may be attached to the Department of Social Security, Child Welfare Departments, or Health Departments. Contact your nearest office for details of when such social workers visit.

6. **Family Welfare Bureaus, The Salvation Army, St Vincent de Paul organizations, and other welfare agencies**. Such organizations care about all people, not just the practical needs of the poverty-stricken. If they are unable to help, they will assist you to find someone who can.

7. **Marriage guidance facilities**.

8. **Government agencies, including Community Health Centres, Psychiatric Clinics, and Child Guidance Clinics**. All such agencies are listed under State Government in the front of the telephone directory.

9. **Private psychiatrists, psychologists and social workers** are also listed in the classified pages of the telephone directory.

10 **Support groups**. Not only do support groups provide emotional support themselves, but they also provide information concerning where help may be sought for persons who feel a need for professional assistance in dealing with their particular difficulties. Many professionals are members of such groups or members of advisory councils of some groups.

Conclusion

Crises in our lives are times when our coping capabilities are stretched to the limit. Child-bearing difficulties, particularly those of a prolonged nature, can erode our emotional resources. For most, grief will pass in time, for they will receive adequate support. For others, the situation can become serious and outside help is needed. A grieving, depressed person is aware of his/her pain, and would like to make some moves toward preventing it worsening. But many don't know where to begin. In this chapter we have tried to provide some starting points. These are not definite answers. As we pointed out at the beginning of this chapter, all anyone can offer is support and suggestions. The final solution rests with you.

References

1. M.L. Free and Tian P.S. Oei, *Biological and Psychological Processes in the Treatment and Maintenance of Depression*, unpublished Masters thesis (University of Queensland, 1987).
2. A modified relaxation and guided imagery program similar to that employed by many mental-health professionals.
3. L.G. Baruth and C.H. Huber, *Counselling and Psychotherapy: Theoretical Analyses and Skills Applications* (Ohio: C.E. Merrell, 1985), 62–68.
4. Free and Oei, *op.cit.*
5. Erich Lindemann, 'Symptomatology and Management of Acute Grief', *American Journal of Psychiatry*, 101 (1944), 141–148; Beverley Raphael, *Anatomy of Bereavement* (New York: Basic Books, 1983), 59–61.
6. David Maddison and Agnes Viola, 'The Health of Widows in the Year Following Bereavement', *Journal of Psychosomatic Research*, 12 (1968), 297–306.

12 You and Your Religion

During times of crisis, not only are a person's emotional and physical capabilities strained, but so are the spiritual. When human intervention is limited or can no longer provide a solution, we look beyond the mortal to the immortal, the omnipotent, to God, whatever we perceive him to be. People have different cultures and religions, but belief in the existence of an omnipotent one helps us make sense of our lives and the incidents that befall us, thereby giving us direction and hope.

Within this chapter we shall concentrate mainly on Christianity, this being the most common religion of Australia. We shall later mention others in a limited manner. We do not have enough knowledge of their teachings to do them justice, but feel that our discussion of Christian beliefs may be of some relevance to all.

Crisis in our lives can draw us closer to, or drive us away from, God. People who have faced a crisis in which they feel powerless, such as bereavement, terminal illness, and false imprisonment, will testify to a struggle with their faith in a God who seems to allow such things to happen. Difficulty in bearing a child is often such a situation. The affected couple, who seem unable to control these events of their lives, struggle with doubts. No matter how strong a faith persons appear to have, none is immune to grief. The Christian and non-Christian alike grieve their losses. Faith may assist in the final resolution of grief, but it cannot prevent it. The pain and confusion of grief are often expressed in crises of faith during such times.

Crises in your faith

It is often difficult to specify particular faith crises, for most feelings are complex, defying separation of the various elements tied together. What we shall try to do here is make arbitrary

separations, by looking at some of the strong feelings and haunting
questions that couples often experience. We do not profess to be
able to answer these questions or rebuild faith, for the very word
'faith' defies such a task. Faith is a confidence and a secure belief in
someone or something that is not necessarily supported by rational
argument or explanation. Faith is personal, and its maintenance is
often beyond reason.

Why us, God?

From earliest childhood, we are taught that there is a reason for
things that happen to us. A child is chastised because he/she fails
to do as told. (You fell off the swing because you didn't hold on
tightly enough. You failed the exam because you didn't study.)
When things happen to us, we go looking for the reason why. We
look for someone or something to blame. Even if we end up
blaming the wrong thing, achieving an explanation is often more
important than what that explanation is. For example, a failure in
an exam can wrongly be attributed to a teacher who was 'out to
get me' rather than to my lack of study. Blaming the teacher may
make us feel better, even if we are only fooling ourselves.

Generally, most crises in our lives indicate, on reflection, the
cause of the problem. We can blame unemployment on the
economy, or the breakdown of a relationship on our possessiveness
or a partner's unfaithfulness. The solution to many such crises may
lie in learning from our mistakes and taking new positive actions.
By our own effort we can succeed, or so it appears.

But there are other crises in our lives in which the cause is
illusive and the solution does not appear within our control. The
question Why? is not followed by a ready answer. Child-bearing
difficulties may be one such crisis. Suddenly our world is
shattered, and we are unable to find adequate reason. In our anger
and depression of grief, we turn and ask: 'Why us, God? What
did we do to deserve this punishment?' If we had been 'bad', we
could see this as punishment; but when we have tried to be 'good',
it doesn't seem fair, particularly when so many 'bad' people seem
to have so few problems in their lives. Why deprive us of a child
whom we would love, when others sexually or emotionally abuse
their children?

We are not the first to ask Why of God! After her brother
Lazarus had died, Mary went out to meet Jesus, and people asked
why:

> 'Lord', she said, 'if you had been here, my brother would not
> have died!' . . . But some of them said, 'He gave sight to the blind
> man, didn't he? Could he not have kept Lazarus from dying?'
> (John 11:32,37 TEV)

Jesus himself asked in his heart why he must die. He had human
feelings of fear and anguish.

> 'Father', he said, 'if you will, take this cup of suffering away
> from me' . . . In great anguish he prayed even more fervently; his
> sweat was like drops of blood falling to the ground.
> (Luke 22:42,44 TEV)

> My God, my God, why hast thou forsaken me?
> (Matthew 27:46 RSV)

Often the answer to our question does not come immediately,
or it may remain obscure. Rabbi Kushner[1] in his book asks the
question why, and tries to find an answer beyond the usual 'It is
God's will'. He feels that perhaps God, after giving man a free
will and providing the processes of nature, then limits his
intervention in these processes. Others believe that God causes or
allows things to happen to lead us in a new direction according to
a preordained plan. Yet others believe that crises are sent to test
our faith. Many even believe that we have no right to question
God's ways. They believe that his ways are perfect, and
questioning indicates a lack of faith.

Many people will accept one of these explanations, while many
more will still be left wondering and asking, not being fully
satisfied with these answers. Perhaps we mortals who don't find a
clear answer may at least find solace in looking around us. We are
not alone in facing crises. Some suffer more than others, and
religion doesn't seem to be the deciding factor. Religious people
are just as likely to face crises. Faith is not some magic act. If faith
promised that there would be no suffering, only joy, would there
be anyone in the world who would not cash in on such a ticket to
Paradise? Suffering, as death, is no respecter of wealth, religion,
social class, previous suffering, sex, or age. Unfortunately, an
innocent baby can be born with a handicap or can die, while a

psychotic killer can be maintained for a lifetime in perfect health. Life is not fair! But we were *never* promised it would be!

The belief that life is fair is a man-made one, which makes us feel safe and secure in a world that we can therefore understand and control. Perhaps the question: 'Why us, God?' should rather be: 'Well, why not us?' In many situations, we do have some control of events. Yet, in others we don't. This is a fact we must accept. Such acceptance does not mean that we must take a pessimistic view of life. We may not be in control of the outcome of events, but in God we have a powerful friend who makes many promises. One of the most powerful of his promises is that, though at times events seem out of control, they are actually in more powerful and wiser hands than ours.

> Look at the birds of the air: they neither sow nor reap nor gather into barns, and yet your heavenly Father feeds them. Are you not of more value than they? (Matthew 6:26 RSV)

> Bad as you are, you know how to give good things to your children. How much more, then, will the Father in heaven give the Holy Spirit to those who ask him! (Luke 11:13 TEV)

We may never receive a definite answer as to why we experience crises in our lives. This is a fact that human beings must accept. Receiving no answer in a flash of inspiration may frighten us, for then life loses some security. We may lose the security of controlling our lives, and yet we can regain a new security in realizing we have not been and never will be abandoned by God, even in the darkest times. Yet, in the depths of grief we may not be able to accept this. As grief heals and confidence returns, the urgency of the question why diminishes, as the stage of acceptance is reached.

I don't have any faith left! I can't pray!

Faith is not just a feeling; it also involves the intellect and a commitment. Sometimes after a disappointment, when depression is our constant companion, our feelings become blunted. That spiritual 'high' can be replaced by a blandness of feeling, and a person begins to doubt his/her faith. He/she feels anything but content, secure, and uplifted; instead, there is anger and sadness. Faith seems to have disappeared, and prayers become hollow and almost impossible to formulate. For the very devout, this can then lead to guilt for having such feelings: 'I keep telling others in trouble to have faith and pray. But now it's my turn, and look what's happened to me. What kind of Christian am I?' No matter how hard one tries to recapture those feelings of serenity, the feelings of being rejected and deserted remain. This is grief, and this is normal.

In marriage, the honeymoon feeling wears off in time. We no longer feel the exhilaration of being 'in love'. This is frightening for some couples. Yet once the honeymoon is over, the real binding of marriage takes over. This is often a matter of the intellect and will, rather than the emotions. We look carefully at our partner, and clarify in our minds the reasons we love him/her and have married. We see his/her good and bad points more realistically. We then must work at developing the skills of communication, caring, and friendship that keep a marriage alive for a lifetime. Considered actions must be combined with the emotional high of love. At times it is determined commitment alone that keeps a marriage together over the rough patches. Faith is similar to marriage. When the feelings are missing, faith has not disappeared. It just needs to be consciously maintained and affirmed until the feelings return. You don't have to 'feel right' to pray.

Prayer is not only the formal words said while in a reverent position with closed eyes and folded hands. Prayer is conversation with God, and can go on continuously, anywhere and at any time.

Pray without ceasing. (1 Thessalonians 5:17 AV)

Prayer is not always a 'pious', respectful activity. Prayer is also the screaming in depression and desperation. Even the words: 'I can't pray, Lord! I've got no faith left!' is prayer. Another father once used them many years ago as his prayer:

Lord, I believe; help thou mine unbelief. (Mark 9:24 AV)

Prayer is discussing your feelings with God, even when you feel anger and resentment toward him. God is not frightened and upset by our anguish. His word says:

Even if I go through the deepest darkness, I will not be afraid, Lord, for you are with me. (Psalm 23:4 TEV)

Even if the feelings are gone, faith hasn't. God understands. Ritual prayer may be tainted, but the pouring out of the heart in prayer can help to regain that lost dimension.

He will be gentle to those who are weak, and kind to those who are helpless. (Matthew 12:20 TEV)

For we know that in everything God works for good with those who love him, who are called according to his purpose. (Romans 8:28 RSV)

I hate God!

Grief often includes anger, and who better to feel angry at than a God who has let this thing happen? As a child throws a tantrum for a parent who refuses a request, we can feel angry at this God who professes to love us but then deprives us of so important a gift as a child. Job knew those feelings of desertion by a God who was supposed to be loving:

If my troubles and griefs were weighed on scales, they would weigh more than the sands of the sea, so my wild words should not surprise you. Almighty God has pierced me with arrows, and their poison spreads through my body. God has lined up his terrors against me. (Job 6:1-4 TEV)

Couples who experience child-bearing difficulties can understand Job's feelings, and feel anger at a God who has done this to them.

If we do not resolve this anger successfully, our faith can be destroyed, and anger toward God may remain with us all our lives. This may happen when this anger toward God is stifled by our own reactions or those of others. Some fear that their being angry with God may provoke him to do something worse to them than has already occurred, so they suppress their outward anger. Others may discourage anger by saying: 'You mustn't say that!' or 'You don't really mean that'. Yet suppression of anger does not make the feeling go away. We are foolish if we think that, by suppressing it outwardly, we are also hiding it from God. He knows our hearts and minds.

Your Father already knows what you need before you ask him. (Matthew 6:8 TEV)

Anger is a normal emotion, which is only a problem when we deal with it in such a way as to hurt others. Even Christ in the temple among the sellers felt anger. God understands and accepts anger. He can take our outbursts. He'll listen quietly while we scream and protest, and be ready to comfort us when our anger is spent. Often our anger is really not at God, but at the situation; he just 'cops it'.

If it means events like this, I don't think I like the plan God has for my life

Many Christians try to comfort the grieving person with words of consolation such as: 'It's God will' or 'He knows what he's doing. It's part of his plan.' Accepting that your life is mapped out in front of you is comforting when all your dreams are coming true. But when suddenly your dearest dream, around which your whole life may be planned, is shattered, the thought of a preordained plan is frightening. It can be a depressing thought, to which one can simply become resigned without hope. One then develops a fatalistic outlook, and becomes depressed. Life can become viewed as something to be endured rather than enjoyed.

God seems to hold out hope by promising to hear our prayers:

> And so I say to you: Ask, and you will receive; seek, and you will find; knock, and the door will be opened to you. (Luke 11:9 TEV)

He promises to answer prayer. Yet we can still be disappointed if we forget that, although he always answers prayer, there are three possible answers, not one. We hope for only a Yes, forgetting that No and Wait are also answers.[2] In fact, Christ received a firm No in Gethsemene as he asked God if he could be relieved of his impending suffering and death.

At the present time in our lives, without the advantage of hindsight, the way ahead may look dark. Yet we have been given some important promises:

> Trust in the Lord with all your heart. Never rely on what you think you know. Remember the Lord in everything you do, and he will show you the right way. (Proverbs 3:5,6 TEV)

> For I know the plans I have for you, says the Lord, plans for welfare and not for evil, to give you a future and a hope. Then you will call upon me and come and pray to me, and I will hear you. (Jeremiah 29:11,12 RSV)

> God keeps his promise, and he will not allow you to be tested beyond your power to remain firm. (1 Corinthians 10:13 TEV)

Take my yoke and put it on you, and learn from me, because I am gentle and humble in spirit; and you will find rest. For the yoke I will give you is easy, and the load I will put on you is light. (Matthew 11:29,30 TEV)

Is God really all-powerful?

'I asked God to save my baby, and he didn't. If he isn't cruel, maybe he just isn't as powerful as I always believed.' These and similar doubts can creep into the mind of the grieving person. We sometimes see others healed, allegedly through the power of prayer. If God saved them, why can't he change this situation? If he made the world, surely he can unblock my tubes? Did he use up all his power on others?

In wrestling with these questions, the grieving person may react in a number of different ways. If God is all-powerful, perhaps it is possible to make a deal with him. Part of grief can be this bargaining: 'God, if you let me have a child (or let my child live, or heal my child), I'll go to church regularly and give regular offerings to the church for the rest of my life.'

A second reaction involves asking for one's needs in prayer: 'If God isn't all-powerful, then even if I ask, he may not be able to help me next time either.' Persons who think this way may develop a fear of trying again, of being a victim of chance. The Psalmist had such doubts:

'Will the Lord always reject us? Will he never again be pleased with us? Has he stopped loving us? Does his promise no longer stand? Has God forgotten to be merciful? Has anger taken the place of his compassion?' Then I said, 'What hurts me most is this — that God is no longer powerful'. (Psalm 77:8–10 TEV)

Yet God is all-powerful. Jesus reassures us:

With God all things are possible. (Matthew 19:26 RSV)

All authority in heaven and on earth has been given to me. (Matthew 28:18 RSV)

We doubt his power when it does not seem directed toward granting our wishes. Yet at night, when the sun disappears from view, we don't doubt its power. Similarly, God's power still exists in our lives, even when things appear out of control. It may simply be present in a different form. Rather than fulfilling our wishes, his power may be present through his giving us the ability to cope with our pain and to grow as people. The power may be flowing through us to others, as they see how we handle a crisis. Power that is not obvious, such as solar power, can still be among the most potent of all. God's power is not limited; only our vision of it is limited.

Is your God big enough?

Our view of God is often as individual as we are. Yet, our particular view can affect our coping with crises in our faith. If one sees God as an angry or cruel God, then a loss in child-bearing will be seen as punishment for some evil of the past or simply as an act of cruelty. Faith is then based on fear. Such a view leaves us with a faith of little joy. It seems strange that such a cruel God would allow his Son to be given as a sacrifice for mortals for whom he cares so little.

Others see God as a just God, totalling up our good and bad points, and awarding blessings according to our balance sheet. With such a God we may be able to bargain! 'The better or more moral the life I lead, the less chance there is of such a terrible event happening in my life again.'

Yet others see a loving God, a friend who feels pain at their sorrow, and provides comfort. He has provided a promise of resurrection. In such loving hands it is easier to place our lives and the life of a beloved child. However, some see this benevolent God of love as also limited in power. They feel that they must still look for control in the events of their life. They ask for help, yet worry and act impulsively, indicating a deep-seated doubt in his ability to answer their prayer. They themselves must try to gain some control, for to be out of control in a world where God is not fully in control is frightening.

We need to consider: Is our God big enough? Do we want a God who fits into our pocket, to be called on only when needed to perform some magic trick? Do we demand a God over whom we have some control, and who will conform to *our* plan for our lives? Most of us, if we are honest, do want such a God!

This picture of a God who is dependent upon our whims is actually a gross distortion of reality. The real picture is probably more of us, a tiny screaming, sulking, tantrum-throwing little creature, standing and beating away at the ankle of an omnipotent,

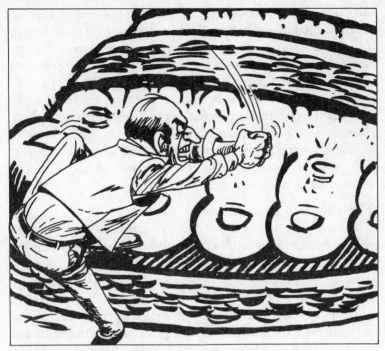

IS YOUR GOD BIG ENOUGH?

huge presence, who with infinite patience and love waits until we exhaust ourselves. When we are at the point of collapse, he stoops down and picks us up, giving us new strength. The view through his eyes then becomes clearer to us than it looked from the depths of our depression. We can see more clearly the future as he has perceived it. Some people call it developing hindsight, being able to find meaning in the seemingly-random past events of our lives. Others see it as a part of the resolution of grief.

To believe in a God who is controlled by man is not comforting when we look around at the mess in the world. It's best if we are able to believe in a God who is in control of us and who loves us, even if we must accept that we may never fully understand his reasoning or his ways.

Is your God big enough?

The hospital chaplain or visitor

The hospital chaplain or visitor often plays a part in the support of the grieving couple early in their grief. His/her role is more obviously noted in cases of death, when couples often seek out religious comfort and funeral rites. In other cases of child-bearing difficulties, couples may seek out the counsel of a member of the clergy or a church elder if depression is weighing upon them heavily. Even couples who are only nominally religious, but who are seeking some solace, may seek out comfort from such people. The reactions of these religious persons are therefore vital. At times, however, the benefits of contact with such people can be dubious. To assume that a person who is educated in matters of religion automatically has at his/her command words of comfort is to court danger.

The chaplain as a person

At times, the hospital chaplain or visitor is expected to deal with people in crisis without having the personal understanding or skills to be successful. As with medical staff, a period of training for a profession does not ensure such skills or understanding. Clergy may still be unsure of their own beliefs, particularly when confronted by people experiencing the crises of faith we have outlined. Many may have been fortunate enough never to have had to face major crises in their own lives and faith. Even their professional contacts with death may have had little impact on them, as they may have been able to keep death and grieving parties at arm's length, so that such persons do not intrude on their personal domain. It can be true that, unless we come face to face with a crisis, we can avoid coming to terms with the issues involved. Where a religious person's life has been maintained on an even keel from Christian home to Christian school to seminary to parish, faith may have been relatively easy to maintain. Such a person may find difficulties in understanding the anger and depression and crises of faith experienced by couples with which they may be confronted. Rather than confront these issues, they may attempt to apply 'first-aid treatment' by retreating to platitudes that supposedly provide automatic support. When the reactions to these platitudes are not favourable, the religious helper can feel threatened.

This is not to deny that a large number of clergy, although they may not have faced major crises themselves, are able, through their deep compassion and sensitivity, to provide immense comfort. To be successful, the chaplain or visitor must be aware of his/her own fears and insecurities about life, himself/herself, and death. The most powerful tool for helpers dealing with grieving persons is a quiet acceptance of themselves and others, their feelings, ideas, and opinions. Combined with this must be a security in the religion they preach, devoid of the need to be able to have all the answers. Another vital component is the development of an ability to communicate in a relaxed friendly manner, combined with a willingness to discuss the whole range of values and beliefs, even those that conflict with their own beliefs or church doctrine. It must be remembered that grieving couples are often questioning couples, whose view of God may be changing and hence can be affected by those they see as representatives of God. A further personal quality of successful chaplains and visitors involves a deeper understanding of what they and others perceive as their role and authority. Clergy, as doctors, are provided by society with a certain status and role. People hold differing expectations of this role. In today's society, the role is changing, and hence the relationship between clergy and laity is changing also. As doctors must recognize and adapt to the expectations of their role as it is perceived by different individuals, so must the clergy.

Finally, the chaplain must also hold honest respect for the individual. Ultimately, the relationship between a person and God is deeply personal. Clergy can guide, but can never force someone to believe a certain way. Even if outward appearances and words seem to indicate a conformity to an acceptable religious pattern, unresolved conflicts that stand between this person and a deeper relationship with God may remain hidden. A conforming flock is of less credit to a clergyman than an honest contented one.

Chaplains are persons first, although this is a fact often forgotten by society. They suffer from the same insecurities and fears as other human beings. Coming to acceptance and understanding of their own needs and motives is the first step for chaplains toward becoming effective in dealing with people in crisis.

Reactions that don't help

Grief, as we have seen, is a mixture of very powerful emotions, involving anger and depression. It is not uncommon for the couple to feel negatively about God and his representatives. Some reactions of clergy or visitors to this grief only serve to make this situation worse. Below are some reactions best avoided.

1. Retreating to clichés and platitudes

In uncomfortable situations, it is often easiest to resort to the common words of comfort:

> It's God's will.
>
> It's all part of God's plan.
>
> He knows what's best for us.
>
> It may really be a blessing in disguise.
>
> Perhaps God's trying to tell you something.
>
> Your baby is God's own little angel now.

If we consider these and other common words of comfort in the light of our knowledge of grief and the faith crises we have discussed, it is not surprising that they generally provide little or no comfort initially. As the grieving couple come to accept their loss, some of these words may have some meaning. Unfortunately, most often they are used initially because the user doesn't know what else to say.

> Sometimes being religious can make it harder, because if you believe in a God and these things keep happening, you ask why he lets it happen or makes it happen. One of the hardest things to cope with is when people say it all happened for some reason.

> I was surprised at how few Christians have really worked out this question of suffering at all. It was quite surprising that the things that people were saying were quite different sometimes. Like 'God doesn't want these sorts of things to happen' and 'God does allow it, but allows it for a purpose'. It's very difficult.

2. Spiritualizing the event before the couple are ready

Pain and suffering are very basic human conditions, eliciting very basic human emotions common to Christian and non-Christian alike. These basic feelings need to be experienced and resolved before the higher intellect and spiritual reasoning can take over. Spiritualizing the event before the couple are ready denies the Christian person the right to human weakness and its honest expression. Christians, too, must feel. Having a faith doesn't destroy the need to feel. Denying the couple the right to feel by trying to make them see the religious aspect of their situation serves only to limit communication and make them feel guilty for their negative feelings, as if they are being 'bad Christians'.

The indiscriminate distributing of tracts and other religious literature is something that must be considered carefully in the initial stages. Many grieving people have taken such tracts and angrily thrown them into the bin after the clergyman has left. Such literature may be seen by the couple as having religion forced on them before they are ready. Literature should be given only when it is appropriate in the context of a deepening relationship between the couple and the chaplain or visitor.

3. Being shocked

Grieving people and those facing crises in their faith often have many confusing thoughts and emotions to deal with. Expressing this confusion can often be the first step in resolving it. Some ideas may sound irreligious and frightening to clergy, who may see them as a challenge to their faith, or an indication that the grieving person is losing his/her faith. Sometimes anger may be expressed: 'I hate God.' 'There is no God of love if he lets this happen.' 'Why be a Christian? It's only meant sadness and deprivation to me. Non-Christians seem to get by all right.' Instead of seeing such statements within the context of grief, some clergy are shocked, and react in panic. They deny the thoughts rather than discuss them.

You don't really mean that, do you?

You mustn't say that!

You know that's not true.

You mustn't feel that way.

Such responses may be met with more anger: 'Yes, I do mean it! I know what I feel!' The anger of grief may then be directed at the chaplain or visitor. It is vital that clergy be comfortable with expressions of anger and confusion.

4. Being uncomfortable

At times the chaplain or visitor must enter the situation feeling inadequate, awkward, and shy. If he/she is uncomfortable with crying or other outward shows of emotions, the job is made even more difficult. Some chaplains enter a room unsure of what to say, yet uncomfortable with silence. A tense atmosphere is created, with both the visitor and patient being lost for words. The grieving person may then feel that he/she has to 'entertain' the chaplain, when it was he/she who sought comfort.

> I had a visitor from the church I go to. She was pretty hopeless. She was an oldish lady, but I don't think she'd had much experience with people who had lost their babies, because she came in and she was surprised not to see the baby. I did get to say that the baby had died, and she quickly changed the subject and talked about this and that and then made a quick exit, which I thought pretty shocking. I thought I deserved more sympathy than that.

The chaplain, who is not at this time experiencing the crisis, may need to take the initiative by seeking out from the grieving person in what direction he/she would like to proceed. The chaplain may have to encourage the person to talk, but must be sensitive to discover the needs of the grieving person. A comfortable acceptance of silence and tears is vital.

5. Pushing religion

At times, a couple may seek out the clergy during a time of crisis, even when their religious practices have otherwise waned. This should not then be used as an opportunity to 'return them to the fold'. Some people, in resolving their grief with the support of clergy, may actually return of their own will. Others may not, and this must be accepted. Trying to push a couple to return to religion or a particular denomination during their time of crisis, while at the same time failing to fulfil the couple's basic present needs of caring and understanding, may drive them further away rather than bring them closer to that goal.

6. Appearing aloof

Sometimes, as a means of protecting themselves from deep involvements, clergy and others remain detached and aloof from the person in crisis. For others, the aloofness comes from the way they see their role as a dignified, controlled, authoritative messenger of God. At a time when their self-esteem is often at a very low ebb, grieving parents are more likely to see this aloofness as a rejection of themselves.

Being of help

Clergy, just like others, can be an important source of support for the grieving couple. In fact, they can provide an extra dimension, the spiritual one, that others may be unable or unwilling to call on.

1. Learn about grief

Knowing about grief and grieving can prevent the chaplain from making obvious mistakes. Such knowledge gives an insight into what feelings and thoughts the couple may have. Not all experience the same problems or have the same feelings, but knowledge and sensitivity can still provide the chaplain with a good place to start in understanding the couple.

2. Listen

The greatest act of love is often the willingness to listen. The grieving person generally needs and wants to talk. Being ready to listen without advising, lecturing, or preaching can provide immense comfort and support. Simply being there, willing and interested, can mean a great deal.

3. See the person as a broken heart before a soul to be saved

Respond as one human being to another, rather than as spiritual shepherd to sheep. Accepting one's own weaknesses and those of others allows one to see the person before the soul. Clergy need to respond to their own feelings and the human reactions of the grieving couple. If they feel that body contact, such as a hug or a hand-squeeze, is appropriate and will deepen the closeness, they should use it. Christ himself responded to the needs of people to be loved before he tried to change their lives. He showed that he loved Mary Magdalene and other afflicted persons by first responding to their humanness, and then giving them food for their soul.

4. Be honest

Being a spiritual leader does not mean having all the answers. Clergy are human beings first. They feel awkward, sad, and depressed for the couple, and are unable to explain fully the mind of God. They must be honest. The grieving couple will not feel less secure because the clergy cannot answer all their queries, or

admit to feeling uneasy or inadequate. They are more likely to
appreciate this display of humanness.

5. Maintain a confidence in your belief

There is a clear but delicate distinction between 'pushing'
religion at people and maintaining a confidence in what you
believe. People in crisis often seek a secure rock to lean on. You
don't need to have all the answers to be able to maintain a
confidence in the basic goodness of God. The grieving couple
don't need the chaplain to adopt their feelings of desolation; they
need him to accept these feelings and share them, and yet maintain
hope and optimism. A person facing a crisis in faith has not
necessarily lost that faith. It is clouded, and needs support from
one whose faith is, at this time at least, steady and secure. Clergy
mustn't force religion on a grieving couple, but neither must they
apologize for their beliefs. Neither approach will help the person
in crisis.

6. Provide rituals and symbols of comfort where appropriate

Oftentimes a simple meaningful act can provide more support
than all the words of wisdom or comfort. Rituals and symbols
don't replace words, but can enhance the words and their
meaning. Religious rituals formalize the church's acceptance of the
seriousness of the situation. Some churches are now recognizing
this, and providing rituals to recognize miscarriage and premature
birth, as well as the death of an infant.

As Kate lay dying, Pastor Renner stood with us beside her
humidicrib in the ICN. As she weakened, at intervals he gave her
the sign of the cross on her head and on her breast, while
commending her to God. He continued with this until she died.
This was very comforting for us. It seemed that we were handing
her from our arms directly across to God.

7. Organize outside support where appropriate

The congregation may include members who have experienced
the pain of a similar situation and the resulting crises of faith.
Clergy do not have to be the sole spiritual support of a
congregation. The clergyman who can draw on the spiritual and
practical resources of a congregation can provide grieving couples

with a much broader network of support that can help in their time of crisis.

What if only one partner is religious?

It is not uncommon for only one partner of the grieving couple to have religious beliefs. This can create difficulties for the couple and for the chaplain who is trying to help them. If the non-religious partner is an accepting person, there may be no real problems. If the partner is hostile, the chaplain must deal with this hostility as well as the reactions and needs of the religious partner. The chaplain must find the fine balance that involves showing acceptance of both partners combined with providing the spiritual support for one. Appearing human and approachable is of vital importance. Listening and caring for a person first can forge a bond between chaplain and individual partners. Being seen as a friend can smooth a great deal of rough water.

> I was really worried when the chaplain came in. I didn't know him. Jim was there, and he doesn't believe. In fact, he really finds it difficult to take clergy. Yet the chaplain came in and just sat and talked about the baby and both of us. He didn't talk religion at all. He was a real person. Soon Jim was talking to him like an old friend. We both cried with him. We'll always appreciate it, particularly me, because later when Jim went, this chaplain came back to see me alone and we talked about how I was feeling about God.

There is no need for chaplains to deny who they are or what they believe in the hope of winning over the non-religious partner. Showing acceptance of him/her will gain more respect than 'playing up' to him/her. The spiritual needs of one must be served, but in such a way as to encourage dialogue between partners rather than drive a wedge between them.

The church and child-bearing

It is dangerous to generalize and talk about 'the church' as if it were a homogeneous group of people and clergy, who believe, think, speak, and react in exactly the same way. Each individual Christian, congregation, and clergy member has unique views, values, beliefs, experiences, and, more importantly, a unique relationship with God. We do not discount this! In discussing 'the church', we are looking more at the establishment called the church as it is viewed by many of the laity and non-believers. Therefore we do not wish our comments to be taken as referring to all who constitute the church; we would prefer the reader to consider our comments open-mindedly rather than defensively.

The church as the family of God

As is the case with society in general, the church places a strong emphasis on the family. It views itself as the family of God, in which Christians are his children. Consider also the emphasis of many churches on the nuclear family, with Family Days, Family Services, Mothers' Unions, Sunday-school, and similar activities. The family is truly an important institution of society, in fact, its basic unit. But have we carefully considered those who are not a family, but would very much like to be one? We refer here particularly to those who through infertility or repeated losses are unable to produce a child of their own, as well as to reluctantly-single people. In many instances, their pain and disappointment can be heightened by a certain sense of isolation from a church in which being a family is recognized as a desirable, accepted goal.

Of course, many will rightly argue that a family is not confined to two parents and their children, and that we are all essentially a human or congregational family. But a couple who face difficulty in bearing a child are generally not ready to see a wider definition, and can often feel isolated from an institution which values highly something they cannot achieve.

Some wedding ceremonies contain prayers for the blessing of children. Later, when a young couple are faced with the possibility of not having children, they may wonder whether they were 'unworthy' of such a blessing. Before a couple have even had the chance to become 'one', we are placing a heavy performance burden on them. A marriage without children is not generally considered a family. In some denominations, the importance of the family is further entrenched with an emphasis on motherood. The Virgin Mary as the Mother of God is a central figure. For many, motherhood has become an idealized state. The statues of the serene Virgin holding and looking lovingly on the baby Jesus can place further subtle strain on the woman who desperately wants to become a mother, but has no success in this area. Many may be unable to see how the church's emphasis on the family could cause distress to a grieving couple, but it must be remembered that these couples suffer from a low self-esteem and a preoccupation with their loss. This is normal.

We do not suggest that the church deny its emphasis on the family. Rather, the church may also have to increase its emphasis on accepting individuals as integral, equal parts of the church in whatever social situation they find themselves — as a single, as part of a couple, or as a family. The family has been highlighted for centuries. Perhaps single people and lone couples must now also be highlighted.

The church's stand on abortion, and the influence of this on child-bearing difficulties

The church in general has been at the forefront of the opposition to abortion on demand. We do not wish to attempt to debate this issue. We only wish to highlight the seeming discrepancy between such a firm stance and the seeming lack of ability to provide real comfort for couples who lose a beloved child through spontaneous abortion.

Many women experience intense guilt upon losing a child through miscarriage. Some search desperately for something they did that may have caused the loss. Others blame some initial ambivalent feelings about the pregnancy for its loss. They wonder if they, although unintentionally, caused the death of their child. Although these beliefs are unfounded, the silence of the church on their plight seems only to heighten their pain. They see that the church fights to save life through an anti-abortion stance, and yet unfortunately it seems to deny this life's very importance by slighting the severity of its loss in miscarriage.

We are pleased to report that many churches are now recognizing this gap in their rituals. Some very beautiful and appropriate orders are being introduced to provide recognition and comfort for those couples who lose a child through miscarriage or at later stages of pregnancy.[3] The church argues that life begins at conception, and hence abortion is murder. It would be hypocritical, with these views, to further fail to recognize and provide support for those who have to face the loss of a child any time after conception.

The church must also face the new issues that are raised as medical science advances. With tests now able to recognize some of the very severe abnormalities in a foetus early in pregnancy, the issue of the induced abortion of such affected babies must be considered. Similarly, the *in vitro* fertilization techniques have introduced many areas for debate within the church. A hard-line stance on such issues by the church is unlikely to see a decline in the use of these procedures by affected couples. Both the issue itself and the grieving couple must be considered as the church struggles to resolve these and the new issues that the future will raise.

The church and its comfort of rituals

The church can play an important role in the areas of baptism and supervision of the final committal of the foetus. Most churches are united in the belief in the importance of emergency baptism for a child born alive but with slim hope of survival. Chaplains, doctors, or nurses will often baptize such babies immediately.

Even many apparent 'non-believers' are comforted by such an action for their child.

When the child is stillborn, the situation is somewhat different. However, here too the church can help the couple by offering a ritual that may provide them with some comfort, particularly when it expresses faith in God and a recognition of the brief life of the child whom he gave.

To further alleviate the pain of many couples who in the future may experience miscarriage or stillbirth, the use of a small ritual of commitment of the child to God when the pregnancy is initially confirmed may provide some sense of relief. This may be of particular significance for couples who experience repeated losses and who embark precariously on each new pregnancy.

Perhaps one area in which the church could provide further support for couples who lose through miscarriage is in the supervision of the final committal of the foetus. If the church recognizes the beginning of life at conception, and the couple also recognize that life, it can be important for the sake of all and as an affirmation of the sanctity of life itself that the church is involved in the final committal of the foetus. For babies born at 20 weeks' gestation and beyond, the law stipulates that appropriate procedures for cremation or burial must be followed. Here the church can provide the rites of a funeral as well.

When a foetus is spontaneously aborted before this time, such final committal procedures have generally not been employed. Although hospital staff usually dispose of the foetus as best they can, it is difficult for a grieving couple to accept that their child was simply disposed of as would be other pieces of tissue. Even when a couple realize that the staff did not simply throw it away as rubbish, it is difficult to accept calmly an unsupervised final committal. Often, many couples won't even think about what happened to their baby until some time later, when the realization of the disposal is difficult.

> One day after the miscarriage I suddenly thought about what had happened to my baby. I asked a nurse friend. She told me that I shouldn't worry about it. I pressed her, and she said that most tissue removed during an operation was burnt in the hospital incinerator. But she said that I shouldn't think that's what happened to my baby; she didn't really know. I know I put her on the spot. It really threw me. I used to drive past the hospital and see the chimney and burst into tears. Even now, six years later, I feel uncomfortable if I see that chimney.

Where it is in accordance with the parents' wishes, the church may be able to provide a more appropriate committal of this child to God, and to supervise its final resting in a dignified manner. Such a procedure then distinguishes this tissue as the body of a lost, beloved child, as opposed to other bodily tissue. We realize that such a procedure may be unpleasant for the clergyman concerned, but the benefits to the couple he is to comfort, and his knowledge that he has contributed meaningfully to the world's view of the sanctity of life, should more than compensate for unpleasantness.

Our son who was lost at 18 weeks was not afforded this type of dignity. Our daughter Kate received a very special and meaningful treatment at her death, which serves to make her death easier to bear. We feel a sense of unresolved loss that we could not even give our son some semblance of a dignified, meaningful farewell. We have decided that if we are ever faced with a similar situation again, we will request such a supervision. Perhaps the church may be able to offer such a service, so that in the future, couples who are unable to think clearly at the time and who see their relationship with God as important, are not later left haunted by the lack of knowledge about the fate of their child's body. Try to tell a couple who lose a child at 17, 18, or 19 weeks that their child, due to a lack of two or three weeks, loses the status of a person and becomes 'only a foetus', and then not provide any security or dignity surrounding the final committal of their child, and you will serve to heighten their pain.

We encourage couples to ask for the type of committal they desire for their child. This is of particular importance for couples who suffer repeated losses. Couples suffering a first loss are generally unaware of the importance and the availability of a dignified committal of their child who is not fully recognized by society. Therefore, hospital staff and clergy may need to offer the couple a variety of options, which they can choose to accept or reject. Couples facing repeated losses, who have decided what they would wish as a final committal for their children, must never be made to feel embarrassed in making requests to clergy for particular rituals. The role of the clergy is to support, guide, and comfort, not to judge or feel embarrassed themselves.

The church and coping with the situation

Thankfully, the concerns of this book involve only a minority of couples. Hence, they remain the exception to the rule. Society in general does not cope well with crises, and the church, as part of that society, may not cope significantly better. Many church members and clergy have never confronted a similar situation. Many have also never thought very deeply about death and loss, let alone infertility and premature labour. When, in addition, we consider that there are very few women clergy, who have inside knowledge of the female's feelings in general, we can see that difficulties may arise.

Many individual clergy, through their own similar experience, some other pain in their lives, or an uncommonly acute sensitivity to others, are able to relate to the kind of couples we are discussing here. Unfortunately, there are many others who are unable to do so appropriately. In general, there is little, if any, discussion on any of these subjects within the seminaries or the churches. Yet we expect the clergy to have the right words at the right time.

It may seem as if we have been putting forward a rather negative view of the church, but this is not our intention. We are simply discussing some issues which affect couples experiencing child-bearing difficulties and which may be addressed by the church.

Many couples have found their faith and the support of the church sources of great comfort:

> No matter how lax you are about your religion, at that stage, without that, I just could not have coped. It was just there to give us that extra strength. I felt that I knew where the baby was going, and that we had to accept the fact that it was for a reason, and in the long term it was the best thing. It was comforting to think there is somebody up there who knows better and who wants him more than we do, and that's it. He's going to have him.

In fact, many couples who have a Christian faith feel that they have a distinct advantage over others who do not have such a security. Many churches and clergy are equipped (or are seeking to equip themselves) with the skills for helping individuals in crisis, whether they be Christians or non-believers. A church willing to recognize and discuss issues involved in life crises is a living, thriving institution, and one that is reflecting the concern for individual pain expressed by Jesus Christ himself.

Although we have confined our discussion so far to the beliefs that embody Christianity, child-bearing difficulties do not similarly confine themselves. They strike peoples of all faiths. However, it would be unrealistic for us to attempt to treat adequately in a few short paragraphs the beliefs of the world's other major religions as they affect couples experiencing child-bearing difficulties. Whole books would be necessary to do justice to this subject. Hence, we apologize for the brevity of the following sections, outlining the general religious influences on couples who are followers of four other major religions: Judaism, Islam, Hinduism, and Buddhism. This brief treatment only intends to show how differences in religious beliefs may affect couples in their grief, and to encourage those who deal with couples who follow different religions to seek out information about their beliefs.

Our thanks is extended to Dr N. Ross Reat, Lecturer, Department of Studies in Religion, University of Queensland,

and to Pastor Paul Renner, whose knowledge provided the basis of these paragraphs.

A Jewish perspective

Jews believe that they, as the children of Abraham, have a special relationship with God, the creator, the originator, and Father. They believe that God is committed to a caring for them and mercy toward them. They in turn are committed to loyalty and obedience to him. The law is seen as God's prescription for human conduct.

Jews have a high degree of trust in God and his steadfast love. Such love may at times be manifest in discipline and chastisement for the benefit of a person. Hence, suffering and misfortune are under the control of the Father; he has the capacity to shape benefit from them. This deep faith in the mercy and love of God should override the feelings of guilt and rejection a Jew may experience when he or she deviates from God's ways.

The Jewish couple experiencing child-bearing difficulties may be comforted in their grief by their belief in God's ability to turn suffering into benefit for the children of Abraham. Although there is a wide variety of beliefs accommodated within the practice of Judaism, there is a solidarity of belief in the Jews' special relationship with God that provides the events of life with meaning and resolution. Jews are often further sustained and comforted by the affirmation of this belief inherent in their rituals.

An Islamic perspective

Muslims believe in a single supreme deity, known as Allah, who is all-powerful, just, and merciful. The followers of Islam believe that Allah has reasons for all events that occur in our lives. Each of us is subject to Allah's justice, and is the beneficiary of his benevolence in the fullness of time. Islamic couples experiencing child-bearing difficulties would, in all likelihood, see such events as the will of Allah, which is not to be questioned. Allah determines all events, and his will is irresistible. The Islamic couple may pray to Allah, yet they recognize that no supplication can alter Allah's divine plan.

Followers of Islam generally believe that death is a dormant state in which we all remain until the end of time, at which moment the faithful will be resurrected to be with Allah in the Garden of Paradise. The death of a child, then, holds the promise of later life with Allah for that child. Malformation or retardation, rather than a curse, may be seen as an indication that Allah has ordained for the child spiritual rather than mundane blessings.

A Muslim couple, through submission to the will of Allah, may be able to accept their loss as part of a divine plan ordained by a just and merciful God.

A Hindu perspective

Hinduism is an extremely diverse religion, composed of many subgroups, each of which tolerate the beliefs of other forms of Hinduism. Therefore, it is impossible to attempt to delineate the beliefs of the religion as if it were a universal whole. However, the doctrine of karma and rebirth is common to all Hindus, and constitutes the basic perspective from which a Hindu couple would view their loss. Hindus believe that all life is intrinsically bound together in a universal movement. Each voluntary action (karma) has results that will accrue in this life or in a future life. This process is mechanical. The inevitable results of good and bad actions are encoded in the very fabric of the universe. No deity controls this process. Hence, a Hindu is less likely to feel that he/she is being punished by a personal moral agent. Instead, misfortune is viewed as the inevitable consequence of actions in this or a previous life. Rather than feeling judged and punished, the Hindu couple may ask the question: What might I have done to have caused this? The question is not self-accusatory, but one of seeking out one's moral responsibility in this present life and situation.

Death or malformation of a baby may then be seen as resulting from past actions on the part of the mother, the father, or both. The Hindu couple may be comforted in the belief that their dead or malformed child has paid off an outstanding debt to the universe and may enjoy a very productive and pleasant afterlife.

A Buddhist perspective

The followers of Buddhism share with the followers of Hinduism the doctrine of the karma and rebirth, with the attendant concept of inevitable moral responsibility. Buddhism is based on the conviction that human life is inherently unsatisfactory. There is always disappointment and suffering because everything is impermanent, including ourselves. Inevitably, the world changes, and we change. Hence, there is no stability or abiding happiness. In the Buddhist couple's crisis of child-bearing, this suffering and impermanence are manifested. The crisis confirms and illustrates the essence of Buddhist doctrine. Suffering is a universal phenomenon, and the individual suffering of such couples may be lessened by contemplation. Such contemplation is seen as the most worthy of all human actions, and the only way to transcend this painful existence by realizing spiritual enlightenment.

References

1. Harold S. Kushner, *When Bad Things Happen to Good People* (London and Sydney: Pan Books, 1981).
2. Harold Lindsell, *When You Pray* (Michigan: Baker Book House, 1969), 77–82.
3. Peter Gagen, 'That You May Have Life: A Baptismal Resource', *Liturgy News* (Bulletin of the Liturgical Commission of the Archdiocese of Brisbane, Queensland, 14(2), April-June, 1984).

13 A Final Word: Suffering

For a couple who dearly want a child, the time of child-bearing difficulties is indeed a period of intense suffering. To suffer is defined as being subjected to pain or defeat or change. Child-bearing difficulties involve all three. The defeat involved in failing to attain the dream of a mature, live child, unaffected by handicap, causes real emotional pain. For many, the prospect of changes in their lives that may divert them from the idealized plan they had of their future, is difficult to contemplate.

Suffering is not new or unique to these couples. Suffering is part of the human condition. Suffering comprises the low points in our lives, which provide a point of comparison for the high points. If our whole lives were filled only with happiness we would become apathetic. What would we have to look forward to? How would we learn gratitude? Perhaps these questions may sound flippant or overly philosophical, but they are not meant to sound this way. Such insights come out of a recognition and acceptance of the changes and growth that have occurred in our own lives and those of others. Suffering has an aspect that is missing from times of happiness. Suffering forces us to accept changes and adapt to these changes. For some, the changes will be too much, and they become bitter and afflicted for life. Suffering has defeated them. This is a sad defeat, but it does not make these persons any less deserving of respect than others who are not defeated. The former's life experiences have generally not equipped them for the fight back from defeat.

For those able to triumph over suffering, there is growth as persons. Most have triumphed, not by reversing the condition that caused their suffering, but rather by modifying their thoughts and attitudes to make the changes work for them. Rather than use emotional energy in prolonged bitterness that is eventually self-destructive, they use this energy to forge new trails toward self-fulfilment.

Many become involved in helping others similarly affected. A new sensitivity to the feelings and needs of others is often noted in those who have suffered. They also experience new feelings of closeness to family, friends, and strangers who have been able to provide meaningful support during the couple's time of crisis. Many believe that they have developed a deeper sense of the meaning of life, and hence a sense of contentment. By being able to accept the precarious balance of life and death, and realizing the often irrational nature of the unfolding of life's events, many couples find greater, not less, peace with life. They surrender the notion that life must be fair, controllable, and predictable. They stop trying to force it to be so. In doing this, they find confidence in realizing that they found the necessary strength to cope with one crisis and will be able to do so in the future if need be.

The ability to triumph over, and gain from, suffering is not something that can be bestowed on one as a gift. It involves hard work on the part of each individual. It is not a condition one would choose voluntarily! It is part of life for all! Whether suffering comes in child-bearing difficulties, loneliness, illness, unemployment, or other circumstance, it is common to all. Suffering that may be dealt with successfully by one person may cause extreme pain to another. Yet what may seem minor or trivial to the former, is still suffering to the latter. To accept it and deal with it is vital in the triumph over suffering. This book has aimed to assist couples experiencing child-bearing difficulties to do this. If the words have not eased tension in supplying information, then at least we hope that the feelings of support we and others have felt for such couples are apparent.

To those professionals and other interested persons who have read this book, we thank you for your interests, concern, and desire to help couples in crisis. To those couples who, like us, have known, are experiencing, or have yet to experience the pain of these type of losses, we pray that time will ease your pain and that you will find the support and strength to triumph over your particular trying circumstances.

Support Groups
of Australia

This section contains a list of *some* of the support groups of Australia which are concerned with the problems of persons experiencing child-bearing difficulties. The groups included here have given their permission to include these details. A few points should be noted:

a) If a support group concerned with your particular need is not mentioned, assistance may be available from the groups that are mentioned. They may have information on groups in your State or area, or may serve your needs themselves.

b) In many cases, support groups for the Northern Territory are under the umbrella of associated South Australian groups. Similarly, Australian Capital Territory groups are often included in New South Wales associations.

c) The social workers of major maternity hospitals will generally have information on these and other groups. Such persons will be only too willing to provide such information.

d) Parents of children with rare congenital problems may not have the advantage of a separate support group. Such parents would be happily embraced by other support groups concerned with congenital abnormalities. Although the abnormality may differ, the practical problems, fears, and insecurities may be very similar.

e) Often, miscarriage support is provided by groups concerned with the death of a child.

f) Smaller groups affiliated with the ones mentioned here are often found throughout the whole of a State. The central group mentioned here will be able to provide information concerning any such groups in your area.

Infertility

Qld: Friends of the Queensland Fertility Group, c/- PO Graceville East, Q 4075 — Susan: (07) 374 2058.

WA: Concern for the Infertile Couple, PO Box 412, Subiaco, WA 6008 — (09) 381 9313, or
c/- 13 Clive Road, Mt Lawley, WA 6050 — Margaret: (09) 272 7491.

SA: Oasis Infertility Support Incorporated, c/- 11 Michael Street, Lockleys, SA 5032 — (08) 43 3886.

Vic: Concern for the Infertile and Childless, PO Box 125, Vermont, Vic 3133 — Wendy and Ron (03) 598 4724.

IVF Friends, GPO Box 482G Melbourne, Vic 3001 (Connected with Monash University/Queen Victoria Medical Centre/Epworth Hospital IVF Program).

The Victoria Endometriosis Association, c/- Lorraine Henderson, 37 Andrew Crescent, South Croydon, Vic 3136 — (03) 879 1276.

Pivot Auxiliary, c/- Reproductive Biology Unit, Royal Women's Hospital, 132 Grattan Street, Carlton, Vic 3053 — (03) 344 1243.

Tas: Encompass: Caring for the Infertile, c/- Dept of Gynaecology and Obstetrics, Queen Alexander Hospital, Argyle Street, Hobart, Tas 7000.

NSW: Concern NSW, PO Box 108, Milsons Point, NSW 2061 — Lindsey (02) 90 3063.

Combined NSW IVF Support Groups, PO Box 69, Round Corner, NSW 2158.

Hope Support Group, PO Box 520, Miranda, NSW 2228 — Kathy 520 7861 (Connected with St George IVF program at Kogarah).

Hunter Invitro (HI) Support Group, PO Box 462, Raymond Terrace, NSW 2324, or D.P. and S. Milne, PO Box 455, Raymond Terrace, NSW 2324 — (049) 87 1607 (Connected with Lingard Hospital IVF program).

IVF Friends (Sydney), PO Box 69, Round Corner, NSW 2158.

Westmead Invitro Self Help (WISH), PO Box 506, Pennant Hills, NSW 2120.

ACT: Concern (ACT), c/- C. and L. O'Keefe, 44 Mackay Crescent, Kambah, ACT 2902 — (062) 31 7860.

Prematurity

Qld: Preterm Infants' Parents' Association (Inc.) (PIPA),
c/- Mrs Judy Wintour, 9 Heathfield Street, Eight Mile Plains, Q 4123 — (07) 341 4856.

Preterm Infants' Parents' Association (Gold Coast), PO Box 5368, Gold Coast Mail Centre, Q 4217.

SA.: Parents of Preterm Infants Association (POPI), PO Box 63, Unley, SA 5061.

Vic: Lightweight Club, PO Box 255, North Mulgrave, Vic 3170.

Prem Support Group of Victoria, c/- Pauline Scrivin, 456 Mountain Highway, Wanterna, Vic 3152.

NSW: Neonatal Intensive Care and Preterm Parents' Association (NIPPA), 161 Lancia Drive, Ingleburn, NSW 2565.

Death (and Miscarriage)

Qld: Pregnancy Loss Support Group, PO Box 771, Milton, Q 4064.
Queensland Sudden Infant Death Research Foundation, GPO Box 1987, Brisbane, Q 4001.
Stillbirth and Neonatal Death Support Group (Inc.) (SANDS)
Brisbane: PO Box 708, South Brisbane,Q 4101.
Toowoomba: c/- Janet Rankin, 2 Lawrence Street, Toowoomba, Q 4350.
South Burnett: c/- Mrs Bev Coutts, 220 Haly Street, Kingaroy, Q — (071) 62 1214.
The Compassionate Friends, c/- Pat Weston (07) 350 2811, or c/- 11 Woodridge Street, Moorooka, Q 4105 —(07) 848 1764.

NT: Loss of Baby Support Group, c/- Childbirth Education Association, 1st Floor, Monteray House, Trower Road, Casuarina, NT 5792 — (089) 27 2575, or
PO Box 42162, Casuarina, NT 5792.
Sudden Infant Death Syndrome Network of the Northern Territory, c/- Miss Debbie Gardiner, PO Box 41482, Casuarina, NT 5792 — (089) 27 5611, or
c/- Mrs Sandra Bond, 5 Amsterdam Court, Wagaman, NT 5792 — (089) 27 8460
(Connected with Bereavement Support Group in Alice Springs).

WA: Stillbirth and Neonatal Death Support Group (WA) (SANDS), Agnes Walsh House, King Edward Memorial Hospital, Bagot Road, Subiaco, WA 6008 —(09) 380 4444.
The Compassionate Friends (Perth Chapter, WA), c/- 45 Todd Avenue, Como, 6152 — (09) 474 1060.
Sudden Infant Death Syndrome Foundation, PO Box 119, Inglewood, WA 6052 — (09) 291 8625.

SA: Stillbirth and Neonatal Death Support Group (SANDS), Parkside House, 109 Young Street, Parkside, SA 5063 — (08) 272 2026, or
(08) 274 1371 (Bronnie), or
(08) 258 8102 (Dianne).
Sudden Infant Death Syndrome Association of South Australia Inc., 2 Wickes Avenue, Campbelltown, SA 5074 — 336 8727.

Vic: Bairnsdale and District Parent Support Group for the Loss of a Child — Stillbirth, Neonatal and Cot Deaths, c/- Mrs Sylvia van den Born, 11 Clara Street, Lakes Entrance, Vic 3909 —
Bairnsdale (051) 56 8387, 52 5676, 52 4760;
Lakes Entrance (051) 55 2504.
Nurture (Gippsland area), c/- Mrs Denise McLure, 14 Brolga Boulevard, Traralgon, Vic 3844 —(051) 74 7112.
Stillbirth and Neonatal Death Support Inc. (SANDS), 27 Sheabrooke Avenue, South Oakleigh, Vic 3167 —(03) 570 2596.
Sudden Infant Death Research Foundation, 2 Barkly Avenue, Malvern, Vic 3144 — (03) 509 7722.

Tas: Stillbirth and Neonatal Death Support (SANDS), North West Group — 3 Wiena Crescent, Devonport, Tas 7310 — (004) 24 7949; 35 4435.

Southern Group — PO Box 120, North Hobart, Tas 7000 (002) 34 5157; 72 6444.

Tasmanian Sudden Infant Death Society Inc., PO Box 370, Hobart, Tas 7000; PO Box 1380, Launceston, Tas 7250.

Unexpected Outcomes Group, c/- Marilyn Jordan, 11 Cormiston Road, North Riverside, Launceston, Tas 7250.

NSW: Stillbirth and Neonatal Death Support (SANDS), c/- Pat Berchtold, 11 Narelle Street, North Epping, NSW 2121 — (02) 869 1431.

Sudden Infant Death Association NSW (SIDA), Building 10A, 92 Seven Hills Road, Baulkham Hills, Sydney, NSW 2153;

PO Box 172, St Ives, 2075 — (02) 639 5343 (Regional branches in Ballina, Casino, Central Coast, Narrabri, Newcastle, New England, Coffs Harbour, Nowra, Parkes, Scone and Wollongong); Newcastle: PO Box 395, Charlestown, NSW 2290 —(049) 46 9392.

ACT: Stillbirth, Miscarriage and Neonatal Death Association of the ACT (SMANDA), c/- 14 Reibey Place, Curtin, ACT 2605.

Sudden Infant Death Association (ACT) Inc. (SIDA), c/- Social Worker, Royal Canberra Hospital —(062) 43 2425, or

PO Box 58, Jamison, ACT 2614.

National Organization:

The Compassionate Friends, Bereaved Parents Support and Information Centre, Rear 205 Blackburn Road, Syndal, Vic 3149 — (03) 232 8222.

Congenital abnormalities
Physically disabled

Qld: Spina Bifida Association of Queensland Incorporated, 387 Old Cleveland Road, Coorparoo, Q 4151, or

PO Box 245, Coorparoo, Q 4151 — (07) 394 3822.

The North Queensland Society for Crippled Children, c/- The Chief Executive Officer, Corner Warburton and Landsborough Streets, North Ward, Townsville, Q 4810 — (077) 72 1460.

The Queensland Society for Crippled Children, Montrose Home, 54 Consort Street, Corinda, Q 4075, or

PO Box 50, Corinda, Q 4075 — (07) 397 9200

(The Society has no affiliations with other organizations in Queensland or interstate).

The Queensland Spastic Welfare League, c/- The Coordinator Childrens Services, PO Box 386, Fortitude Valley, Q 4006, or Oxlade Drive, New Farm, Brisbane, Q 4005 —(07) 358 3011.

NT: Northern Territory Spastics Association (Inc.), PO Box 41066, Casuarina, NT 5792 — (089) 27 1166.

WA: a) Muscular Dystrophy Research Association of Western Australia Incorporated.
b) The Neuromuscular Foundation Incorporated.
Both of the above are found at: The Neuromuscular Research Institute, 4th Floor, 'A' Block, Verdun Street, Nedlands, WA 6009, or
PO Box 328, West Perth, WA 6005 — (09) 382 2067; (09) 382 2700
(Sister Margaret Mears of the Royal Perth Hospital Department of Neuropathology provides liaison between affected persons and agencies of assistance).
The Spastic Welfare Association of Western Australia Incorporated, c/- Mrs Carla Baron, Clinical Services Manager, PO Box 61, Mt Lawley, WA 6005, or
106 Bradford Street, Coobinia, WA — (09) 443 0211.
The Spina Bifida Association of Western Australia Incorporated, PO Box 159, Wembley, WA 6014, or
364 Cambridge Street, Wembley, WA — (09) 387 3431 on Thursdays only.
The Western Australian Society for Crippled Children Incorporated, 60 McCabe Street, Mosman Park, WA 6012, or
PO Box 53, Mosman Park, WA 6012 —(09) 384 1855.

Vic: The Osteogenesis Imperfecta Foundation, Rear 606 Canterbury Road, Vermont, Vic 3133, or
PO Box 34, Vermont, Vic 3133 — (03) 874 8883.
The Spina Bifida Association of Victoria, 52 Thistlethwaite Street, South Melbourne, Vic 3205 —(03) 699 2066.
Yooralla Society of Victoria, 52 Thistlethwaite Street, South Melbourne, Vic 3205, or
PO Box 88, South Melbourne, Vic 3205 —(03) 698 5222.

Tas: Spina Bifida Association of Tasmania, PO Box 114, Rosny Park, Tas 7018.

NSW: Osteogenesis Imperfecta Society of New South Wales (Brittle Bones), PO Box 401, Epping, NSW 2121 —(02) 80 4488.
Muscular Dystrophy Association of New South Wales, Corner Bedford and Chalmers Streets, Sydney, or
PO Box 10, Strawberry Hills, NSW 2012 —(02) 698 9555.
The New South Wales Society for Crippled Children, PO Box 10, Strawberry Hills, NSW 2012 —(02) 698 9555.
The Paraplegic and Quadriplegic Association of New South Wales, Paraquad Centre, 33-35 Burlington Road, Homebush, NSW 2140 — (02) 764 4166.
The Spastic Centre of New South Wales, c/- The Medical Director, 6 Queen Street, Mosman, NSW 2088 — (02) 969 1666.

(Referrals should be made to the Medical Director *only* through a patient's doctor).

NSW and national:

Australian Quadriplegic Association Limited, 1 Jennifer Street, Little Bay, NSW 2036 — (02) 661 8855.

Intellectually disabled

Qld: The Endeavour Foundation, 38 Jordan Terrace, Bowen Hills, Q 4006, or PO Box 40, Newstead, Brisbane, Q 4006 — (07) 52 7000.

WA: Irrabeena Division for the Intellectually Handicapped, 53 Ord Street, West Perth, WA 6005, or
PO Box 441, West Perth, WA 6005 — (09) 322 2499.
Slow Learning Children's Group of Western Australia Incorporated, 313 Churchill Avenue, Subiaco, WA 6008 — (09) 381 9574.

NSW: Challenge Foundation of New South Wales, 8 Junction Street, Ryde, NSW 2112 (63 branches throughout NSW).

Physically/intellectually disabled

Qld: Friends of Brain Injured Children of Queensland, c/- Mr Ray Johnson, 54 Royston Street, Brookfield, Q 4069, or
PO Box 69, Stafford, Q 4053 — (07) 374 1629.

WA: Association for the Advancement of Brain Injured Children WA Incorporated, Kara Educational Centre, Chessell Drive, Duncraig, WA 6023 — (09) 447 3590.

Vic and national:

Australian Centre for Brain Injured Children, 15 Powlett Street, Mordialloc, Vic 3195, or
PO Box 353, Mordialloc — (03) 580 1056
(Each state has a parent support group known as Friends of Brain Injured Children).

Down's syndrome

Qld: Down's Syndrome Association of Queensland, GPO Box 1556, Brisbane 4001, or 101 Highgate Street, Coopers Plains, Q 4108 — (07) 275 1947.

NT: Down's Syndrome Association of the Northern Territory, PO Box 41545, Casuarina, NT 5792 —(089) 27 9408.

SA: Down's Syndrome Association of South Australia Incorporated, PO Box 65, Burnside, SA 5066 —(08) 275 5326.

Vic: Down's Syndrome Association of Victoria, 55 Victoria Parade, Collingwood, Vic 3066 — (053) 419 1653.

Tas: Down's Syndrome Association of Tasmania, 1 Tower Road, Newtown, Tas 7008 — (002) 28 4196, (AH) (002) 72 4779.

NSW: Down's Syndrome Association of New South Wales, PO Box 2356, North Parramatta, NSW 2151 —(02) 683 4333.

Epilepsy

Qld: Epilepsy Association of Queensland Incorporated, Room 322, Penneys Building, 210 Queen Street, Brisbane, 4000 — (07) 229 3606.

WA: West Australian Epilepsy Association Incorporated, 14 Bagot Road, Subiaco, WA 6008 — (09) 381 1187 (Mothers' support group meets first Wednesday of each month).

SA: Epilepsy Association of South Australia Incorporated, 471 Regency Road, Prospect, SA 5082 —(08) 269 3511.

Vic: Epilepsy Foundation of Victoria Incorporated, Kintore Epilepsy Centre, 818-822 Burke Road, Camberwell, Vic 3124, or PO Box 88, Camberwell Vic 3124 — (03) 813 2866.

Tas: Epilepsy Association of Tasmania Incorporated, 86 Hampden Road, Battery Point, Tas 7000, or PO Box 421, Sandy Bay, Tas 7005 — (002) 34 6967.

NSW: Epilepsy Association of New South Wales, 468 Pennant Hills Road, Pennant Hills, NSW 2120, or PO Box 521, Pennant Hills, NSW 2120 (02) 875 1855.

ACT: Epilepsy Association of the Australian Capital Territory Incorporated, SHOUT Office, Hughes Community Centre, Wisdom Street, Hughes, ACT 2605 —(062) 81 2983.

National:

National Epilepsy Association of Australia, PO Box 554, Lilydale, Vic 3140 — (03) — 735 0211.

Hearing impaired

Qld: Queensland Deaf Society Incorporated, 34 Davidson Street, Newmarket, Q 4051 — (07) 356 8255.

WA: The Western Australian Deaf Society Incorporated, 16 Brentham Street, Leederville, WA 6007 —(09) 443 2677.

SA: Royal South Australian Deaf Society Incorporated, 262 South Terrace, Adelaide, SA 5000 — (08) 223 3335; (08) 223 6530.

Vic: Deafness Foundation (Victoria), 340 Highett Road, Highett, Vic 3190 — (03) 555 8777.
(This is the Victorian division of the Australian Deafness Council).

NSW: Deaf and Blind Children's Centre, 361-365 North Rocks Road, North Rocks, NSW 2151
(Run by the Royal NSW Institute for Deaf and Blind Children).
The Adult Deaf Society of New South Wales Deaf Centre, 123 Cambridge Street, Stanmore, NSW 2048 — (02) 560 6433.
The Shepherd Centre (For Deaf Children and their Parents), University of Sydney, Sydney, NSW 2006 —(02) 692 9788.

Visually impaired

Tas: Royal Tasmanian Society for the Blind and Deaf, Corner Argyle and Lewis Streets, Hobart, Tas 7000, or PO Box 82, North Hobart, Tas 7002 — (002) 34 4666.

Vic.: Royal Victoria Institute for the Blind, 333 Burwood Highway, Burwood, Vic 3125 — (03) 288 6422.

NSW: Royal Blind Society of New South Wales, c/- The Director, Child and Adolescent Services Department, 4 Mitchell Street, Enfield, NSW 2136 — (02) 747 6622.

Cleft palate and lip

National:

(Australian support groups have requested that all enquiries be addressed to the National body)

The Cleft Palate and Lip Society, National Headquarters, PO Box 475, Lane Cove, NSW 2066 —(02) 331 3880; (02) 427 1843.

Autism

NSW: Autistic Association of New South Wales, 41 Cook Street, Forestville, NSW 2087 — (02) 452 4041.

WA: Association for Autistic Children in Western Australia (Inc), Suite 114, 396 Scarborough Beach Road, Osbourne Park, WA 6017 — (09) 444 6933.

Heart defects

Qld: 'Heart to Heart' — Parents' Cardiac Support Group, c/-Mrs Karen Daniel, 39 Rinora Street, Corinda, Q 4075 — (07) 379 8474 (Supported by Prince Charles Hospital, Brisbane).

WA: 'Heart Beat', c/- Mrs L. Quinlivan, 85 North Road, Bassendean, WA 6054 — (09) 279 6590 (Supported by Princess Margaret Hospital for Children).

Vic and national:

'Heart Beat', c/- Congenital Abnormality Support Association, c/- Mrs Susan Wright, 7 Loongana Avenue, Oak Park, Vic 3046 — (03) 306 8124.

Cystic fibrosis

Qld: Cystic Fibrosis Association of Queensland, 32 School Street, Kelvin Grove, Q 4059, or
PO Box 225, Paddington, Q 4064 — (07) 352 6322
(The Queensland Association can provide information on the National Federation).

WA: Cystic Fibrosis Association of Western Australia, PO Box 7271, Cloisters Square, Perth, WA 6001 —(09) 321 9422.

Tas: Cystic Fibrosis Association of Southern Tasmania Incorporated, GPO Box 245C, Hobart, 7001.

NSW: Cystic Fibrosis Association of New South Wales, Suite 4, First Floor, 21-23 Belmore Street, Burwood, NSW 2134, or
PO Box 241, Burwood 2134 — (02) 745 1288.

Miscellaneous
WA & NSW: Diabetes

> Diabetic Association of Western Australia Incorporated, 48 Wickham Street, East Perth, WA 6000 —(09) 325 7699.
>
> Diabetic Association of New South Wales, 9th Floor, National Building, 250 Pitt Street, Sydney, NSW 2000, or
>
> PO Box A6, Sydney South 2000 — (02) 264 6851.

Qld, WA, SA, Tas, Vic, NSW, national:

> The Association for the Welfare of Children in Hospital (AAWCH)
>
> Qld — c/- Mrs Joan Cifuentes, PO Box 2101, Southport Q 4215.
>
> WA — 'Meerilinga', 1186 Hay Street, West Perth, WA 6005 — (09) 321 4821, (09) 321 6277.
>
> SA — Florence Knight Nurses Home, Room 9, Adelaide Children's Hospital, North Adelaide, SA 5006 (08) 267 7347.
>
> Vic — 25 Banool Road, Balwyn, Vic 3103.
>
> Tas — PO Box 273, Moonah, Tas 7009.
>
> NSW & National — Floor 78-80 Phillip Street, Parramatta, NSW 2150 — (02) 635 4785.

WA: Australian Huntington's Disease Association Incorporated, Marjorie Guthrie Centre, 81 Manning Road, Bentley, WA 6102 — (09) 350 5444.

Vic: Thalassaemia Society of Victoria, 50 Cardigan Street, Carlton, Vic 3053 — (03) 663 6000.

National:

> Congenital Abnormality Support Association (CASA), c/- Mrs Susan Wright, 7 Loongana Avenue, Oak Park, Vic 3046 — (03) 306 8124.

Assistance to the disabled
Qld: Queensland Parents of the Disabled, GPO Box 1466, Brisbane, Q 4001 — (07) 391 6912.

WA: Parents and Friends of Spastics, 85 Fitzroy Road, Riverdale, WA 6103.

Vic: Action Group for Disabled Children, PO Box 69, Chadstone, Vic 3148.

> Disabled Persons Information Bureau, Health Commission of Victoria, Ground Floor, 555 Collins Street, Melbourne, Vic 3000, or
>
> GPO Box 4013, Melbourne, Vic 3001 —(03) 616 7746.
>
> Parent Support For Parents of Children with Disabilities, c/- Lee Llewellyn, 2/105 Severn Street, Box Hill, Vic 3129 — (03) 898 6559.

Tas: Action Group for Children with Disabilities, c/- Mrs Maxine Griffiths, 28 Carcoola Street, Chigwell, Tas 7011 — (002) 49 4757.

> Support Group for Parents of Young Handicapped Children, c/-

Douglas Parkes Rehabilitation Centre, 31 Tower Road, Newtown, Tas 7008 — (002) 38 1801.

Relationships

Qld: Queensland Marriage Guidance Council, 159 St Pauls Terrace, Brisbane 4000 — (07) 221 2005 (Branches also in: Rockhampton, 114 Fitzroy Street, 4700 —(079) 27 4238; Townsville, 24 Paxton Street, 4810 —(077) 71 3780; Ipswich; Wynnum; Redcliffe; Mt Gravatt; Toowoomba; Bundaberg; Gladstone; Mackay; Cairns; Mt Isa).

WA: Marriage Guidance Council of Western Australia Incorporated, 32 Richardson Street, West Perth, WA 6005 — (09) 322 4755, or 1 Ord Street, Fremantle, WA 6160 — (09) 336 2144.

NT: Marriage Guidance Council of the Northern Territory Incorporated, Second Floor, Centrepoint, The Mall, Darwin, NT 5792 — (089) 81 6676.

SA: Marriage Guidance Council of South Australia Incorporated, 55 Hutt Street, Adelaide, SA 5000 —(08) 223 4566.

Vic: The Marriage Guidance Council of Victoria, 46 Princess Street, Kew, Vic 3101, or
PO Box 132, Kew, Vic 3101 — (03) 861 8512; (03) 861 5354; (03) 861 5794.

NSW: The Marriage Guidance Council of New South Wales, Coughlan House, 226 Liverpool Road, Enfield, NSW 2136, or
PO Box 245, Enfield, NSW 2136 — (02) 745 4411 (Branches in: Newcastle — (049) 69 3977; Wollongong — (042) 28 7711).

ACT: Canberra Marriage Counselling Service Incorporated, Second Floor, Savings House, 8 Petrie Plaza, ACT 2601 — (062) 48 0530 (Branch at Wagga Wagga).

General coping

Qld: Anglican Family Care, 162 Vulture Street, South Brisbane, Q 4101 — (07) 44 5927.
Centre Care, Catholic Family Welfare, Morgan Street, Fortitude Valley, Q 4006, or
PO Box 289, Fortitude Valley, Q 4006 —(07) 52 4371.
Kalparrin Family Welfare Centre, Valley Uniting Church, Warner Street, Fortitude Valley, Q 4006, or
PO Box 780, Fortitude Valley, Q 4006 —(07) 52 4545.
The Relaxation Centre of Queensland Limited, Corner Brookes and Wickham Streets, Fortitude Valley, Q 4006 — (07) 52 3574.

NT: Childbirth Education Association — Darwin Incorporated, First Floor, Monterey House, Trower Road, Casuarina, NT 5792 — (089) 27 2575.

WA: Childbirth and Parenthood Education Association of Perth WA Incorporated, PO Box 230, Subiaco, WA 6008, or
'Meerilinga' 1186 Hay Street, West Perth, WA 6005 — (09) 321 4821
(Includes Post Natal Depression Support Group; Caesarean Birth Support Group; Meet a Mum Association).
Western Institute of Self Help (WISH), 80 Railway Street, Cottesloe, WA 6011 (WISH has an excellent text compiled by Tina Jezewski, called 'Not Common Knowledge Self Help Groups').

Vic: Post and Ante Natal Depression Association Incorporated (PANDA), c/- 14 Lillimur Road, Ormond, Vic 3163 — (03) 578 8261.

Qld,WA,SA,NSW,national:
GROW (Providing general assistance for people experiencing emotional difficulties)

Qld: Room 240, Second Floor, 20 Duncan Street, Fortitude Valley, Q 4006, or
PO Box 740, Fortitude Valley, Q 4006 (07) 52 5701.

WA: 146 Beaufort Street, Perth, WA 6000 —(09) 328 3344.

SA: 354 Marion Road, Plympton, North Adelaide, SA 5037 — (08) 297 6933.

NSW: 46 Marion Street, Harris Park, NSW 2150 — (02) 635 7112.

National: 209A Edgeware Road, Marrickville, NSW 2204 — (02) 516 3733.

Bibliography

Adamson, M. 'The 24-26 Week Infant', in Proceedings of the Inaugural Congress of the Australian Perinatal Society, in Excerpta Medica and Asia Pacific Congress Series 18, *Journal of Australian Perinatal Society*, March 12–14, 1983.

Adelstein, A.M., Isobel M. Macdonald Davies, and Josephine A.C. Weatherall. *Perinatal and Infant Mortality: Social and Biological Factors 1975-77*, Studies on Medical and Population Subjects No. 41, Office of Population Answers and Surveys. London: Her Majesty's Stationery Office, 1980.

Alberman, Eva, M. Creasy, Maureen Elliott, and C. Spicer. 'Maternal Factors Associated with Fetal Chromosomal Anomalies in Spontaneous Abortions', *British Journal of Obstetrics and Gynaecology*, 83 (1976), 621–627.

Alberman, Eva, Maureen Elliott, M. Creasy, and R. Dhadial. 'Previous Reproductive History in Mothers Presenting with Spontaneous Abortions', *British Journal of Obstetrics and Gynaecology*, 82 (1975), 366–373.

Aring, Charles D. 'Intimations of Mortality: An Appreciation of Death and Dying', *Annals of Internal Medicine*, 69 (1968), 137–152.

Awan, A.K. 'Some Biologic Correlates of Pregnancy Wastage', *American Journal of Obstetrics and Gynaecology*, 119 (1974), 525–532.

Baird, D., J. Walker, and A.M. Thomson. 'The Causes and Prevention of Stillbirths and First Week Deaths', *The Journal of Obstetrics and Gynaecology of the British Empire*, 61(4) (1954), 433–448.

Barnes, Cyril G. *Medical Disorders in Obstetric Practice*. 4th ed. London: Blackwell Scientific Publications, 1974.

Barr, Peter A., Julie C. Dunsmore, and Glynis J. Howard. *Premature Babies* and *The Death of Your Baby*. Booklets produced by the Department of Neonatology, Royal North Shore Hospital, St Leonards, New South Wales.

Bell, Stephen J. 'Psychological Problems among Patients Attending an Infertility Clinic', *Journal of Psychosomatic Research*, 25 (1981), 1–3.

Benfield, D. Gary, Susan A. Leib, and Jeanette Reuter. 'Grief Responses of Parents after Referral of the Critically Ill Newborn to a Regional Center', *The New England Journal of Medicine*, 294 (1976), 975–978.

Benfield, D. Gary, Susan A. Leib, and John H. Vollman. 'Grief Responses of Parents to Neonatal Death and Parent Participation in Deciding Care', *Pediatrics*, 62(2) (1978), 171–177.

Berezin, Nancy. *After a Loss in Pregnancy: Help for Families Affected by a Miscarriage, a Stillbirth or the Loss of a Newborn*. New York: Simon and Schuster, 1982.

Billings, Evelyn L., and Ann Westmore. *The Billings Method: Controlling Fertility without Drugs or Devices*. Victoria: Anne O'Donovan, 1980.

Blischer, Norman A., and Eric V. Mackay. *Obstetrics and the Newborn: For Midwives and Medical Students*. New South Wales: Holt-Saunders, 1976.

Blum, Barbara L., ed. *Psychological Aspects of Pregnancy, Birthing and Bonding.* New York: Human Sciences Press, 1980.

Borg, Susan, and Judith Lasker. *When Pregnancy Fails: Families Coping with Miscarriages, Stillbirth and Infant Death.* Boston: Beacon Press, 1981.

Bourne, Gordon. *Pregnancy.* Revised. London: Pan Books, 1975.

Bourne, S. 'Stillbirth, Grief and Medical Education', *British Medical Journal*, April 30, 1977, 1157.

Brammer, Lawrence M. *The Helping Relationship: Process and Skills.* New Jersey: Prentice Hall, 1973.

Braunstein, Glenn D., William G. Karow, William D. Gentry, and Maclyn E. Wade. 'Subclinical Spontaneous Abortion', *Obstetrics and Gynaecology*, 50 (1977), Supplement, 41s–44s.

Brody, Jane E. 'Miscarriage: Myths Often Add to Grief', *The New York Times*, March 5, 1980.

Bugen, Larry A. 'Human Grief: A Model for Prediction and Intervention', *American Journal of Orthopsychiatry*, 47(2) (1977), 196–206.

Cain, Albert C., Irene Fast, and Mary E. Erickson. 'Children's Disturbed Reactions to the Death of a Sibling', *American Journal of Orthopsychiatry*, 34 (1964), 741–752.

Callan, Victor. 'Coping with Infertility', talk given to and published in the newsletter of the Friends of the Queensland Fertility Group, Number 7 (August 1985), 11,12.

Callan, V.J. *The Experience of Infertility: A Guide for Couples.* In press.

Cameron, Bob. 'The "Miracle" That Turns Men into Fathers', *New Idea*, September 14, 1985, 29.

Carlson, Dimity B., and Richard C. Labarba. 'Maternal Emotionality during Pregnancy and Reproductive Outcome: A Review of the Literature', *International Journal of Behavioural Development*, 2 (1979), 343–376.

Case, Ronna. 'When Birth Is Also a Funeral', *The Journal of Pastoral Care*, 32 (1978), 6–21.

Chalmers, John. Talk given to Inaugural Meeting of Stillbirth and Neonatal Death Support Group (Queensland), March, 1984.

Clarke, Ann M., and A.D.B. Clarke, eds. *Readings from Mental Deficiency — The Changing Outlook.* London: Methuen, 1974.

Clayton, Paula J. 'Weight Loss and Sleep Disturbance in Bereavement', in Schoenberg, Bernard, *et al*, *Bereavement — Its Psychological Aspects.* New York: Columbia University Press, 1975.

Clyman, Ronald I., Charlotte Green, Cynthia Mikkelson, Jane Rowe, and Linda Ataide. 'Do Parents Utilize Physician Follow-up after the Death of Their Newborn?', *Pediatrics*, 64(5) (1979), 665–667.

Coleman, James, C., James N. Butcher, and Robert C. Carson. *Abnormal Psychology and Modern Life.* 6th ed. Illinois: Scott, Foresman and Co., 1964.

Combined Newsletter of the Combined New South Wales IVF Support Groups, Spring '85, Summer '86, and Autumn '86.

Compassionate Friends (Australia). Pamphlets and Information Sheets produced by the Bereaved Parent Support and Information Centre, Melbourne.

Corney, Robert T., and Frederick T. Horton. 'Pathological Grief Following Spontaneous Abortion', *American Journal of Psychiatry*, 131(7) (1974), 825–827.

Cornwall, Joanne, Barry Nurcombe, and Leslie Stevens. 'Family Response to Loss of a Child by Sudden Infant Death Syndrome', *The Medical Journal of Australia*, April 30, 1977, 656–658.

Crandon, Alex J., 'Maternal Anxiety and Obstetric Complications', *Journal of Psychosomatic Research*, 23 (1979), 109–111.

Cruikshank, W.M., ed. *Psychology of Exceptional Children and Youth*. 4th ed. New Jersey: Prentice Hall, 1980.

Cystic Fibrosis: A Summary of Symptoms, Diagnosis and Treatment. Booklet produced by Cystic Fibrosis Association of New South Wales.

Daly, C., J.A. Heady, and J.N. Morris. 'Social and Biological Factors in Infant Mortality: The Effects of Mother's Age and Parity on Social-class Differences in Infant Mortality', *The Lancet*, February 26, 1955, 445–448.

Donaghy, Bronwyn. 'Thursday's Child: A Story of Down's Syndrome', *Parents and Children*, January/July 1985, 89–95.

Down's Syndrome Association of Victoria. *Down's Voice*, Volume 7(2) (June 1985).

Duff, Raymond S., and A.G.M. Campbell. 'Moral and Ethical Dilemmas in the Special-care Nursery', *The New England Journal of Medicine*, 289 (1973) 890–894.

Dunlop, Joyce L. 'Bereavement Reactions Following Stillbirth', *The Practitioner*, 222 (1979), 115-118.

Earl, W.J.H., 'Help for Parents after Stillbirth', *British Medical Journal*, February 25, 1978, 505, 506.

Edmondson, Kate. 'A Grieving Couple — a Gap in the Liturgy', *The Leader*, February 27, 1983, 10,11.

Elliott, Barbara A. 'Neonatal Death: Reflections for Parents', *Pediatrics*, 62(1) (1978), 100–102.

Endometricosis. Pamphlet prepared by the Women's Health Resource Centre, Brunswick, Victoria, 1983.

Fedrick, J., and Philippa Adelstein. 'Influence of Pregnancy Spacing on Outcome of Pregnancy', *British Medical Journal*, 4 (1973), 753–761.

Fischhoff, J., and N. O'Brien. 'After the Child Dies', *The Journal of Pediatrics* 88(1) (1976), 140–146.

Francis, Vida, Barbara M. Korsch, and Marie J. Morris. 'Gaps in Doctor-Patient Communication — Patients' Response to Medical Advice', *The New England Journal of Medicine*, 280 (1969), 535–540.

Fraser, Jane. 'Women Who Grieve for a Wanted Baby', *The Australian*, May 22, 1984.

Free, M.L., and Tian P.S. Oei. *Biological and Psychological Processes in the Treatment and Maintenance of Depression*. Unpublished Masters thesis, University of Queensland, 1987.

Friedman, Standford B. 'Psychological Aspects of Sudden Unexpected Death in Infants and Children', *Pediatric Clinics of North America* 21(1) (1974), 103–111.

From Us to You When Your Baby Dies. Booklet produced by Stillbirth and Neonatal Death Support Group (Queensland), 1984.

Funderburk, S.J., D. Guthrie, and D. Meldrum. 'Outcome of Pregnancies Complicated by Early Vaginal Bleeding', *British Journal of Obstetrics and Gynaecology*, 87 (1980), 100–105.

Furlong, R.M., and J.C. Hobbins. 'Grief in the Perinatal Period', *Obstetrics and Gynaecology*, 61 (1983), 497–500.

Gagen, Peter. *That You May Have Life: A Baptismal Resource*, Liturgy News Bulletin of the Liturgical Commission of the Archdiocese of Brisbane, Queensland, 14:2 (1984), 37–72.

Gibson, George J. 'Care of the Family Who Has Lost a Newborn', *Post Graduate Medicine*, 60(6) (1976), 67–70.

Gibson, Pam. *Community Resources*. Booklet used as part of telephone counsellors' training program of Lifeline, Brisbane, 1975.

Giles, P.F.H. 'Reactions of Women to Perinatal Death', *Australia and New Zealand Journal of Obstetrics and Gynaecology*, 10 (1970), 207–210.

Goodlin, R.C. *Care of the Foetus*. New York: Masson Publishing, 1979.

Gordeuk, A. 'Motherhood and a Less Than Perfect Child: A Literary Review', *Maternal-Child Nursing Journal*, 5 (1976), 57–68.

Graham, F.M., and J. Ellis. 'The Social Relevance of Infertility', *Patient Management*, 10 (1986), 19–31.

Greenhill, J.P. 'Emotional Factors in Female Infertility', *Journal of the American Academy of Obstetrics and Gynaecology*, 7 (1956), 602–606.

'Grief and Stillbirth', *British Medical Journal*, January 15, 1977, 126.

Guerrero, Rodrigo, and Oscar I. Rojas. 'Spontaneous Abortion and Aging of Human Ova and Spermatozoa', *New England Journal of Medicine*, 293 (1975), 573–575.

Gunn, Alex. 'Miscarriage', *Mother and Baby*, August 1973, 10,11.

Hales, Dianne. 'Will Your Baby Wait Nine Months?', *New Idea*, July 30, 1983, 49–59.

Halpern, Werner I. 'Some Psychiatric Sequelae to Crib Death', *American Journal of Psychiatry*, 129(4) (1972), 398-402.

Hardy, J.B. 'Viral Infection in Pregnancy: A Review', *American Journal of Obstetrics and Gynaecology*, 93 (1965), 1052–1065.

Harlap, S., and P.H. Shiono. 'Alcohol, Smoking and Incidence of Spontaneous Abortion in the First and Second Trimester', *The Lancet*, July 26, 1980, 173–180.

Harvey, David, ed. *The New Life: Pregnancy, Birth and Your Child's First Year*. London: Marshall Cavendish, 1979.

Haves, L.F. *Recognizing Emotional or Mental Illness*. Booklet used as part of telephone counsellors' training program of Lifeline, Brisbane, 1975.

Hawthorne, Desleyanne. 'Pain, Grief, Hope: A Premature Baby', *Courier Mail*, May 26, 1984.

Heady, J.A., C. Daly, and J.N. Morris. 'Social and Biological Factors in Infant Mortality: Variation of Mortality with Mother's Age and Parity', *The Lancet*, February 19, 1955.

Heady, J.A., C.F. Stevens, C. Daly, and J.N. Morris. 'Social and Biological Factors in Infant Mortality: The Independent Effects of Social Class, Region, the Mother's Age and Her Parity', *The Lancet*, March 5, 1955, 499–502.

Helmrath, Thomas A., and Elaine M. Steinitz. 'Death of an Infant: Parental Grieving and the Failure of Social Support', *The Journal of Family Practice*, 6(4) (1978), 785–790.

Hertig, Arthur T., and Robert G. Livingstone. 'Spontaneous Threatened and Habitual Abortions: Their Pathogenesis and Treatment', *The New England Journal of Medicine*, 230 (1944), 797-806.

Hoenk Shapiro, Constance. 'The Impact of Infertility on the Marital Relationship', *Social Casework: The Journal of Contemporary Social Work*, 63(7) (1982), 387–393.

Horowitz, Nancy Heller. 'Adolescent Mourning Reactions to Infant and Fetal Loss', *Social Casework: The Journal of Contemporary Social Work*, 59 (1978), 551–559.

Howard, Donald. *Christians Grieve Too*. Sydney: Chio Publishing, 1979.

Howell, Deborah. 'Help for Parents after Stillbirth', *British Medical Journal*, March 25, 1978, 787,788.

'Infertility: Men Who Can't Be Fathers', *Parents and Children*, April/May 1986, 109–111.

Javert, Carl T. *Spontaneous and Habitual Abortion*. New York: McGraw-Hill-Blakeston Division, 1957.

Johns, Nan. 'Family Reactions to the Birth of a Child with a Congenital Abnormality', *The Medical Journal of Australia*, January 30, 1971, 277–281.

Jolly, Hugh. 'Family Reactions to Stillbirth', *Proceedings of the Royal Society of Medicine*, 69 (1976), 835–837.

Kaij, L., A. Malinquist, and A. Nilsson. 'Psychiatric Aspects of Spontaneous Abortion — II. The Importance of Bereavement, Attachment and Neurosis in Early Life', *Journal of Psychosomatic Research*, 13 (1969), 53–59.

Kaplan, David M., and Edward A. Mason. 'Maternal Reactions to Premature Birth Viewed as an Acute Emotional Disorder', *American Journal of Orthopsychiatry*, 30 (1960), 539–552.

Keirse, M.J.N.C., R.W. Rush, A.B.M. Anderson, and A.C. Turnbull. 'Risk of Pre-term Delivery in Patients with Previous Pre-term Delivery and/or Abortion', *British Journal of Obstetrics and Gynaecology*, 85 (1978), 81–85.

Kenihan, Kerry. *How to Be the Parents of a Handicapped Child and Survive*. Victoria: Penguin, 1981. (This book provides a comprehensive list of Australian support groups dealing with handicap.)

Kennell, John H., and Marshall H. Klaus. 'Care of the Mother of the High Risk Infant', *Clinical Obstetrics and Gynecology*, 14(3) (1971), 926–954.

Kennell, John H., Howard Slyter, and Marshall H. Klaus. 'The Mourning Response of Parents to the Death of a Newborn Infant', *The New England Journal of Medicine*, 283 (1970), 344–349.

Kimball, Anne C., B.H. Kean, and Fritz Fuchs. 'The Role of Toxoplasmosis in Abortion', *American Journal of Obstetrics and Gynecology*, 111 (1971), 219–226.

Kitchen, W., M. Ryan, A. Richards, and J. Rissenden. *Premature Babies — A Guide for Parents*. Melbourne: Hill of Content Publishing, 1983.

Klaus, Marshall H., and John H. Kennell. 'Care of the Mother, Father and Infant.' In Behrman, Richard E., ed., *Neonatal-Perinatal Medicine* (2nd ed.), St Louis: C.V. Mosby, 1977.

Klaus, Marshall H., and John H. Kennell. *Maternal Infant Bonding: The Impact of Early Separation or Loss on Family Development*. St Louis: C.V. Mosby, 1976.

Klemesrud, Judy. 'Helping Couples Cope with the Loss of an Infant', *The New York Times*, May 29, 1978.

Kline, Jennie, Zena A. Stein, Mervyn Susser, and Dorothy Warburton. 'Smoking: A Risk Factor for Spontaneous Abortion', *The New England Journal of Medicine*, 297 (1977), 793-796.

Knapp, Ronald J., and Larry G. Peppers. 'Doctor-patient Relationships in Foetal/Infant Death Encounters', *Journal of Medical Education*, 54 (1979), 775-780.

Koocher, Gerald P. 'Talking with Children about Death', *American Journal of Orthopsychiatry*, 44(3) 404-411.

Kovacs, Gabor T. 'Artificial Insemination by Donor', *Patient Management*, 10 (1986), 65-77.

Krell, Robert, and Leslie Rabkin. 'The Effects of Sibling Death on the Surviving Child: A Family Perspective', *Family Process*, 18 (1979), 471-477.

Kretser, David de, and Robert McLachlan. 'Causes and Management of Male Infertility', *Patient Management*, 10 (1986), 47-64.

Kübler-Ross, Elizabeth. *On Death and Dying*. London: Tavistock, 1969.

Kushner, Harold S. *When Bad Things Happen to Good People*. London and Sydney: Pan Books, 1981.

Lawrence, Joan. *Emotional Aspects of Miscarriage*. Paper presented at the meeting of the Association for Loss and Grief, Brisbane, June 1984.

Leeton, John. Talk given by Professor Leeton and reprinted in Newsletter of IVF Friends, Melbourne, June 1985, 7-15.

Lewis, Emanuel. 'Mourning by the Family after a Stillbirth or Neonatal Death'. *Archives of Disease in Childhood*, 54 (1979), 303-306.

Lewis, Emanuel. 'The Management of Stillbirth — Coping with an Unreality', *The Lancet*, September 18, 1976, 619,620.

Lewis, Emanuel, and Anne Page. 'Failure to Mourn a Stillbirth: An Overlooked Catastrophe', *British Journal of Medical Psychology*, 51 (1978), 237-241.

Lewis, Thomas H. 'A Culturally Patterned Depression in a Mother after Loss of a Child', *Psychiatry*, 38 (1975), 92-95.

Limerick, Lady. 'Support and Counselling Needs of Families Following a Cot Death Bereavement', *Proceedings of the Royal Society of Medicine*, 69 (1976), 839-844.

Lindemann, E. 'Symptomatology and Management of Acute Grief', *American Journal of Psychiatry*, 101 (1944), 141-148.

Lindsell, Harold, *When You Pray*. Michigan: Baker House, 1969.

Llewellyn-Jones, Derek. *Everywoman — A Gynaecological Guide for Life*. 3rd ed. London: Faber and Faber, 1982.

Llewellyn-Jones, Derek, *Fundamentals of Obstetrics and Gynaecology*. Volume 1 — *Obstetrics*. 3rd ed. London: Faber and Faber, 1982.

MacCarthy, Dermod. 'The Repercussions of the Death of a Child', *Proceedings of the Royal Society of Medicine*, 62 (1969), 553,554.

Machin, G.A. 'Chromosome Abnormality and Perinatal Death', *The Lancet*, March 30, 1974, 549-551.

Maddison, David, and Agnes Viola. 'The Health of Widows in the Year Following Bereavement', *Journal of Psychosomatic Research*, 12 (1968), 297-306.

Maddison, David, and Wendy L. Walker. 'Factors Affecting the Outcome of Conjugal Bereavement', *British Journal of Psychiatry*, 113 (1967), 1057–1067.

Malmquist, A., L. Kaij, and A. Nilsson. 'Psychiatric Aspects of Spontaneous Abortion — I. A Matched Control Study of Women with Living Children', *Journal of Psychosomatic Research*, 13 (1969), 45–51.

Mann, Edward C. 'Psychiatric Investigation of Habitual Abortion', *Journal of the American Academy of Obstetrics and Gynecology*, 7(6) (1956), 589–601.

'Maternal Blocking Antibodies, the Foetal Allograft and Recurrent Abortion', *The Lancet*, November 19, 1983, 1175,1176.

McBride, William, consultant ed. *The Complete Book of Babycare*. London: Octopus, 1978.

Mead, Barbara. 'How Small Is Too Small?', *The Catholic Leader* — Mater Jubilee Supplement, March 16, 1986, 9.

Miller, J.F., E. Williamson, J. Glue, Y.B. Gordon, J.G. Grudzinokas, and A. Sykes. 'Foetal Loss after Implantation: A Prospective Study', *The Lancet*, 2 (September 13, 1980), 554–556.

Miscarriage. Booklet produced by the National Childbirth Trust, London, 1983.

Mishinski, Judy. 'Epilepsy', *The Sunday Mail*, October 13, 1985.

Mishinski, Judy. 'Special Sense of Grief for Death of a Baby', *The Sunday Mail*, March 23, 1986.

Mooney, Joan. 'Infertility: Medical Advances Bring Joy to Many', *Woman's Day*, March 4, 1985, 44–47.

Morris, David. 'Parental Reactions to Perinatal Death', *Proceedings of the Royal Society of Medicine*, 62 (1969), 837,838.

Mudd, Emily H. 'The Couple as a Unit: Sexual, Social and Behavioural Considerations to Reproductive Barriers', *Journal of Marital and Family Therapy*, 6 (1980), 23–28.

Murray, J.A. *Parental Reactions to Perinatal Death*. Unpublished thesis in Department of Psychology, University of Queensland, 1986.

Muscular Dystrophy Association of New South Wales, Information Sheet, Volume 3(7) (July 1985).

Nicholas, Anthony M., and Terry J. Lewin. 'Grief Reactions of Parental Couples: Congenital Handicap and Cot Death', *The Medical Journal of Australia*, 144 (March 17, 1986), 292–295.

Nicol, Margaret T., Jeffrey R. Tompkins, Norman A. Campbell, and Geoffrey J. Syme. 'Maternal Grieving Response after Perinatal Death', *The Medical Journal of Australia*, 144 (March 17, 1986), 287–289.

Niswander, Kenneth R., and Myron Gordon. *The Women and Their Pregnancies: The Collaborative Perinatal Study of the National Institute of Neurological Diseases and Stroke*. Philadelphia: W.B. Saunders, 1972.

Norbeck, Jane S., and Virginia Peterson Tilden. 'Life Stress, Social Support, and Emotional Disequilibrium in Complications of Pregnancy: A Prospective Multivariate Study', *Journal of Health and Social Behaviour*, 24 (1983), 30–46.

Oakley, Ann, Ann McPherson, and Helen Roberts. *Miscarriage*. Glasgow: Fontana, 1984.

Parkes, C. Murray. 'Bereavement and Mental Illness', *British Journal of Medical Psychology*, 38 (1965), 1–26.

Parkes, C. Murray. 'Recent Bereavement as a Cause of Mental Illness', *British Journal of Psychiatry*, 110 (1964), 198–204.

Parkes, Colin Murray. *Bereavement: Studies of Grief in Adult Life*. London: Tavistock, 1972.

Pepperell, Roger J. 'Female Infertility: Tuning the Diagnosis for Effective Treatment', *Patient Management*, 10 (1986), 35–45.

Peppers, Darcy G., and Ronald J. Knapp. *Motherhood and Mourning: Perinatal Death*. New York: Praeger, 1980.

Pollack, George H. 'Anniversary Reactions, Trauma, and Mourning', *The Psychoanalytic Quarterly*, 39 (1970), 347–371.

Potter, Anne. *Having a Baby: An Essential Handbook for Australian Parents*. Melbourne: Sphere Books, 1983.

Poznanski, Elva Orlow. 'The "Replacement Child": A Saga of Unresolved Parental Grief', *The Journal of Pediatrics*, 81(6) (1972), 1190–1193.

Preece, Anna, 'Heart Baby Hollie Roffey Didn't Die in Vain', *Woman's Day*, October 29, 1984, 42,43.

Pryer, Hank, and Christine O'Brien Palinski. *Coping with a Miscarriage*. London: Jill Norman, 1980.

Raphael, Beverley. 'Grieving over the Loss of a Baby', leading article, *The Medical Journal of Australia*, 144 (March 17, 1986), 281,282.

Raphael, Beverley. 'Preventive Intervention with the Recently Bereaved', *Archives of General Psychiatry*, 34 (1977), 1450–1454.

Raphael, Beverley, *The Anatomy of Bereavement*. New York: Basic Books, 1983.

Raphael, Beverley. 'The Management of Bereavement.' In Burrows, G., ed., *Handbook of Depression*, Amsterdam: ASP Biological Press, 1976.

Raphael, Beverley. 'The Management of Pathological Grief', *Australia and New Zealand Journal of Psychiatry*, 9 (1975), 173–180.

Richardson, B. 'Children's Reactions to the Death of a Sibling', Newsletter of Stillbirth and Neonatal Death Support Group (Queensland), No. 7 (June 1984).

Richardson, Stephen A., and Alan F. Guttmacher, eds. *Childbearing — Its Social and Psychological Aspects*. New York: Williams and Wilkins, 1967.

Roberts, C.J., and C.R. Lowe. 'Where Have All the Conceptions Gone?', *The Lancet*, March 1, 1975, 498,499.

Rosenblatt, Paul C. 'Uses of Ethnography in Understanding Grief and Mourning'. In Schoenberg, Bernard, *et al, Bereavement — Its Psychological Aspects*, New York: Columbia University Press, 1975.

Rowe, Jane, Ronald Clyman, Charlotte Green, Cynthia Mikkelsen, Jeanette Haight, and Linda Ataide. 'Follow-up of Families Who Experience a Perinatal Death', *Pediatrics*, 62(2) (1978), 166–170.

Sanders, Catherine M. 'A Comparison of Adult Bereavement in the Death of a Spouse, Child and Parent', *Omega*, 10(4) (1979–80), 303–322.

Schoenberg, Bernard, Irwin Gerber, Alfred Wiener, Austin H. Kutscher, David Peretz, and Arthur C. Carr, eds. *Bereavement: Its Psychological Aspects*. New York: Columbia University Press, 1975.

Shereshefsky, Pauline M., and Leon J. Yarrow. *Psychological Aspects of a First Pregnancy and Early Postnatal Adaptation*. New York: Raven Press, 1973.

Sillence, D.O., ed. *Osteogenesis Imperfecta: A Handbook for Medical Practitioners and Health Care Professionals*. Booklet produced by the Osteogenesis Imperfecta Society of New South Wales, Ims Publishing.

Slade, Margot. 'Infant Death and Parental Grief: Debunking the Old Notions', *The New York Times*, September 13, 1980.

Snow, Rose, ed. *Understanding Adoption*. Sydney: Fontana Books, 1983.

Solnit, Albert J., and Morris Green. 'Psychologic Considerations in the Management of Death on Pediatric Hospital Services', *Pediatrics*, 24 (1959), 106–112.

Speck, William T. 'Commentary: The Tragedy of Stillbirth', *Journal of Pediatrics*, 93 (1978), 869,870.
Spina Bifida: A Handbook for Parents. Book produced by the Australian Spina Bifida Association. South Australia, 1982.
Staff of the Mt Sinai Hospital, New York City. Ravensky, J.J., and A.F. Guttmacher, eds. *Medical, Surgical and Gynecologic Complications of Pregnancy*. 2nd ed. Baltimore: Williams and Williams, 1965.

Stringham, Jean G., Judith Hotham Riley, and Ann Ross. 'Silent Birth: Mourning a Stillborn Baby', *Social Work* 27 (1982), 322–327.

Suchy, Sherene, and Simone Cahill. *The Infertility Resources Handbook*. Victoria: The Citizen's Welfare Service of Victoria, 1981.

Swinton, Alan. 'Grief and Stillbirth', *British Medical Journal*, 1 (April 9, 1977), 971.

Taylor, Colin, and W. Page Faulk. 'Prevention of Recurrent Abortion with Leucocyte Transfusions', *The Lancet*, 2 (July 11, 1981), 68,69.

Tengbom, Mildred. *Help for Bereaved Parents*. St Louis: Concordia Publishing House, 1981.

'The Abhorrence of Stillbirth', *The Lancet*, June 4, 1977, 1188–1190.

Tudehope, David I., Jon Iredill, David Rodgers, and Andrew Gunn. 'Neonatal Death: Grieving Families', *The Medical Journal of Australia*, 144 (March 17, 1986), 290–292.

Tudehope, D.I., and M.J. Thearle. *A Primer of Neonatal Medicine*. Queensland: William Brooks, 1984.

Tudehope, David, Judith Wintour, and John Chalmers, *Special Care for Newborn Babies: An Introduction to the Special Care Nursery*. Booklet produced by the Mater Misericordiae Mothers Hospital, South Brisbane, 1982.

Vessey, M., Laura Meisler, Rosemary Flavel, and D. Yeates. 'Outcome of Pregnancy in Women Using Different Methods of Contraception', *British Journal of Obstetrics and Gynaecology*, 86 (1979), 548-556.

Welu, Thomas C. 'Pathological Bereavement: A Plan for Its Prevention', in Schoenberg, Bernard, *et al.*, *Bereavement — Its Psychological Aspects*, New York: Columbia University Press, 1975.

Whittaker, P.G., A. Taylor, and T. Lind. 'Unsuspected Pregnancy Loss in Healthy Women', *The Lancet*, May 21, 1983, 1126,1127.

Williams, Howard. 'On a Teaching Hospital's Responsibility to Counsel Parents Concerning Their Child's Death', *The Medical Journal of Australia*, 2 (October 19, 1963), 643–645.

Wolf, Penny. 'Chorionic Villus Biopsy: The Earlier Test for Genetic Disorders', *Parents and Children*, January/July 1985, 13–15.

Wolff, John R., Paul E. Nielson, and Patricia Schiller. 'The
    Emotional Reaction to a Stillbirth', *American Journal of Obstetrics and Gynecology*,
    108(1) (1970), 73-77.
Wood, Carl, and Ann Westmore. *Test-tube Conception*. Melbourne:
    Hill of Content, 1983.
Wright, James. *Women's Problems*. Sydney: Golden Press, 1981.

Index